Diabetes
and
Atherosclerosis

Diabetes and Atherosclerosis
Molecular Basis and Clinical Aspects

Edited by

Boris Draznin, MD, PhD

Chief, Section of Endocrinology
Veterans Affairs Medical Center;
Professor of Medicine and
Vice Chairman for Research Affairs
Department of Medicine
University of Colorado Health Sciences Center
Denver, Colorado

Robert H. Eckel, MD

Professor of Medicine
Division of Endocrinology, Metabolism, Diabetes
Department of Medicine
University of Colorado Health Sciences Center
Denver, Colorado

Elsevier

New York • Amsterdam • London • Tokyo

Elsevier Science Publishing Co., Inc.
655 Avenue of the Americas, New York, New York 10010

Sole distributors outside the United States and Canada:
Elsevier Science Publishers B.V.
P.O. Box 211, 1000 AE Amsterdam, The Netherlands

© 1993 by Elsevier Science Publishing Co., Inc.

This book has been registered with the Copyright Clearance Center, Inc. For further information, please contact the Copyright Clearance Center, Inc., Salem, Massachusetts.

All inquiries regarding copyrighted material from this publication, other than reproduction through the Copyright Clearance Center, Inc., should be directed to: Rights and Permissions Department, Elsevier Science Publishing Co., Inc., 655 Avenue of the Americas, New York, New York 10010. FAX 212-633-3977.

This book is printed on acid-free paper.

Library of Congress Cataloging-in-Publication Data

Diabetes and atherosclerosis : molecular basis and clinical aspects /
    edited by Boris Draznin, Robert H. Eckel.
        p.   cm.
    Includes bibliographical references and index.
    ISBN 0-444-01665-1 (hard cover : alk. paper)
    1. Atherosclerosis—Pathogenesis. 2. Diabetes—Complications.
    3. Dyslipoproteinemias—Molecular aspects. I. Draznin, Boris.
    II. Eckel, Robert H.
    [DNLM: 1. Atherosclerosis—complications. 2. Diabetes Mellitus—complications.
    3. Hypertension—complications. 4. Lipids—metabolism.   WK 835 D5334]
    RC692.D5   1993
    616.1'36071—dc20
    DNLM/DLC
                                                                                92-48854
                                                                                CIP

Current Printing (last digit):
10 9 8 7 6 5 4 3 2 1

Manufactured in the United States of America

Contents

PART 3   Diabetes and Hypertension

Preface

Although the life expectancy of many patients with diabetes mellitus has been extended to virtually match that of the general population, and the quality of life of these patients has improved, atherosclerosis has emerged as the major complication of this complex and chronic disease. Despite advances in the treatment of many diabetic complications, atherosclerosis is a significant contributor to the mortality and morbidity that accompany this disorder.

Multiple factors underlie the pathogenetic mechanisms of dyslipidemia, atherosclerosis, and hypertension in diabetes. In order to elucidate these factors, many investigators have devoted their resources to study specific aspects of these complications. Numerous separate discoveries have begun to shed light on the overall picture of the pathogenesis of atherosclerosis in diabetes.

Our book summarizes these recent advances. This volume is divided into three parts: Diabetes and Lipids, Diabetes and Atherosclerosis, and Diabetes and Hypertension. Each section contains several chapters written by experts in the field. A concluding chapter in each part summarizes the clinical applications and practical implications of the research presented.

It is our hope that this approach will enable clinicians to integrate a vast array of new knowledge into their practices. In addition, as an up-to-date compendium of a developing area, we envision this work to be beneficial to academicians and researchers in a variety of related fields.

Boris Draznin, M.D., Ph.D.
Robert H. Eckel, M.D.

Contributors

John D. Bagdade, MD
Department of Medicine, Rush Medical College, 1653 W. Congress Parkway, Chicago, Illinois 60612

Nirmal K. Banskota, MD
Joslin Diabetes Center, One Joslin Place, Boston, Massachusetts 02215

Boris Draznin, MD, PhD
Chief, Section of Endocrinology, Medical Research Service and Department of Medicine, Veterans Affairs Medical Center; Professor of Medicine and Vice Chairman for Research Affairs, Department of Medicine, University of Colorado Health Sciences Center, 1055 Clermont Street, Denver, Colorado 80220

Robert H. Eckel, MD
Professor of Medicine, Division of Endocrinology, Metabolism, and Diabetes, Department of Medicine, University of Colorado Health Sciences Center, 4200 E. 9th Ave, Denver, Colorado 80262

Christopher J. Fielding, PhD
Neider Professor of Cardiovascular Physiology, Cardiovascular Research Institute, University of California Medical Center, San Francisco, California 94143

Simona Frontoni, MD
Post-doctoral Fellow, Division of Endocrinology, Department of Medicine, Albert Einstein College of Medicine, 1300 Morris Park Avenue, Bronx, New York 10461

Abhimanyu Garg, MD
Assistant Professor of Internal Medicine and Clinical Nutrition, Center for Human Nutrition, University of Texas Southwestern Medical Center, 5323 Harry Hines Boulevard, Dallas, Texas 75235

Scott M. Grundy, MD, PhD
Professor of Internal Medicine, Biochemistry, and Clinical Nutrition, University of Texas Southwestern Medical Center, 5323 Harry Hines Boulevard, Dallas, Texas 75235

Steven M. Haffner, MD
Division of Clinical Epidemiology, Department of Medicine, University of Texas Health Science Center at San Antonio, 7703 Floyd Curl Drive, San Antonio, Texas 78284

Barbara V. Howard, PhD
Medlantic Research Foundation, 108 Irving Street, N.W., Washington, D.C. 20010

Toyoshi Inoguchi, MD, PhD
Joslin Diabetes Center, One Joslin Place, Boston, Massachusetts 02215

George L. King, MD
Senior Investigator and Section Head, Joslin Diabetes Center, One Joslin Place, Boston, Massachusetts 02215

Andrzej S. Krolewski, MD, PhD
Chief, Section of Epidemiology and Genetics, Joslin Diabetes Center, One Joslin Place, Boston, Massachusetts 02215

Ching Fai Kwok, MD
Joslin Diabetes Center, One Joslin Place, Boston, Massachusetts 02215

Thomas Ledet, MD, PhD
Research Laboratory for Biochemical Pathology, Kommunehospitalet, 8000 Aarhus C, Denmark

Gary F. Lewis, MD
Division of Endocrinology, Department of Medicine, University of Toronto, The Toronto Hospital, General Division, 200 Elizabeth Street, Toronto, Ontario M5G 2C4 Canada

Maria F. Lopes-Virella, MD, PhD
Professor of Medicine, Division of Endocrinology, Metabolism and Nutrition, Medical University of South Carolina, 171 Ashley Avenue, Charleston, South Carolina 29425

Timothy J. Lyons, MD
Assistant Professor of Medicine, Division of Endocrinology, Metabolism and Nutrition, Medical University of South Carolina, 171 Ashley Avenue, Charleston, South Carolina 29425

Caroline Michel, MD
Royal Victoria Hospital, Cardiology Division, 687 Pine Avenue West, Montreal, Quebec, Canada H3A 1A1

F. Javier Oliver, PhD
Joslin Diabetes Center, One Joslin Place, Boston, Massachusetts 02215

Sylvie Picard, MD
Division of Endocrinology and Metabolism, Department of Medicine, University of California, San Diego, 9500 Gilman Drive, La Jolla, California 92093

Normand Racine, MD
Royal Victoria Hospital, Cardiology Division, 687 Pine Avenue West, Montreal, Quebec, Canada H3A 1A1

Jeffrey L. Ram, PhD
Associate Professor, Department of Physiology, Wayne State University, Detroit, Michigan 48201

Peter D. Reaven, MD
Assistant Adjunct Professor of Medicine, Division of Endocrinology and Metabolism, Department of Medicine, University of California, San Diego, 9500 Gilman Drive, La Jolla, California 92093

Marian Rewers, MD
Department of Preventive Medicine and Biometrics, University of Colorado Health Sciences Center, 4200 East 9th Avenue, Denver, Colorado 80262

Mary Richardson, PhD
Associate Professor of Pathology, McMaster University, 1200 Main Street West, Hamilton, Ontario, Canada L8N 3Z5

Luciano Rossetti, MD
Associate Professor of Medicine, Division of Endocrinology, Department of Medicine, Albert Einstein College of Medicine, 1300 Morris Park Avenue, Bronx, New York 10461

Susan Savage, MD
Assistant Professor of Medicine, Department of Medicine, University of Colorado Health Science Center, 4200 East 9th Avenue, Denver, Colorado 80262

Robert W. Schrier, MD
Professor and Chairman, Department of Medicine, University of Colorado Health Science Center, 4200 East 9th Avenue, Denver, Colorado 80262

Teruo Shiba, MD, PhD
Joslin Diabetes Center, One Joslin Place, Boston, Massachusetts 02215

Allan Sniderman, MD
Royal Victoria Hospital, Cardiology Division M4.76, 687 Pine Avenue West, Montreal, Quebec, Canada H3A 1A1

James R. Sowers, MD
Veterans Administration Medical Center, Allen Park, Michigan 48201; and Professor and Director, Division of Endocrinology and Hypertension, Wayne State University, Detroit, Michigan 48201

Paul R. Standley, PhD
Research Associate, Department of Physiology, Wayne State University, Detroit, Michigan 48201; Veterans Administration Medical Center, Allen Park, Michigan 48101

George Steiner, MD
Professor of Medicine and Physiology, Division of Endocrinology and Metabolism, Department of Medicine, University of Toronto, The Toronto Hospital, General Division, 200 Elizabeth Street, Toronto, Ontario M5G 2C4 Canada

Michael P. Stern, MD
Division of Clinical Epidemiology, Department of Medicine, University of Texas Health Science Center at San Antonio, 7703 Floyd Curl Drive, San Antonio, Texas 78284

Karl E. Sussman, MD
Associate Chief of Staff for Research and Development, Veterans Administration Medical Center, 1055 Clermont Street, Denver, Colorado 80220

Michael L. Tuck, MD
Professor of Medicine, Chief, Department of Endocrinology, Sepulveda VA, Sepulveda, California 91343

James H. Warram, MD
Section of Epidemiology and Genetics, Joslin Diabetes Center, One Joslin Place, Boston, Massachusetts 02215

Peter D. Winocour, PhD

Associate Professor of Pathology, McMaster University, 1200 Main Street West, Hamilton, Ontario, Canada L8N 3Z5

Robert W. Wissler, MD, PhD

Department of Pathology, University of Chicago, 5841 South Maryland Avenue, Chicago, Illinois 60637

Joseph L. Witztum, MD

Division of Endocrinology and Metabolism, Department of Medicine, University of California, San Diego, 9500 Gilman Drive, La Jolla, California 92093

Part **1**

Diabetes and Lipids

Chapter 1

Lipoproteins: Structure and Function

Barbara V. Howard, PhD

Atherosclerotic complications are by far the leading cause of morbidity and mortality among individuals with diabetes mellitus. In order to understand this phenomenon, it is important to understand the structure and metabolism of lipoproteins, because lipoprotein abnormalities undoubtedly play a central role in the atherosclerotic process. Their role is partly related to their levels of cholesterol, the lipid that accumulates in the atherosclerotic plaque. However, as knowledge of lipoproteins increases, it is evident that they also play a more subtle and complex role in the atherosclerotic process through their interactions both with each other and with other components of the vessel wall.

There has been literally an explosion of knowledge concerning the structure and function of lipoproteins over the last 40 years. Prior to the 1940s, it was simply known that blood fats were carried in plasma attached to unspecified proteins, a requirement dictated by their physical and chemical characteristics.[1] After the introduction of ultracentrifugation procedures by Gofman and co-workers,[2] investigators were able to isolate and quantify major classes of lipoproteins; since then, major advances have been made rapidly in understanding the structure of the major lipoprotein classes and their complexity, the genetics of their production, and the activity and regulation of enzymes involved in lipoprotein metabolism. This chapter outlines the current knowledge of the structure of the major lipoprotein classes and summarizes the current information concerning their metabolism and its regulation.[3-10] In individuals with diabetes mellitus, abnormalities in both composition and metabolism have been identified in many aspects of lipoprotein composition and metabolism. These are discussed in subsequent chapters.

Structure and Classification of Lipoproteins

Since lipids are insoluble in aqueous solutions, they cannot circulate freely in plasma. Lipoproteins are macromolecular complexes containing lipids and proteins. The latter are referred to as apolipoproteins or apoproteins. The function of these microemulsions is to transport cholesterol and triglyceride in plasma. The structure of all lipoprotein particles follows a similar pattern. They are

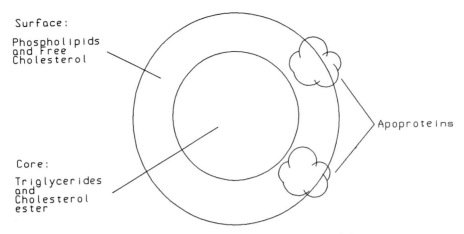

Surface:

Phospholipids
and Free
Cholesterol

Apoproteins

Core:

Triglycerides
and
Cholesterol
ester

Figure 1.1 General structure of lipoprotein particles.

spherical particles containing a central core of nonpolar lipids (primarily triglycerides and cholesteryl esters). The surface is a monolayer of phospholipids into which are inserted free cholesterol and apoproteins. The orientation of the phospholipids, cholesterol, and proteins in the outer layer resembles that of the outer leaflet of the plasma membrane, with the polar components facing outward and the nonpolar fatty acid chains and nonpolar portions of the proteins oriented toward the inner nonpolar lipid core (Figure 1.1).

Lipoproteins have been classified based on their density after ultracentrifugation (Table 1.1). Their names are based on their density, although older names corresponded to their electrophoretic mobility. Chylomicrons are mainly triglyceride-bearing particles; they are produced by the intestine after digestion of exogenous fat[11] and have a density of less than 1. Chylomicrons range widely in size from 1,000 to 4,000 Å. The major apoprotein of chylomicrons is B-48, which is only produced by the intestine. Chylomicrons also contain apo Cs, apo E, and apo A-I.

Very-low-density lipoproteins (VLDLs) are also triglyceride-bearing lipoproteins. They are secreted by the liver and carry endogenously produced triglycerides.[11] On electrophoresis, they show pre-β mobility. VLDLs actually represent a heterogeneous range of particles widely varying in size from 400 to 700 Å. They are often separated into subclasses on the basis of their rate of flotation,

Table 1.1 Major Lipoprotein Classes

Name	Size (Å)	Density	Electrophoretic Mobility	Major Apoproteins
Chylomicrons	1,000–4,000	<1.0	Origin	B-48, C-II, C-III, E, A-I
VLDL	400–700	<1.0006	Pre-β	B-100, C-II, C-III, E
IDL	300–400	1.006–1.019	Pre-β	B-100, C-II, C-III, E
LDL	225–275	1.019–1.063	β	B-100
HDL	75–100	1.063–1.210	α	A-I, A-II, C-II, C-III, E
Lp(a)	300–400	1.040–1.063	β	apo (a)

but there is no standard definition of the subclasses of VLDLs. The main apolipoprotein of VLDL is apo B = 100. VLDLs also contain lesser amounts of apolipoproteins E, C-I, C-II, and C-III. VLDLs may also be subdivided into particles that have the presence or absence of apolipoprotein E.

Intermediate-density lipoproteins (IDLs) are a poorly understood class representing remnants of the metabolism of triglyceride-rich lipoproteins and are intermediates in the conversion of VLDL to low-density lipoproteins (LDLs).[11] The major apolipoprotein in IDL is apolipoprotein B-100. IDL also contains apolipoproteins C and E, but in lesser proportions than VLDL.

LDLs are the main cholesterol-bearing lipoproteins and the most strongly related to the occurrence of cardiovascular disease.[12] LDLs show β mobility on electrophoresis and range from 225 to 275 Å. Virtually the only apoprotein in LDL is apo B-100. LDLs have recently been recognized to be a heterogeneous group of particles that can be separated, by either ultracentrifugation or gradient gel electrophoresis, into at least seven subfractions. These subfractions vary in their density and their proportion of lipid to apoprotein.

Lipoprotein (a), or Lp(a), is a subclass of the LDL fraction that consists of LDL complexed to a large glycoprotein resembling plasminogen. This complex has also been associated with atherosclerosis.[13]

High-density lipoproteins (HDLs) are the smallest (75 to 100 Å), most dense lipoproteins. Although they also transport substantial amounts of cholesterol, they have been negatively associated with cardiovascular disease.[14] They have α electrophoretic mobility. They are derived from the liver and the intestine. HDLs can be divided into subfractions on the basis of density; the most common subfractions are HDL_2 (between densities 1.063 and 1.125) and HDL_3 (between densities 1.125 and 1.210).[15] The major apolipoproteins in HDL are apolipoproteins A-I and A-II. HDLs also contain C apoproteins, apo A-IV, and apo E. HDLs may also be subdivided according to the content of their apoprotein into particles that contain only A-I (LpA-I), particles containing A-I and A-II (LpA-I/A-II), and, to a lesser extent, particles containing A-I and the C or E apoproteins.

The production and metabolism of all the lipoproteins are largely controlled by the apoprotein portion of the complex (Table 1.2). All of these proteins have been sequenced and their genes localized.[16] Of the four major categories of apoproteins, those with the highest molecular weight are the apoprotein Bs. In

Table 1.2 Apoproteins and Their Function

Name	Molecular Weight	Lipoprotein	Function
A-I	28,000	Chylomicrons, HDL	Efflux of cell cholesterol receptor binding ACAT activator
A-II	17,000	HDL	Efflux of cell cholesterol
A-IV	46,000	HDL	Not clear
B-100	550,000	VLDL, IDL, LDL	Binding to B/E receptor
B-48	264,000	Chylomicrons	Binding to LRP
C-I	5,800	VLDL, IDL, HDL	Not clear
C-II	9,100	VLDL, IDL, HDL	Activate LPL
C-III	8,750	VLDL, IDL, HDL	Inhibit LPL
E	35,000	VLDL, IDL, HDL	Binds to B/E receptor and liver LRP
(a)	200,000–500,000	Lp(a)	Interferes with fibrinolysis

Table 1.3 Major Enzymes of Lipoprotein Metabolism

Name	Function
Lipoprotein lipase	Hydrolysis of triglycerides on chylomicrons and VLDL
Hepatic lipase	Hydrolysis of triglycerides on VLDL Hydrolysis of phospholipids on HDL
Lecithin:cholesterol acyltransferase (LCAT)	Esterification of plasma cholesterol; associated with HDL
Cholesteryl ester transfer protein (CETP)	Transfer of cholesteryl ester and triglycerides between lipoproteins
Acyl-coenzyme A cholesterol acyltransferase (ACAT)	Esterification of cellular cholesterol

humans, apo B-48 is produced by the intestine and present only on chylomicrons, whereas apo B-100 is synthesized by the liver and is the major apoprotein in VLDL and IDL, and virtually the only one in LDL. Apo Cs and Es are synthesized in the liver; in the circulation, they are found on chylomicrons, VLDL, IDL, and HDL. Three major forms of apolipoprotein E have been identified, coded by alleles ε2, ε3, and ε4. These differ by only one or two amino acids, but these differences confer marked effects on receptor recognition. Since each person inherits two alleles for apo E, six major phenotypes are possible. The relative frequency for phenotype E3/E3 (the most common) is approximately 60% of the population, and that for E2/E2 (the least common) is approximately 1% of the population.

Most of the apolipoproteins are hydrophobic and serve as ligands for specific receptors involved in the metabolism of the various lipoproteins, or as cofactors for enzymatic activities involved in lipoprotein metabolism. Several other proteins play key roles in plasma lipoprotein transport (Table 1.3). These include lipoprotein lipase[17] and hepatic lipase,[18] which catalyze the delipidation of triglyceride-rich particles; lecithin:cholesterol acyltransferase (LCAT),[19] which is responsible for the synthesis of virtually all cholesteryl esters in plasma lipoproteins; cholesteryl ester transfer protein (CETP),[20] which facilitates the transfer of cholesterol and cholesteryl ester between lipoproteins during their metabolism; and acyl-coenzyme A cholesterol acyltransferase (ACAT), which esterifies cellular cholesterol. These enzymes are discussed further in the following sections.

Formation and Metabolism of Chylomicrons (Figure 1.2)

Chylomicrons are responsible for the transport of dietary triglycerides and cholesterol from the intestine to the liver. Dietary triglycerides are hydrolyzed in the gut to release free fatty acids. Micelles are formed containing the released fatty acids and monoglycerides, lecithin, lysolecithin, and bile acids. From these, the lipids enter the intestinal mucosal cells. Within the intestinal mucosal cell, fatty acid is re-esterified to reform triglycerides. These triglycerides are assembled together with the absorbed cholesterol, apo B-48 and apo A-I. On secretion from the enterocyte, they enter the lymphatic circulation and then the bloodstream, where they acquire C apoproteins and apo E by transfer from HDL. As

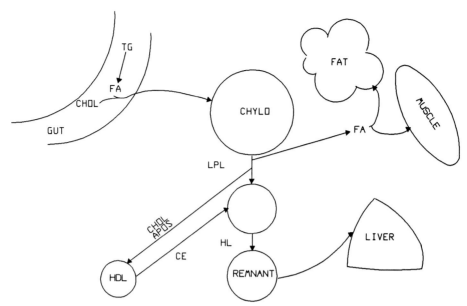

Figure 1.2 Metabolism of chylomicrons (CHYLO). TG = triglyceride; FA = fatty acids; CHOL = free cholesterol; LPL = lipoprotein lipase; HL = hepatic lipase; CE = esterified cholesterol.

chylomicrons enter the plasma, triglyceride is rapidly hydrolyzed by the enzyme lipoprotein lipase, which resides on the surface of capillary endothelial cells. Lipoprotein lipase is synthesized mainly in adipose tissue and in striated muscle. It is then secreted and transported to the endothelial surface, where it acts on triglyceride-rich particles. Its action requires the presence of apo C-II on the surface of lipoproteins, whereas apo C-III inhibits lipoprotein lipase. The enzyme appears to be induced in adipose tissue by insulin.[21]

When chylomicrons or other triglyceride-rich lipoproteins interact with lipoprotein lipase, fatty acids are released and bind to circulating albumin for transport in plasma, to meet the oxidative needs of muscle and other peripheral cells. The excess free fatty acid is stored, mainly in adipose tissue, by being taken up and resynthesized into triglycerides. This triglyceride serves as a future source for free fatty acids. A portion of free fatty acids can also be taken up by the liver, where they can be a source of fuel or resynthesized into triglycerides.

As the core triglyceride in chylomicrons is depleted, surface phospholipids and A and C apoproteins are transferred to HDL. The residual particle, which has lost 80% to 90% of its triglycerides and is now relatively cholesterol enriched, is called a chylomicron remnant. During the course of its formation, this remnant is believed to take on additional amounts of apo E, which then facilitates its recognition by a receptor in the liver, termed the LDL receptor–related protein (LRP).[22] The binding to this receptor is enhanced in the presence of lipoprotein lipase. The remnants then are incorporated into liposomes, from which cholesterol can enter into all metabolic pathways of hepatocytes, including excretion into the bile. The remaining triglyceride enters the hepatic triglyceride stores.

Much of hepatic cholesterol is secreted into the bile, and hence into the intestine, either as free cholesterol or, after conversion, as bile acid. The process by which cholesterol and also bile acids cycle between the intestine and the liver is known as the enterohepatic circulation. When biliary cholesterol enters the intestine, approximately 50% is absorbed and returned to the liver; the remainder is excreted. Over 97% of bile acids are reabsorbed and very little excreted. This amount of biliary cholesterol and bile acids returning to the liver, supplemented by the constant influx of dietary cholesterol, regulates the amount of synthesized cholesterol. A high rate of flux of cholesterol to the liver, either by high dietary intake or efficient reabsorption, suppresses the activity of cholesterol synthesis. If less cholesterol returns to the liver, production is increased.

VLDL Metabolism (Figure 1.3)

VLDLs are synthesized in the endoplasmic reticulum of hepatocytes. They are composed of endogenous triglycerides derived from plasma free fatty acids, from chylomicron and VLDL remnants, and from de novo lipogenesis. Apo B-100 is synthesized in the ribosomes of the rough endoplasmic reticulum. Triglyceride components, along with small amounts of cholesteryl ester, are synthesized by enzymes in the smooth endoplasmic reticulum. Lipids and apoproteins join at the junction of the smooth and rough endoplasmic reticula and VLDL particles are formed. These pass to the Golgi apparatus, where secretory vesicles containing large numbers of VLDL particles bud off and migrate to the surface of the cell.

VLDL production is influenced by glucose, fatty acid, and insulin levels. Concentrations of circulating free fatty acids govern rates of triglyceride esterification in the liver, and concentrations of free glucose, especially when glycogen synthesis is impeded, may stimulate de novo production of free fatty acid.

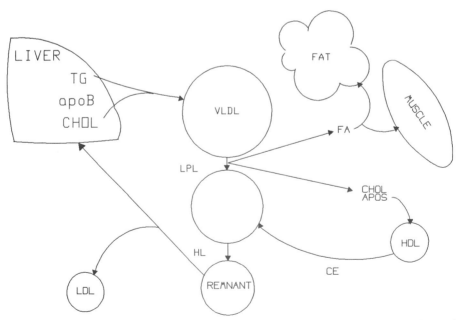

Figure 1.3 Metabolism of VLDL. TG = triglyceride; FA = fatty acids; CHOL = free cholesterol; LPL = lipoprotein lipase; HL = hepatic lipase; CE = esterified cholesterol.

Insulin is required for VLDL production both for apoprotein synthesis and also because it regulates several enzymes involved in lipogenesis.[23] However, increasing insulin has been shown to inhibit VLDL secretion and hepatocytes by phosphorylating apo B, which impedes its assembly with lipids in the endoplasmic reticulum.[24]

Nascent VLDLs that are secreted in the circulation contain apo B-100 and small amounts of apo C and apo E. As they circulate, they are transformed into mature VLDLs by the acquisition of cholesteryl esters and apoproteins C and E, which are transferred from HDLs. This process is assisted by two cofactors: the enzyme LCAT, which esterifies the free cholesterol in HDL; and CETP, which facilitates the exchange of both cholesteryl ester and triglycerides. VLDLs are metabolized in the same manner as chylomicrons by the enzyme lipoprotein lipase, with the liberated fatty acids following the same fate as that of chylomicrons. Free cholesterol is progressively exchanged into HDL, where it is esterified and the cholesteryl esters returned to VLDL. As the VLDL becomes depleted of triglycerides, a portion of the surface, including apolipoproteins C and E and phospholipids, is transferred to HDL.

Hepatic lipase also plays a role in the metabolism of smaller VLDLs during the latter stages of the VLDL catabolic cascade.[25] The remnants of VLDL are triglyceride-depleted, cholesterol-rich particles, some of which are isolated in the IDL density range and some of which still remain in the VLDL compartment. The relative proportion of apolipoprotein E appears to decline when VLDL is metabolized, and its size decreases. It is not known whether all VLDL particles initially have apoprotein E and it then remains in some during catabolism or there are initially two classes of VLDL.

VLDL remnants can have two fates: they can be taken up by the liver or they can be transformed into LDLs. In humans, at least half of VLDL remnants are removed from the circulation without conversion to LDL. Remnant particles are cleared from the circulation primarily by receptors in the liver. The predominant receptor is the B/E receptor, which also clears LDL (see below). However, VLDL remnants, especially those containing apo E and perhaps associated with lipoprotein lipase, are cleared by LRP, which was described above for chylomicrons. A portion of the VLDL remnant is further metabolized, possibly by a process involving hepatic lipase within the liver sinusoids, to form LDL. During this process, more triglyceride and the remainder of apolipoproteins other than apo B are lost.

The mechanisms that determine which and what portion of VLDLs are converted to LDLs are not clearly understood. VLDLs are believed to be secreted in a spectrum of sizes with various proportions of triglyceride. The larger VLDL particles appear to be more rapidly cleared and less likely to be converted to LDL.[26] In contrast, smaller, more cholesterol-rich VLDL may be preferentially converted to LDL. The phenotype of apo E also influences the fate of these remnants. The apo E2 is not recognized by the B/E receptor. In individuals with the ε2 allele, chylomicrons and VLDL remnants are cleared more slowly than normal and can accumulate in the plasma (as in type III hyperlipidemia). Because of their lack of affinity for the B/E receptor, and their consequent removal from liver-mediated processes, the VLDL remnants of individuals with E2 phenotype are less likely to be converted to LDL, and these individuals have lower LDL concentrations. In contrast, the E4 phenotype has the highest affinity for the receptor; this appears to be associated with more efficient conversion to LDL, and these individuals have higher LDL concentrations.

LDL Metabolism (Table 1.4)

As indicated above, LDL is a product of the metabolism of VLDL. The only apolipoprotein present in LDL is apo B, and there is only one molecule of apo B per particle. There are a varying number of cholesteryl ester molecules, ranging from approximately 1,000 to 1,500, depending on the size and density of the particle and the triglyceride content. LDL can be removed either by the liver or by extrahepatic tissues. Current estimates in humans indicate approximately 75% of LDL is cleared by the liver. Clearance by either the liver or extrahepatic tissues can occur by both receptor- and non-receptor-mediated pathways. In healthy humans, approximately two thirds of the circulating pool of LDL is cleared by the receptor pathway.

Receptor-mediated clearance is mediated by the B/E receptors present on the surface of cells.[10] When these receptors are synthesized by cells, they are transported to the surface, where they cluster in special regions on the cell surface referred to as coated pits. After LDL binds to the receptor, the lipoprotein is internalized by an endocytotic process. The vesicle then fuses with lysosomes, where enzymes degrade the apo B and hydrolyze the cholesteryl ester to free cholesterol. Triglycerides and phospholipids may also be hydrolyzed. The cholesterol can have several fates. It can serve as a constituent for cell membrane, it can be re-esterified into cholesteryl ester for storage, or it can be converted to steroid hormones in tissues such as the adrenal; in the liver, it can leave the cell into bile either as free cholesterol or after to conversion to bile acids.

The influx of free cholesterol from LDL sets into motion a cascade of regulatory events that control the cell cholesterol content. Esterification of cholesterol is stimulated by activation of ACAT. Cholesterol production is inhibited on the cholesterol influx by the inhibition of hepatic hydroxymethylglutaryl-coenzyme A reductase, the rate-limiting enzyme for cholesterol biosynthesis. Finally, accumulation of intracellular cholesterol limits the further uptake of cholesterol-rich lipoproteins by inhibiting synthesis of the B/E receptor and its migration to the cell surface.

The LDL receptor is a molecule of approximately 120,000 daltons. It has several functional domains. The receptor binding region, which is required for binding LDL, is located external to the plasma membrane. It recognizes both apo B and apo E. The second domain is homologous to epidermal growth factor; the functional significance of this is unknown. The third domain, most proximal to the cell membrane, is the segment where carbohydrate residues are linked. The next segment of only 22 amino acids spans the cell membrane and is hy-

Table 1.4 Events Associated With LDL Receptor Binding

1. Internalization and degradation of LDL in lysozomes; release of free cholesterol
2. Activation of ACAT—esterification of cholesterol
3. Inhibition of hepatic hydroxymethylglutaryl-coenzyme A reductase and, therefore, cholesterol production
4. Down-regulation of surface LDL receptors

drophobic. The fifth, or cytoplasmic, domain is responsible for the recognition of coated pits and, thus, the transport of receptors to and from the cell membrane. It also governs the clustering of receptors on the apical surfaces of polarized cells, such as in the liver and in the kidney.

The regulation of the amount of B/E receptor synthesis in response to the amount of cell cholesterol is a critical process in controlling both cellular and plasma cholesterol. It is postulated that a portion of cellular cholesterol is converted to an oxysterol that enters the cell nucleus, interacts with the regulatory protein, and directly suppresses the transcription of the LDL receptor gene. Thus, when cell cholesterol content increases, the number of receptors decreases; conversely, when cell cholesterol content declines, receptor number is activated. This, in turn, has an influence on plasma cholesterol concentrations for two reasons. First, increased amounts of receptors clear a greater proportion of VLDL remnants, which are precursors of LDL, thus decreasing LDL production (Figure 1.3). Second, increasing receptors lead to increased receptor-mediated clearance of LDL.

For the internal economy of the cell, the down-regulation of the receptor halts the internal cellular accumulation of cholesterol. Conversely, LDL receptors are up-regulated when cell cholesterol content declines, thus making free cholesterol available for cells' needs. With regard to the economy of the whole body, understanding this practice is critical in both the maintenance of plasma cholesterol levels and strategies for their lowering.

The influx of dietary cholesterol and, thus, the influx of cholesterol to the liver results in down-regulation of hepatic receptors, the main avenue for clearance of plasma LDL; therefore, plasma LDL concentrations increase. In contrast, strategies that deplete hepatic cholesterol, either by inhibition of cholesterol synthesis or by interruption of the enterohepatic circulation by agents such as bile acid binding resins, result in depletion of hepatic cholesterol concentrations. This, in turn, will up-regulate hepatic LDL receptors, increasing clearance of plasma LDL, and this results in declines in LDL concentrations.

An understanding of this pathway can further elucidate the potential effect of variations in apo E isoforms. Individuals with apo E2 phenotype have impaired clearance of VLDL remnants. This results in the depletion of hepatic cholesterol, up-regulation of LDL receptors, and thus lower LDL concentrations. Conversely, in individuals with the E4 phenotype, the remnants bind much more avidly; thus more remnants are cleared, hepatic cholesterol increases, and LDL receptors down-regulate, resulting in higher plasma LDL concentrations.

Many other physiologic processes are also believed to influence this regulation of LDL receptor activity. These include thyroid hormone, which stimulates LDL receptors, and the presence of saturated fat in the plasma membrane, which appears to inhibit LDL receptors.

LDL may also be cleared by non-B/E receptor-mediated clearance mechanisms, which occur in phagocytic cells. This includes both nonspecific endocytotic uptake and a receptor-mediated process by macrophages that recognize altered LDL.[27] This process, thought to be responsible for cholesterol deposition in the vesicle wall, becomes increasingly important when either defects in the LDL receptor are present or there are abnormalities in LDL composition. The latter include oxidation and glycation of LDL, which may be accelerated by injury or alterations of endothelial cell function.

Lp(a)

Although the existence of the particle has been known for some time, only recently have aspects of the metabolism of Lp(a) and its importance in the atherogenic process been investigated. Lp(a) consist of an LDL particle to which apolipoprotein (a) is attached through a disulfide link. Apo (a) is a large molecule that resembles plasminogen. There are at least seven major isoforms of apoprotein (a). A large portion of the structure of apo (a) consists of repeat sequences of Kringle IV of the plasminogen molecule. The isoforms appear to differ in their number of these repeat sequences and vary widely in molecular weight, from 400,000 to over 600,000. Plasma concentration of Lp(a) varies widely, averaging from 3 to over 100 mg/dL. Individuals with the smallest isoforms of Lp(a) tend to have higher plasma concentrations.

Lp(a) appears to be synthesized in the liver. The recent observation that a portion of apo (a) appears to be associated with triglyceride-rich particles suggests that it might be secreted with VLDL and then be converted to an LDL-like particle in a manner similar to that in which LDL is produced from VLDL.

Clearance of Lp(a) is poorly understood; it has a residence time longer than that of LDL. There appears to be some binding to the B/E receptor, but it also appears to accelerate LDL binding and uptake. Other pathways for degradation are not currently understood. The mechanism of the association between Lp(a) and atherosclerosis is also only partly understood. Lp(a) appears to be deposited in atherosclerotic plaques in the same areas as apo B. One possibility is that Lp(a) competes with the binding of plasminogen to endothelial cells and therefore inhibits fibrinolysis. This inhibition of fibrinolysis may also be enhanced through an inhibition of plasminogen activator inhibitor-1.

HDL Metabolism (Figure 1.4)

The steps involved in the production and metabolism of HDL are complex. The first step in HDL production is the secretion into the circulation of nascent HDL. This is a discoid particle that contains phospholipids, cholesterol, some cholesteryl ester, and either apo A-I or apo A-I plus apo A-II. Apo E is usually contained on the apo A-I particle. The apo A-I–containing particle may be secreted by both the intestine and the liver, whereas the A-I/A-II particle is secreted only by the liver. Through the action of LCAT, the free cholesterol in the particle is rapidly esterified to cholesterol ester and the particle is transformed into a small spherical particle in the HDL_3 density range.

During the metabolism of triglyceride-rich lipoproteins, these small HDLs serve as a source of cholesteryl ester for transfer to the triglyceride-rich lipoproteins, and as a receptor for the free cholesterol, apo C, apo E, and surface components of the triglyceride-rich particles that are removed as their core is depleted. Thus, the HDL compartment is augmented during the action of lipoprotein lipase. This process is also enhanced by the constant activity of LCAT, which esterifies the free cholesterol as it is received. As cholesteryl esters begin to accumulate in the HDL particle, they grow in size and become less dense, HDL_2 particles. Thus, during the lipolytic process, HDL particle size increases.

The cross-transfer of triglycerides and cholesteryl esters between HDL and triglyceride-rich particles is facilitated by CETP. The exchange of triglyceride and cholesteryl ester between triglyceride-rich particles and HDL is accelerated

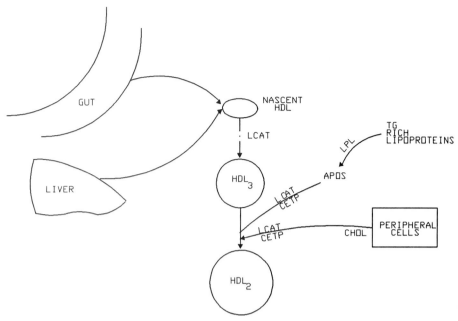

Figure 1.4 Metabolism of HDL. LCAT = lecithin:cholesterol acyltransferase; TG = triglyceride; LPL = lipoprotein lipase; CETP = cholesteryl ester transfer protein; CHOL = free cholesterol.

by the presence of free fatty acid on HDL. Thus, situations in which free fatty acids are elevated may result in lower concentrations of HDL cholesterol and higher proportions of HDL triglyceride.

It is believed that HDL, along with LCAT and CETP, is also involved in the flux of cholesterol between cells and plasma lipoproteins.[20,28] Cholesterol substrate for LCAT also can be derived from cell membranes, especially under conditions in which HDL is relatively depleted of cholesterol and the cell cholesterol content is elevated. It has been proposed that the A-I–containing HDL particles, especially those also containing apo E, may serve as efficient receptors for this reverse cholesterol transfer.

Cholesterol can only be removed from the body through the liver; therefore, to remove excess cholesterol from peripheral tissue, cholesterol must be transported back to the liver. Unesterified cholesterol can exchange between cell membranes and HDL through the action of LCAT, but if cholesterol is esterified, a portion of that cholesteryl ester is then shuttled to VLDL and to LDL by CETP. This cholesteryl ester can then be returned to the liver by the direct uptake of VLDL remnants or after their conversion to LDL. Also, whole HDL particles are believed to be removed intact by the liver. The sum total of these processes represents a pathway for "reverse cholesterol transport," in which cholesterol from peripheral cells can be removed and transported to the liver for excretion in bile.

The mechanisms that control clearance of HDL are not well understood. Cholesteryl esters from HDL may be taken up by hepatic cells without endocytosis of the HDL particles per se. In addition, hepatic lipase may hydrolyze HDL phospholipids, which, in turn, may promote net transfer of cholesterol to the surface of the liver. The LpA-I particles appear to be more rapidly hydrolyzed than those containing both A-I and A-II. Finally, there are specific HDL receptors on peripheral cells that may be involved not only in the cholesterol efflux process, but also in specific uptake and degradation of the HDL particles.[29]

Summary

As more information becomes available concerning lipoprotein metabolism, it is increasingly evident that each lipoprotein class consists of a complex and heterogeneous group of particles whose metabolism is tightly regulated. Although the biochemistry of the apolipoproteins and the enzymology of the catalytic activities involved have been partially elucidated, it is clear that much information is still lacking. From the perspective of the diabetologist, it will become increasingly evident in subsequent chapters that multiple sites in the lipoprotein metabolic cascade may be influenced by diabetes, and that diabetics may contain lipoproteins with significant alterations in composition. Detailed mechanisms for these changes and how these changes lead to atherosclerosis must be elucidated so that effective preventive therapy can be developed.

References

1. Bloor WR: *J Biol Chem* 1916;25:577–599.
2. Gofman JW, Lindgren FT, Elliott H: *J Biol Chem* 1949;179:973–979.
3. Gotto AM Jr, Pownall HR, Havel RJ: Introduction to the plasma lipoproteins. *Methods Enzymol* 1986;128:3.
4. Havel RJ: Origin, metabolic fate and metabolic function of plasma lipoproteins, in Steinberg D, Olefsky JM (eds): *Comptemporary Issues in Endocrinology and Metabolism.* New York, Churchill Livingstone, 1987, vol 3, p 117.
5. Assmann G: *Lipid Metabolism and Atherosclerosis.* New York, Schattauer, 1982.
6. Grundy SM: *Cholesterol and Atherosclerosis: Diagnosis and Treatment.* Philadelphia, JB Lippincott, 1990.
7. Edelstein C, Kezdy F, Scanu AM, et al: Apopipoproteins and the structural organization of plasma lipoproteins: Human plasma high density lipoprotein-3. *J Lipid Res* 1979; 20:143.
8. Havel RJ, Kane JP: Introduction: Structure and metabolism of plasma lipoprotein, in Scriver CR, Beaudet AL, Sly WS, et al (eds): *The Metabolic Basis of Inherited Disease,* ed 6. New York, McGraw-Hill, 1989, pp 1129–1138.
9. Kane JP, Havel RJ: Disorders of the biogenes and secretion of lipoproteins containing the B apolipoproteins, in Scriver CR, Beaudet AL, Sly WS, et al: *The Metabolic Basis of Inherited Disease,* ed 6. New York, McGraw-Hill, 1989, pp 1139–1164.
10. Goldstein JL, Brown MS: Familial hypercholesterolemia, in Scriver CR, Beaudet AL, Sly WS, et al (eds): *The Metabolic Basis of Inherited Disease,* ed 6. New York, McGraw-Hill, 1989, pp 1215–1250.
11. Havel RJ: Metabolism of triglyceride-rich lipoproteins, in Schettler FD (ed): *Atherosclerosis VI.* Berlin, Springer-Verlag, 1983, p 480.
12. Grundy SM: Cholesterol and coronary heart disease—a new era. *JAMA* 1986;256:2849–2858.
13. Scanu AM, Fless GM: Lipoproteins (a)—heterogeneity and biological relevance. *J Clin Invest* 1990;85:1709–1715.

14. Castelli WP, Garrison RJ, Wilson PWF: Incidence of coronary heart diseae and lipoprotein cholesterol levels. The Framingham Study. *JAMA* 1986;256:2835–2838.

15. Eisenberg S: High density lipoprotein metabolism. *J Lipid Res* 1984;25:1017.

16. Brewer HB Jr, Santamarina-Fojo S, Hoeg JM: The molecular biology of the human plasma apolipoproteins, lipoprotein receptors and lipoprotein lipase, in Steiner G, Shafir E (eds): *The Hyperlipidemias.* New York, McGraw-Hill, vol 11: *Primary Hyperlipidemias,* 1991.

17. Garfinkel AS, Schotz MC: Lipoprotein lipase, in Gotto AM (ed): *Plasma Lipoproteins.* Amsterdam, Elsevier, 1987, p 335.

18. Jackson RL: Lipoprotein lipase and hepatic lipase, in Boyer PD (ed): *The Enzymes.* New York, Academic Press, 1984, vol 16, p 141.

19. Jauhiainen M, Dolphin PJ: Human plasma lecithin–cholesterol acyl transferase. *J Biol Chem* 1986;261:7032.

20. Fielding CJ, Fielding PE: Cholesterol transport between cells and body fluids. *Med Clin North Am* 1982;66(2):353.

21. Yki-Jarvinen H, Taskinen MR, Koivisto VA, et al: Response of adipose tissue lipoprotein lipase activity and serum lipoproteins to acute hyperinsulinemia in man. *Diabetologia* 1984;27:364.

22. Havel RJ, Hamilton RL: Hepatocytic lipoprotein receptors and intracellular lipoprotein catabolism. *Hepatology* 1988;8:1689–1704.

23. Schonfeld G: Diabetes, lipoproteins and atherosclerosis. *Metabolism* 1985;32(suppl 1):45–50.

24. Sparks CE, Sparks JD, Bolognino M, et al: Insulin effects apolipoprotein B lipoprotein synthesis and secretion by primary cultures of rat hepatocytes. *Metabolism* 1986; 35(suppl 12):1128–1136.

25. Goldberg IJ, Le NA, Paterniti JR Jr, et al: Lipoprotein metabolism during acute inhibition of hepatic triglyceride lipase in the cynomolgus monkey. *J Clin Invest* 1982; 70:1184–1192.

26. Packard CJ, Munro A, Lorimer AR, et al: Metabolism of apolipoprotein B in large triglyceride-rich very low density lipoproteins of normal and hypertriglyceridemic subjects. *J Clin Invest* 1984;74:2178–2192.

27. Steinberg D, Parthasarathy S, Carew TE, et al: Beyond cholesterol: Modifications of low-density lipoprotein that increase its atherogenicity. *N Engl J Med* 1989;320:915–924.

28. Gwynne JT: Reverse cholesterol transport. *Am J Cardiol* 1989;64:10G–17G.

29. Graham DL, Oram JF: Identification and characterization of a high density lipoprotein-binding protein in cell membranes by ligand blotting. *J Biol Chem* 1987;262:7439–7442.

Chapter 2

Low-Density Lipoprotein Metabolism in Diabetes

Peter D. Reaven, MD, Sylvie Picard, MD, and Joseph L. Witztum, MD

Atherosclerosis is the major cause of death in diabetic subjects. For this reason there have been extensive attempts to determine the prevalence of cardiovascular risk factors in this population.[1] Special attention has been focused on the possibility that differences in plasma lipoprotein levels may play an important role in the increased prevalence of coronary artery disease (CAD) in diabetics. Although diabetes may affect all lipoproteins (reviewed elsewhere in this book), this chapter focuses on the role that alterations in the levels of low-density lipoproteins (LDLs) or modifications of LDLs may play in the atherogenic process.

Levels of LDL Cholesterol in Diabetes

LDL Cholesterol Levels in Insulin-Dependent Diabetes Mellitus

Uncontrolled insulin-dependent diabetes mellitus (IDDM) is associated with a variety of lipid abnormalities. In this situation of profound insulin deficiency, a marked decrease of lipoprotein lipase (LPL) activity contributes to impaired chylomicron and very-low-density lipoprotein (VLDL) catabolism. Consequently, VLDLs and chylomicrons accumulate, and high-density lipoprotein (HDL) and LDL levels are greatly decreased. However, this is the exception, and most studies of *treated* IDDM reveal little difference in LDL cholesterol levels compared to appropriately matched nondiabetics. The ratio of LDL cholesterol levels in diabetics to that in nondiabetics is close to 1:1 in the majority of reported studies (Table 2.1).[2–10] These reports, from many different countries, have evaluated subjects over a wide range of ages and frequently included both men and women. Perhaps the largest study to date is the ongoing Diabetes Control and Complications Trial (DCCT).[4] In this multicenter study involving over 1,500 men and women with IDDM, lipid values at baseline were measured and compared to age- and sex-matched nondiabetics in the Lipid Research Clinic (LRC) prevalence study. Lipoprotein measurements were performed by tech-

Table 2.1 Comparison of Lipoprotein Values in IDDM Subjects Versus Controls in Various Countries

Country	Study Group	Age Range (or Mean)	No. of Diabetics	Ratio of Diabetic to Control Values				Correlation of LDL-Chol with HbA$_{1c}$	Comments	Ref. No.
				LDL-Chol	HDL-Chol	VLDL-Chol	TG			
Spain	Clinic patients	(36)	24	0.93	1.15	1.58	1.04	—	Age, weight, smoking hx matched	2
Germany	Prevalence study	50–65	M—302 F—84	0.97 1.04	0.95 0.84	NA	1.41 1.58	—		3
US	Volunteers	13–14 15–19 20–24	F—761	1.13* 1.18* 1.12*	0.93* 0.89* 0.98	1.09 1.25* 1.00	1.09 1.25* 1.00	0.2	LDL-Chol levels similar at all other ages (vs. LRC data). In men with IDDM, LOL-Chol lower ages 25–39	4
	Clinic patients	10–33	105	[a]1.02–1.11	[a]0.97–0.93	[a]1.3*–1.9*	[a]1.07–1.67*	Increases with HgbA$_{1c}$	Age and gender adjusted	5
	Clinic patients	2–22	106	[b]1.17–1.60*	[b]1.14–0.70*	1.1–1.9*	0.92–1.9*	M—0.35 F—0.43	Age adjusted, stratified by glucose "control"	6
	Diabetic register	33 34	M—63 F—48	1.05 1.24*	1.14* 1.11*	0.87 1.33*	1.01 1.66	—	Similar-age controls	7
Finland	Diabetic register	35–55	M—84 F—86	0.98 0.106	1.18* 1.17*	1.00 0.82	0.93 0.106	LDL chol. increased with FBG	Nondiabetic sibling controls	8
	Diabetic register	45–64	M—43 F—44	0.97 0.90*	1.14* 1.16*	1.04 0.89	1.05 0.97	—	No differences in alcohol, cigarette use	9
	Diabetic register	45–64	M—32 F—31	0.97 0.95	1.12 1.24*	0.96 0.85	1.01 0.82	NS	Age matched, CHD free patients only	10

Abbreviations: F: female; M: male.

* Significantly different from nondiabetic values.

[a] First value of each pair refers to diabetics with HbA$_{1c}$ <13%, whereas the second value is for HbA$_{1c}$ values >15%.

[b] First value is for subjects in "good control," whereas second value is for subjects in "poor control."

Country	Population	Age	Group	Value	Comparison	Ref
US	Caucasian volunteers	20–78	*NIDDM* M—69	0.96	Age adjusted	25
			F—58	0.98		
			IGT M—14	1.01		
			F—27	0.99		
US	Free-living population	M—(65)	*NIDDM* M—52	0.96	Age-matched incl. hormone HDL adjusted	26
		F—(63)	F—40	0.97		
US	Diabetic register & clinic patients	20+	M—62	1.02	Age-matched controls	7
			F—35	1.12		
			Men D—43	0.91		
			S—38	0.90		
			I—79	0.88*		
			Women D—39	0.94		
			S—25	1.01		
			I—46	0.95		
US	Community screening of Pima Indians	Above age 15	*IGT* M—57	NS	Age adjusted	29
			F—126	Sig. increase		
			NIDDM M—179	NS		
			F—328	Sig. increase		
Finland	Registered diabetics	45–64	M—126	0.94	Age-matched controls	9
			F—138	0.91		
England	Unselected consecutive volunteers	M—(52)	*NIDDM* M—16	1.10	Similar-age controls	92
		F—(50)	F—29	1.00		
		M—(55)	*IGT* M—26	1.17		
		F—(45)	F—28	0.82		

Abbreviations: S: treated with sulfonylureas; D: treated with diet; I: treated with insulin.
* Significant compared to nondiabetic values.

elevated triglycerides and low HDL cholesterol. Although hypercholesterolemia is quite common, with possibly as many as 40% of patients meeting the National Cholesterol Education Program criteria for hyperlipidemia,[23] LDL cholesterol levels are usually similar to those in nondiabetics. This appears true for nearly all races and nationalities (Table 2.2). In the 15 studies that included a control comparison group, with a total of nearly 2,500 diabetic subjects, only one small study from China ($n = 23$) showed a significantly higher LDL cholesterol level in diabetic women.[24] In studies that adjusted for age and/or other variables known to influence lipoprotein levels,[20,25,26] LDL cholesterol levels were nearly identical in diabetics and nondiabetics. In several studies[2,27,28] in which subjects were subdivided by the mode of current treatment (diet, sulfonylureas, or insulin), LDL cholesterol levels were still similar to those of nondiabetics.

A number of studies also looked at LDL cholesterol levels in IGT populations. In nearly all of these there was no difference in LDL cholesterol levels compared to subjects with normal glucose tolerance. In a large study of older free-living people with IGT, LDL cholesterol levels were similar to controls in both men and women, both before and after adjusting for relevant variables such as age, body mass index (BMI), smoking, alcohol intake, exercise, and hormone use.[20] An exception to these consistent findings was a study of the Pima Indians[29] that found that women with IGT had, overall, significantly higher LDL cholesterol levels than nondiabetic controls. However, this difference was actually evident only in a small number of subjects in the oldest age group. Although few studies have prospectively determined the effect of glucose control on LDL cholesterol levels, a number of studies have compared the effect of glucose-lowering modalities, whether insulin, oral agents, or weight loss. In general, these studies have shown no change or only a modest tendency to lower LDL cholesterol levels[22,30,31] in addition to their effects on plasma triglyceride and HDL cholesterol levels.

In summary, increased triglyceride and decreased HDL cholesterol levels are the most common lipid abnormalities in both IGT and NIDDM. LDL levels, although frequently elevated in an absolute sense, are similar to those found in appropriately matched nondiabetic populations. Improvement in glucose control may have a modest beneficial effect on LDL cholesterol levels in addition to its effects on triglyceride and HDL cholesterol levels.

A final caveat must be made about the data presented in Tables 2.1 and 2.2. These tables have presented the ratio of LDL levels in diabetics to those of control populations presumably subjected to the same environmental influences in an attempt to isolate the effect that diabetes alone may have on LDL levels. However, this type of analysis overlooks the profound impact of environmental influences on *absolute* differences in LDL levels, and the important impact this has on expression of CAD. For example, the studies of Kawate et al[32] demonstrated that Japanese diabetics living in Japan (probably most were NIDDM) had an incidence of CAD of 10% to 13%, whereas Japanese living in Hawaii had an incidence of 32%, similar to the rate of CAD among caucasians in Hawaii (33%) or the United States (40%). These differences were ascribed to marked differences in cholesterol and triglyceride values in the different populations. Similarly, an increased incidence of CAD in eastern Finnish diabetic populations, compared to western Finnish populations, was ascribed in part to a more atherogenic lipoprotein profile.[33] Comparable differences in the nondiabetic population were also seen. Thus, although it is clear that many other factors must be taken into account in explaining the enhanced risk of atherosclerosis in diabetic subjects, it must not be forgotten that *absolute* LDL levels have a profound impact on the development of vascular disease in diabetics, just as in the nondiabetic population.

LDL Levels in Diabetics With Vascular Disease

Several investigators have compared lipid levels in diabetic subjects with and without large vessel disease. Laakso et al showed that LDL cholesterol levels were higher in IDDM men with CAD[10] and in IDDM and NIDDM subjects with claudication symptoms[9] compared to asymptomatic diabetic subjects. In diabetic patients with claudication symptoms the differences were statistically significant only in the NIDDM population, and this difference persisted even after adjustment for BMI. In a study of 657 IDDM subjects by Maser et al,[34] LDL cholesterol levels were significantly higher in those with lower extremity arterial disease, but not in those with coronary heart disease. The relationship between LDL cholesterol levels and lower extremity arterial disease was independent of other lipoprotein levels and vascular disease risk factors. No association was found between LDL cholesterol levels and CAD in 139 male and 145 female NIDDM patients evaluated by Laakso et al.[35] In a community-based study of Japanese men with glucose intolerance, LDL levels were not higher in those with CAD.[36] In summary, data are limited on this topic and more information is needed. There is certainly no reason to think that the risk factors that apply to nondiabetic populations will not also apply to diabetics, and, if this is correct, undoubtedly elevated LDL levels are a risk factor for vascular disease in diabetics, as in euglycemic populations. However, clearly, levels of LDL cannot explain the accelerated atherosclerosis seen in diabetic populations.

LDL Levels in Diabetics of Diverse Ethnic Origin

A few investigators have tried to compare diabetic lipoprotein levels in diabetics of different races. To ascertain whether differences in lipoproteins may explain the lower coronary heart disease prevalence in Chinese NIDDM populations compared to comparable American diabetics, a direct comparison was made between their lipoproteins levels.[24] The two diabetic groups and their respective controls were matched for age, BMI, and glucose tolerance. Although Chinese men (diabetic and normal) had significantly higher HDL cholesterol levels, their LDL cholesterol levels were only modestly lower (borderline significance) than those of their American counterparts. Pacy et al[37] also found no statistical difference in LDL cholesterol levels among caucasian, black, and Asian NIDDM patients, although blacks had lower triglyceride and higher HDL cholesterol levels. Similarly, there were no differences in LDL levels between Hispanic and Anglo NIDDM patients in the large population-based San Luis Valley Diabetes Study.[25] LDL cholesterol levels were also similar in caucasian and black IDDM patients.[12,38] It seems clear from these studies that differences in LDL levels alone do not explain any differences in CAD that exist between diabetics of different racial backgrounds.

In summary, it is important to realize that many of the published studies to date comparing diabetic to nondiabetic subjects suffer from design or analysis problems. These problems include:

1. Use of controls who do not always match diabetic subjects in appropriate variables such as age, weight, exercise, diet, coronary heart disease, and other drug use.

2. Use of selected clinic patients rather than randomly recruited patients.

3. Use of control patients who were not fully evaluated for mild glucose intolerance (thus, the values obtained from these control populations may have been influenced by the inclusion of subjects with mild degrees of glucose intolerance).

4. Use of historical controls.

Despite these problems the results are generally consistent among studies. Overall, differences in LDL levels in diabetics compared to controls are not uniformly present, and, when present, are small in extent. This makes the higher CAD prevalence in diabetic populations less likely to be explained by differences in LDL levels alone. Although other lipoprotein abnormalities such as changes in triglyceride or HDL cholesterol levels or lipoprotein composition differences are very important, LDL undoubtedly contributes to the development of heart disease through mechanisms discussed below. It is likely that, in the face of several different types of LDL modifications that can take place in diabetes, as well as the presence of many other (nonlipoprotein) predisposing atherogenic factors, a "normal" LDL cholesterol level in diabetics is still far too high. In this context LDL levels typical of the American population may be regarded as "hypercholesterolemic" for diabetic subjects, and LDL values well below 100 mg/dL, as typified by Japanese populations, should be considered appropriate levels to achieve. Similar conclusions were recently reached by Garg and Grundy.[39]

LDL Metabolism in Diabetes

The metabolism of LDL in diabetics has been intensively investigated by numerous individuals and has been the subject of several excellent reviews.[40-42] Because of the heterogeneity of the subjects studied, confounding medical problems, and variability in degree of hyperglycemia at the time of study, as well as differences in methodologies used, it is difficult to define patterns of change that characterize diabetic populations. Although there is considerable heterogeneity in the composition and metabolism of LDL and LDL subfractions even in the nondiabetic population, this heterogeneity is clearly exaggerated in diabetics. Some authors have reported that LDLs from diabetics are skewed toward small and dense subpopulations,[41] but whether this is due to genetic influences or to the so-frequently-associated hypertriglyceridemia and obesity is unknown. In addition, when one considers the multiple modifications of LDL that occur in diabetic populations (eg, triglyceride enrichment and nonenzymatic glycosylation), there is an almost bewildering degree of complexity involved in trying to define the kinetics of LDL metabolism in diabetes.

In diabetes, the LDL particles are frequently triglyceride enriched and cholesterol depleted. Hence, whereas LDL cholesterol levels are relatively normal (eg, Tables 2.1 and 2.2), in fact the LDL apolipoprotein B levels are frequently elevated.[41-44] Thus, in actuality there is the accumulation in plasma of an increased number of smaller and more dense LDL particles. As noted by several investigators, this pattern in the nondiabetic population is typical of that found in familial combined hyperlipidemia and/or hyperbetalipoproteinemia.[45,46] Such a pattern appears to be an inherited trait[47] and in general is associated with an increased risk for CAD. Whether there is enrichment of the genetic pool in diabetics for this pattern, or this pattern is a product of the altered VLDL metabolism characteristic of diabetes (eg, the hypertriglyceridemia), or combinations of these factors is as yet unknown. However, the metabolism of such dense LDL particles almost certainly differs from that of lighter LDL particles, and this calls into question the interpretation of LDL kinetics in previous studies using whole LDL fractions as tracers. In other words, kinetic homogeneity of the LDL tracer, a key assumption of most modeling techniques, is almost certainly not present in many diabetic subjects, particularly those with hypertriglyceridemia.

Patients with IDDM may have numerous alterations in apo B metabolism. In hepatocyte cell culture, free fatty acids (FFAs) may drive apo B synthesis and VLDL output,[48,49] whereas insulin clearly diminishes apo B synthesis,[50] possibly by increasing its intrahepatocyte degradation of apo B by decreasing apo B phosphorylation.[51] In vivo, this would suggest that insulin deficiency would favor apo B synthesis. When this is coupled with increased FFA delivery to the liver, driving triglyceride synthesis as well, then VLDL triglyceride and apo B production would be enhanced, leading to hypertriglyceridemia.[52] If one assumes that all LDL apo B is derived from VLDL apo B (a controversial point to be sure[53]), a priori this would predict increased LDL apo B levels. However, a deficiency in LPL activity also occurs in this setting, leading to plasma enrichment of large VLDLs, which in fact have a low rate of conversion to LDL. Furthermore, glycosylation of apo E[54] may further impair hepatic removal of VLDL/IDL and/or conversion to LDL. Thus, during insulin deficiency VLDLs accumulate and LDL levels generally decline. In fact, the finding of relatively "normal" LDL levels in many diabetics despite hypertriglyceridemia (when one might have expected low LDL levels) is probably a reflection of the impaired LDL catabolism that also occurs in this situation. The decreased LDL catabolism[55] is probably multifactorial and due to (1) down-regulation of hepatic LDL receptors as a result of insulin deficiency[56] and possibly also enhanced return (in absolute terms) to the liver of VLDL remnants; (2) enhanced nonenzymatic glycosylation of LDL apo B[54,57]; and (3) abnormal composition of LDL secondary to hypertriglyceridemia[58] (described in more detail below). Clearly, with restoration of euglycemia achieved by intensive insulin therapy, LDL levels decrease still further.[14–17,59,60]

The situation with NIDDM subjects is even more complicated because these subjects have confounding problems of obesity and insulin resistance associated with hyperinsulinemia. These patients usually overproduce VLDL apo B in the form of triglyceride-enriched particles.[41,61,62] This overproduction is most likely due to the influence of high FFA flux, obesity, insulin resistance, and possibly decreased relative insulin secretion. In turn, VLDL catabolism may be impaired because of relative LPL deficiency[63] (as noted above), leading to a decreased fractional conversion to LDL. As noted above for IDDM, LDL cholesterol levels are not frequently elevated in these subjects, although again the caveat should be noted that these levels are probably higher than expected for the degree of hypertriglyceridemia seen. Again, many of these subjects have an increased *number* of LDL particles, despite the "normal" LDL cholesterol levels (ie, they have an increased LDL apo B level).[41] According to the extensive studies of

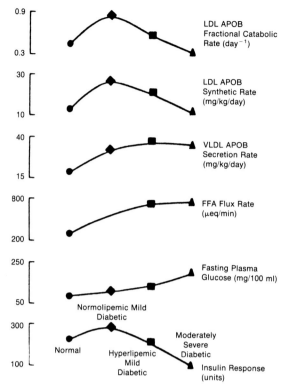

Figure 2.1 Relationship of apo B metabolism to parameters of metabolic control in normal and diabetic subjects with varying degrees of hyperglycemia. *(Reprinted, by permission, from Kissebah AH: Low density lipoprotein metabolism in non-insulin-dependent diabetes mellitus. Diabetes Metab Rev 1987; 3:619–651.)*

Kissebah,[41] NIDDM patients frequently have increased LDL apo B flux, either because of overproduction of apo B–containing particles or increased VLDL-to-LDL conversion. As noted, this may or may not lead to increased LDL cholesterol levels, depending on the rate of LDL clearance and the degree of abnormality in LDL composition (ie, the extent to which the individual LDL particles are depleted of cholesterol). This suggests that LDL cholesterol concentrations are not always a good index of LDL particle number. Because the degree of hyperglycemia may also profoundly affect LDL catabolism, the effect on LDL kinetics of multiple factors must be considered. Figure 2.1, taken from the work of Kissebah, attempts to integrate the multiple influences on LDL kinetics.[41]

Atherogenic Modifications of LDL That May Make It Atherogenic

It is now clear that LDLs isolated from patients with diabetes may be altered in a number of ways that could affect their metabolism and their atherogenicity. These include enhanced nonenzymatic glycosylation, alterations in composition secondary to hypertriglyceridemia, and the potential for enhanced susceptibility to oxidative modification.

Metabolic Consequences of Nonenzymatic Glycosylation of LDLs

In the presence of hyperglycemia, nearly all plasma proteins undergo enhanced nonenzymatic glycosylation. For many proteins such a modification may not be of functional consequence, but for LDL there was a theoretical reason to think that nonenzymatic glycosylation would be an adverse modification. Weisgraber et al[64] showed that lysine residues of LDL apo B were critical for the specific recognition of LDL by the LDL receptor. It was shown that a number of modifications that blocked the ε amino group of lysine residues of apo B, such as by methylation, also inhibited the ability of LDL to bind to its receptor. The degree of inhibition was proportional to the extent of lysine modification, and even when as few as 3% of lysine residues of apo B were modified, inhibition of LDL binding could be demonstrated. Because nonenzymatic glycosylation is known to involve the ε amino group of lysine on hemoglobin and other proteins, it seemed likely that LDL apo B lysine residues would also be glycosylated in vivo in diabetics and that this would also inhibit the ability of LDL to bind to its receptor. Extensive glycosylation of lysine residues of LDL was achieved by incubating LDL with glucose in the presence of cyanoborohydride, yielding LDL in which 20% to 70% of lysine residues were glycosylated. This glc-LDL failed to bind to the LDL receptor, as predicted.[57] Furthermore, when such glc-LDL preparations were injected intravenously into guinea pigs, their clearance from plasma was greatly delayed, consistent with the predicted role of the LDL receptor in mediating clearance of LDL in vivo.[57]

At the time these initial studies were performed, the degree to which LDL was cleared by the LDL receptor pathway in humans was undefined. Because the extensively glycosylated LDL did not bind to the LDL receptor at all, its plasma clearance was accounted for solely by non-LDL receptor-mediated mechanisms.[65] Thus, by simultaneously injecting radiolabeled native LDL (cleared by both LDL receptor and non-LDL receptor pathways) with heavily glycosylated LDL (cleared only by nonreceptor pathways), one could estimate the extent of the LDL receptor pathway as the difference in clearance between the two tracers. When such studies were performed in guinea pigs, rabbits, and humans, it was demonstrated that approximately 75% of LDL clearance was accounted for by the LDL receptor pathway.[57,65–67] Because the LDL receptor pathway is so important for mediating LDL clearance, it follows that factors altering hepatic LDL receptor activity will have a profound affect on LDL plasma levels. For example, it is known in cell culture that insulin up-regulates LDL receptor activity.[56] This implies that, in vivo, in an insulinopenic state, LDL receptor activity would be reduced, leading to increased LDL levels. Our data[57,65–67] also suggested that anything decreasing the ability of LDL to be an effective ligand for the LDL receptor would also delay its clearance and consequently also raise plasma LDL levels.

The lysine modification of apo B produced for the studies described above was extensive and not physiologic. In other studies, using amino acid analysis of apo B, we determined that in euglycemic individuals only 2% to 3% of lysine residues were modified, whereas in diabetics the values were 3% to 5%, with occasional patients showing values up to 7%.[57] To determine if this much smaller degree of modification could alter in vivo LDL clearance, LDL was modified in vitro by incubation with glucose to prepare glc-LDL with varying degrees of

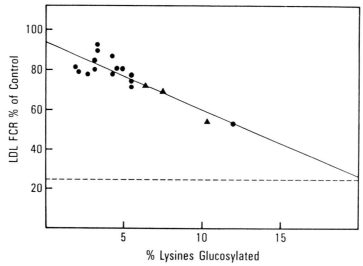

Figure 2.2 Relationship between extent of glycation of LDL and inhibition of its fractional rate of clearance (FCR) from plasma. ● are studies in which the LDL was glycated by incubations with glucose alone; while ▲ represent LDL samples glycated by incubations with glucose and cyanoborohydride. The dotted line represents the fraction of the total FCR that is accounted for by LDL receptor independent mediated mechanisms. *(Reprinted, by permission, from Steinbrecher UP and Witztum JL: Glucosylation of low-density lipoprotein to an extent comparable to that seen in diabetes slows their catabolism. Diabetes 1984; 33:130–134.)*

lysine modification.[68] Conditions were used to produce glc-LDL that were modified to a degree similar to that observed in LDL isolated from diabetic subjects. The degree of lysine modification was then determined, and both native and glc-LDL preparations were labeled differentially with radioiodine and simultaneously injected into guinea pigs, and their respective fractional catabolic rates (FCRs) determined. In Figure 2.2, the FCR of each glc-LDL is presented as a percentage of the simultaneously determined FCR of native LDL and related to the percentage of lysine residues modified. It can be seen that, even when the glc-LDL had only 3% to 6% of its lysine residues modified, clearance was inhibited by 10% to 30%. Higher degrees of lysine modification, achieved by incubating the LDL with glucose in the presence of cyanoborohydride (the solid triangles), produced even greater degrees of inhibition of plasma clearance. It is of interest that extrapolation of the regression line to approximately 20% of lysine residues modified would predict total inhibition of LDL receptor-mediated clearance (ie, 75% of total plasma clearance), and indeed these data are in good agreement with the earlier report of Weisgraber et al from cell culture studies[64] and our own data in vivo in animals and humans.[65–67] Recently Nordestgaard and Zilversmit[69] have shown that LDLs isolated from diabetic rabbits are cleared more slowly than LDLs isolated from euglycemic rabbits, similar to our findings. Of practical importance, these studies suggested that the degree of nonenzymatic glycosylation of lysine residues found in LDLs in some diabetic patients could slow LDL clearance by as much as 20% to 30%. It should be noted that a number of investigators who have prospectively treated IDDM subjects with intensive insulin regimens to achieve near euglycemia have reported decreases in LDL levels of 5% to 27%.[14–17,61,62] Of course, in such studies other variables may have been altered as well, as noted below.

Lopes-Virella et al[70] directly tested the ability of LDLs isolated from IDDM subjects to be a ligand for the LDL receptor of fibroblasts. LDLs were isolated during a baseline period when subjects were in poor control and subsequently during a period of improved control while undergoing intensive insulin therapy. It was found that the LDLs isolated during the tight control period were bound and degraded by the fibroblast's LDL receptor pathway 20% to 25% more efficiently than the LDLs isolated during the poor control period. We have also made similar observations.[71] Figure 2.3 shows a similar study in which LDL was isolated from a subject during an "out of control" period and then during a period of tight control. The extent of nonenzymatic glycosylation of his LDL was decreased 50% by the tight control. As seen in the left panel, the LDL isolated during the tight control period was taken up and degraded more avidly by the LDL receptor of fibroblasts, and, when injected in vivo into a guinea pig, its clearance was increased markedly compared to the simultaneously determined clearance of the LDL isolated from the poorly controlled period.

These data suggest that nonenzymatic glycosylation may indeed play an important role in lowering the affinity of LDL for its receptor and thereby increasing its residence time in plasma. Assuming no alteration in production rates, this should lead to enhanced plasma LDL levels. Furthermore, other compositional changes occur in diabetic LDLs that also adversely affect their ability to bind to the LDL receptor.

Alterations in LDL Composition Secondary to Hypertriglyceridemia

Hypertriglyceridemia is a common problem in diabetic subjects, particularly in the poorly controlled and/or NIDDM patient. In such situations profound alterations in LDL composition occur, leading to more dense and triglyceride-enriched particles. As shown by Aviram, Chait, and colleagues, these changes also decrease the ability of LDL to bind to the fibroblast's LDL receptor.[72] However, these compositional changes in LDLs only occurred if the LDLs were isolated from plasma in which triglyceride levels were greater than about 500 mg/dL.[58] It should be noted that the LDL depicted in Figure 2.3 was isolated from a diabetic subject whose triglyceride level was below 300 mg/dL, and thus it is likely that the changes seen in that subject were related in large part to the degree of nonenzymatic glycosylation. However, the subjects with the most extensive degrees of nonenzymatic glycosylation frequently also have marked hypertriglyceridemia, and for many diabetic subjects it is likely that LDL is a less effective ligand for the LDL receptor because of both nonenzymatic glycosylation and compositional differences. Thus, a decreased ability to bind to the LDL receptor, coupled with down-regulated cellular LDL receptor activity (as a result of insulin deficiency) would lead to increased plasma LDL levels, which would be expected to be atherogenic. In addition, as noted above, the small, dense LDL profile in itself has been reported to be an atherogenic risk factor, perhaps because of an increased ability to penetrate the arterial wall[69] or an increased susceptibility to oxidative modification.[73]

30

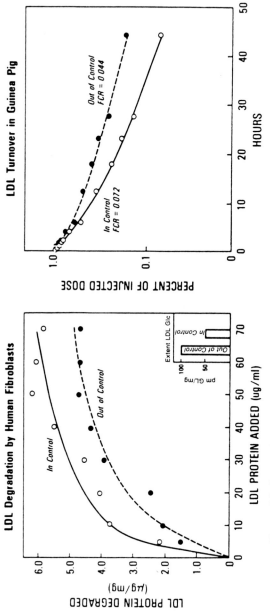

Figure 2.3 Comparison of the metabolism of LDL isolated from the same subject during an "out of control" and "in control" period. The left panel shows LDL degradation by human fibroblasts and the right panel shows the *in vivo* plasma clearance of the same LDL samples which were simultaneously injected into a guinea pig. *(Reprinted, by permission, from Witztum JL and Koschinsky T: Metabolic and immunological consequences of glycation of low density lipoproteins, in Baynes JW, Monnier VM (eds): The Maillard Reaction in Aging, Diabetes, and Nutrition, New York, Alan R. Liss, Inc., 1989, pp 219–234.)*

Enhanced Susceptibility of LDLs to Oxidative Modification

LDLs may be more atherogenic in diabetics because of other mechanisms as well. As noted above, LDL isolated from diabetics is more extensively glycosylated than LDL isolated from euglycemics,[74] and Lyons et al previously reported that such LDLs have enhanced uptake by macrophages.[75] Lopes-Virella et al further demonstrated that LDL incubated with glucose in vitro to mimic diabetic LDL also had enhanced macrophage uptake,[76] but the mechanism(s) accounting for the enhanced uptake were not defined. It is possible that glc-LDL more readily aggregates, and aggregated LDL is now clearly known to have enhanced macrophage uptake, in part mediated by the LDL receptor pathway.[77] Additionally, glc-LDL may be more susceptible to oxidative modification (see below). Further experiments are indicated to evaluate these possibilities.

The atherogenicity of LDL undoubtedly comes after it has penetrated into the artery wall. Much evidence has now accumulated to suggest that modification of LDL that occurs within the artery wall greatly enhances its atherogenicity.[78,79] Chief among these modifications is oxidative modification initiated by lipid peroxidation of the unsaturated fatty acids present in the LDL. Not only does oxidized LDL have enhanced uptake in macrophages, potentially leading to foam cell formation, but increasingly it is clear that a wide variety of products are formed during the oxidation process that may have important biologic consequences.[79] For example, oxidized LDL is chemotactic for monocytes, inhibits mobility of macrophages, is cytotoxic to a variety of arterial cells, may alter coagulation pathways, and, importantly, may interfere with endothelial-dependent mediated relaxation of coronary artery smooth muscles. In addition, products of oxidized LDL may alter gene expression of arterial cells, such as stimulation of gene transcription of MCP-1 and colony-stimulating factors and induction of adhesion molecules on overlying endothelium. Thus, oxidized LDL may be atherogenic by multiple mechanisms and, in fact, by the time it has been taken up by the macrophages via the scavenger receptor, it may already have produced many pathogenic processes that lead to plaque formation. Furthermore, several different lines of evidence suggest that oxidation of LDL does occur in vivo both in experimental animal models and in humans.[79] Most importantly, agents that inhibit the oxidative modification of LDL inhibit atherogenesis in hypercholesterolemic rabbits. Thus, any process that would enhance oxidative modification might increase the atherogenicity of LDL.

Diabetes may contribute to this process in several ways. First, as noted above, changes in LDL composition and nonenzymatic glycosylation may prolong the half-life of LDL in plasma. Although it is unlikely that extensive modification of LDL can occur in plasma because of the many antioxidants present, it is nevertheless conceivable that subtle degrees of lipid peroxidation do occur, and then, when such LDLs enter the subintimal space of the artery, they are "primed" for more rapid oxidation. Furthermore, there are numerous reports of an enhanced content of lipid peroxides in plasma of diabetic subjects. Morel and Chisolm[80] have clearly demonstrated that the VLDL and LDL fractions of diabetic rats have enhanced lipoperoxides and that these lipoproteins are cytotoxic. Both the enhanced lipoperoxide content and the cytotoxicity were reversible by administration of antioxidants such as vitamin E or probucol. A definitive demonstration of a similar phenomenon in diabetic humans has not yet been accomplished.

Second, prolongation of the residence time of LDL *in the artery wall* itself may also enhance the opportunity for oxidative modification. Not only does nonenzymatic glycosylation occur, but advanced glycosylation end product (AGE) formation also occurs in the artery wall.[81] Trapping of LDL to matrix proteins via such glucose adducts would undoubtedly prolong the residence time of LDL and thus render it more susceptible to oxidation.[82]

Third, there is an ever-growing body of evidence to suggest that the reactions leading to AGE formation and oxidation are closely related, and in fact that the two processes can potentially mutually accelerate each other (excellently reviewed by Baynes[83]). Thus, free radicals generated from autoxidative decomposition of sugars or sugar adducts to proteins may accelerate lipid peroxidation in LDL, and the lipid peroxidation initiated in LDL may accelerate AGE-like products. In fact, we have recently produced immunocytochemical evidence for the presence of one AGE, FFI, in atherosclerotic lesions of euglycemic WHHL rabbits but not in normal rabbit aortas (Palinski et al, unpublished data). It is possible that the increased "oxidative stress" that may be present in diabetics as a result of the extensive and widespread nonenzymatic glycosylation/AGE formation may make even "normal" levels of LDL atherogenic. If so, antioxidant therapy may prove of particular value for the diabetic subject. It is of considerable interest that several investigators have reported that antioxidant therapy decreased HbA_{1c} levels,[84,85] suggesting that the nonenzymatic glycosylation modification of hemoglobins, conventionally thought to involve only Amadori reactions, is in fact more complicated and involves free radical intermediates as well.

Finally, it should be mentioned that even minor modifications of LDL render it immunogenic.[86] Nonenzymatic glycosylation and AGE formation both render LDL immunogenic, and autoantibodies to these modifications have been observed in both normal and diabetic subjects.[71,87] Because many arterial wall structures are also similarly modified, it is possible that immune complex deposition in the artery—made up of antibodies directed against nonenzymatic glycosylation/AGE epitopes and proteins so modified—could also contribute to immune-mediated injury.

The process of AGE formation appears to play an important role in mediating the toxicity of hyperglycemia. For this reason, considerable efforts are being made to inhibit AGE formation. Recently aminoguanidine has been advocated because of its ability to trap aldehydes (and possibly lipoperoxides) formed as intermediates in AGE formation.[88] The process of oxidative modification of LDL involves the lipid peroxidation of unsaturated fatty acids, which decompose to yield highly reactive aldehydes. In turn, these complex with lysine residues of apo B to yield novel epitopes that form the ligand on oxidized LDL that is recognized by the scavenger receptor of macrophages. Because aminoguanidine traps aldehydes efficiently, we thought is might also be effective in inhibiting the oxidative modification of LDL.[89] To test this, LDLs were incubated with endothelial cells or with copper (conditions that initiate oxidative modification of LDL) in the absence or presence of increasing concentrations of aminoguanidine. Subsequently, the LDLs were tested for their ability to be taken up and degraded by macrophages (Figure 2.4). Compared to LDLs oxidized in the absence of aminoguanidine, LDLs oxidized in the presence of varying amounts of aminoguanidine showed inhibited modification in a dose-dependent manner. Other studies demonstrated that in large part this was due to prevention of

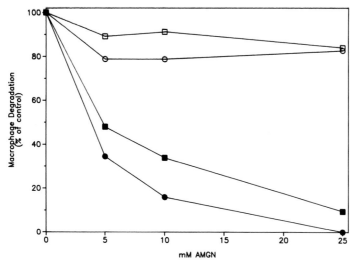

Figure 2.4 Aminoguanidine (AMGN) inhibits modification of LDL. ^{125}I-LDL (100 μg/ml) was incubated with endothelial cells (○, ●) or with 5 μM copper (□, ■) for 20 hr at 37°C in the absence (○, □) or presence (●, ■) of the indicated concentration of aminoguanidine and then the degradation of ^{125}I-LDL by macrophages was detemined. To demonstrate that the aminoguanidine did not directly alter macrophage function, aminoguanidine was added directly to macrophage cultures (○, □). Results are expressed as the percentage of the value obtained for the LDL sample oxidized in the absence of aminoguanidine and after substraction of the amount of native LDL degraded. *(Reprinted, by permission, from Picard S, Parthasarathy S, Fruebis J, Witztum JL: Aminoguanidine inhibits the oxidative modification of low density lipoprotein and the subsequent increase in macrophage uptake via scavenger receptor. Proc Natl Acad Sci USA 1992;89:6876–6880.)*

formation of the lysine adducts, as predicted.[89] Thus aminoguanidine may inhibit atherogenesis by inhibiting AGE formation as well as inhibiting the oxidative modification of LDL.

Summary

Although LDL levels are usually not elevated in most diabetics when compared to normal populations, intensive treatments that produce near-euglycemic conditions normalize LDL composition and lower LDL levels, most likely by several mechanisms. This may be of considerable importance because LDL is likely more atherogenic in diabetics than in nondiabetics. Hyperglycemia, leading to enhanced rates of nonenzymatic glycosylation and AGE formation, as well as enhanced free radical formation because of autoxidation of sugar and sugar adducts, may lead to enhanced trapping of LDL within the arterial matrix, enhanced oxidation of LDL (in plasma and in the artery wall), and thus, enhanced atherosclerosis. Therefore, achievement of euglycemia may directly decrease atherogenesis. Because AGE formation presumably occurs in the artery wall with aging even in euglycemics, therapies designed to inhibit AGE formation may be of benefit not only to diabetics but euglycemic individuals as well.

References

1. Pyörälä K, Laakso M, Uusitupa M: Diabetes and atherosclerosis: An epidemiologic view. *Diabetes Metab Rev* 1987;3:463–524.

2. Joven J, Vilella E, Costa B, et al: Concentrations of lipids and apolipoproteins in patients with clinically well-controlled insulin-dependent and non-insulin dependent diabetes. *Clin Chem* 1989;35:813–816.

3. Assmann G, Schulte H: The prospective cardiovascular Munster (PROCAM) study: Prevalence of hyperlipidemia in persons with hypertension and/or diabetes mellitus and the relationship to coronary heart disease. *Am Heart J* 1988;00:1713–1724.

4. The DCCT Research Group: Lipid and lipoprotein levels in patients with insulin-dependent diabetes mellitus: The Diabetes Control and Complications Trial (DCCT) experience. *Diabetes Care,* 1992;15(7):886–894.

5. Sosenko JM, Breslow JL, Miettinen OS, et al: Hyperglycemia and plasma lipid levels: A prospective study of young insulin-dependent diabetic patients. *N Engl J Med* 1980; 302:650–654.

6. Lopes-Virella MF, Wohltmann HJ, Loadholt CB, et al: Plasma lipids and lipoproteins in young insulin-dependent diabetic patients: Relationship with control. *Diabetologia* 1981;21:216–223.

7. Walden CE, Knopp RH, Wahl PW, et al: Sex differences in the effect of diabetes mellitus on lipoprotein triglyceride and cholesterol concentrations. *N Engl J Med* 1984;311: 953–959.

8. Nikkila EA, Hormila P: Serum lipids and lipoproteins in insulin-treated diabetes: Demonstration of increased high density lipoprotein concentrations. *Diabetes* 1978;27: 1078–1086.

9. Laakso M, Pyorala K: Lipid and lipoprotein abnormalities in diabetic patients with peripheral vascular disease. *Atherosclerosis* 1988;74:55–63.

10. Laakso M, Pyorala K, Sarlund H, et al: Lipid and lipoprotein abnormalities associated with coronary heart disease in patients with insulin-dependent diabetes mellitus. *Arteriosclerosis* 1986;6:679–684.

11. Reckless JPD, Betteridge DJ, Wu P, et al: High-density and low-density lipoproteins and prevalence of vascular disease in diabetes mellitus. *BMJ* 1978;1:883–886.

12. Semenkovich CF, Ostlund RE, Schechtman KB: Plasma lipids in patients with type I diabetes mellitus. Influence of race, gender, and plasma glucose control: Lipids do not correlate with glucose control in black women. *Arch Intern Med* 1989;149:51–56.

13. Gonen B, White N, Schoenfeld G, et al: Plasma levels of apoprotein B in patients with diabetes mellitus: The effect of glycemic control. *Metabolism* 1985;34:675–679.

14. Pietri A, Dunn FL, Raskin P: The effect of improved diabetic control on plasma lipid and lipoprotein levels. A comparison of conventional therapy and continuous subcutaneous insulin infusion. *Diabetes* 1980;29:1001–1005.

15. Dunn FL, Pietri A, Raskin P: Plasma lipid and lipoprotein levels with continuous subcutaneous insulin infusion in type I diabetes mellitus. *Ann Intern Med* 1981;95: 426–431.

16. Lopes-Virella MF, Wohltmann HJ, Mayfield RK, et al: Effect of metabolic control on lipid, lipoprotein and apolipoprotein levels in 55 insulin-dependent diabetic patients. A longitudinal study. *Diabetes* 1983;32:20–25.

17. Pietri AO, Dunn FL, Grundy SM, et al: The effect of continuous subcutaneous insulin infusion on very-low-density lipoprotein triglyceride metabolism in type I diabetes mellitus. *Diabetes* 1983;32:75–81.

18. Zavaroni I, Mazza S, Luchetti L, et al: High plasma insulin and triglyceride concentrations and blood pressure in offspring of people with impaired glucose tolerance. *Diabetic Med* 1990;7:494–498.

19. Barakat HA, Carpenter JW, McLendon VD, et al: Influence of obesity, impaired glucose

tolerance, and NIDDM on LDL structure and composition: Possible link between hyperinsulinemia and atherosclerosis. *Diabetes* 1990;39:1527–1533.

20. Laakso M, Barrett-Connor E: Asymptomatic hyperglycemia is associated with lipid and lipoprotein changes favoring atherosclerosis. *Arteriosclerosis* 1989;9:665–672.

21. Dunn FL: Hyperlipidemia in diabetes mellitus. *Diabetes Metab Rev* 1990;6:47–61.

22. Laker MF, Winocour PF: Plasma lipids and lipoproteins in diabetes mellitus. *Diabetes Annu* 1991;6:431–456.

23. Stern MP, Haffner SM: Dyslipidemia in type II diabetes, implications for therapeutic intervention. *Diabetes Care* 1991;14:1144–1159.

24. Pan XR, Walden CE, Warnick GR, et al: Comparison of plasma lipoproteins and apo-proteins in Chinese and American non-insulin-dependent diabetic subjects and controls. *Diabetes Care* 1986;9:395–400.

25. Burchfiel CM, Hamman RF, Marshall JA, et al: Cardiovascular risk factors and impaired glucose tolerance: The San Luis Valley Diabetes Study. *Am J Epidemiol* 1990;131:57–70.

26. Barrett-Connor E, Witztum JL, Holdbrook M: A community study of high density lipoproteins in adult noninsulin-dependent diabetics. *Am J Epidemiol* 1983;117:186–192.

27. Yoshino G, Iwai M, Kazumi T, et al: Cholesterol-enrichment of low density lipoprotein fraction is absent in Japanese normolipidemic diabetes. *Horm Metab Res* 1989;21:152–153.

28. Iwai M, Yoshino G, Matsushita M, et al: Abnormal lipoprotein composition in nor-molipidemic diabetic patients. *Diabetes Care* 1990;13:792–795.

29. Howard BV, Knowler WC, Vasquez B, et al: Plasma and lipoprotein cholesterol and triglyceride in the Pima Indian population: Comparison of diabetics and nondiabetics. *Arteriosclerosis* 1984;4:462–471.

30. Billingham MS, Milles JJ, Bailey CJ, et al: Lipoprotein subfraction composition in non-insulin-dependent diabetes treated by diet, sulphonylurea, and insulin. *Metabolism* 1989;38:850–857.

31. Hughes TA, Clements TS, Fairclough PK, et al: Effect of insulin therapy on lipoproteins in non-insulin dependent diabetes mellitus (NIDDM). *Atherosclerosis* 1987;67:105–114.

32. Kawate R, Yamakido M, Nishimoto Y, et al: Diabetes mellitus and its vascular complications in Japanese migrants on the island of Hawaii. *Diabetes Care* 1979;2:161–170.

33. Laakso M, Rönnemaa T, Pyörälä K, et al: Atherosclerotic vascular disease and its risk factors in non-insulin-dependent diabetic and nondiabetic subjects in Finland. *Diabetes Care* 1988;11:449–463.

34. Maser RE, Wolfson SK Jr, Ellis D, et al: Cardiovascular disease and arterial calcification in insulin-dependent diabetes mellitus: Interrelations and risk profiles. *Arterioscler Thromb* 1991;11:958–965.

35. Laakso M, Voutilainen E, Pyorala K, et al: Association of low HDL and HDL$_2$ cholesterol with coronary heart disease in noninsulin-dependent diabetics. *Arteriosclerosis* 1985;5:653–658.

36. Bergstrom RW, Leonetti DL, Newell-Morris LL, et al: Association of plasma triglyceride and C-peptide with coronary heart disease in Japanese-American men with a high prevalence of glucose intolerance. *Diabetologia* 1990;33:489–496.

37. Pacy PJ, Dodson PM, Kubicki AJ, et al: Differences in lipid and lipoprotein levels in White, Black and Asian non-insulin dependent (type 2) diabetics with hypertension. *Diabetes Res* 1987;4:187–193.

38. Levitsky LL, Scanu AM, Gould SH: Lipoprotein(a) levels in black and white children and adolescents with IDDM. *Diabetes Care* 1991;14:283–287.

39. Garg A, Grundy SM: Management of dyslipidemia in NIDDM. *Diabetes Care* 1990;13:153–169.

40. Ruderman NB, Haudenschild C: Diabetes as an atherogenic factor. *Prog Cardiovasc Dis* 1984;XXVI:373–412.

41. Kissebah AH: Low density lipoprotein metabolism in non-insulin-dependent diabetes mellitus. *Diabetes Metab Rev* 1987;3:619–651.

42. Ginsberg HN: Lipoprotein physiology in nondiabetic and diabetic states. Relationship to atherogenesis. *Diabetes Care* 1991;14:839–855.

43. Schonfeld G, Birge C, Miller JP, et al: Apolipoprotein B levels and altered lipoprotein composition in diabetes. *Diabetes* 1974;23:827–834.

44. Fisher WR: Heterogeneity of plasma low density lipoproteins: Manifestations of the physiologic phenomenon in man. *Metabolism* 1983;32:283–291.

45. Teng B, Thompson GR, Sniderman AD, et al: Composition and distribution of low density lipoprotein fractions in hyperapobetalipoproteinemia, normolipidemia, and familial hypercholesterolemia. *Proc Natl Acad Sci USA* 1983;80:6662–6666.

46. Austin MA, Brunzell JD, Fitch WL, et al: Inheritance of low density lipoprotein subclass in familial combined hyperlipidemia. *Arteriosclerosis* 1990;10:520–530.

47. Austin MA, Krauss RM: Genetic control of low density lipoprotein subclasses. *Lancet* 1986;2:592–594.

48. Witztum JL, Schonfeld G: Carbohydrate diet-induced changes in very low density lipoprotein composition and structure. *Diabetes* 1978;27:1215–1229.

49. Cianflone K, Dahan S, Monge JC, et al: Pathogenesis of carbohydrate-induced hypertriglyceridemia using HepG2 cells as a model system. *Arterioscler Thromb* 1992; 12:271–277.

50. Durrington PN, Newton RS, Weinstein DB, et al: The effects of insulin and glucose on very low density lipoprotein triglyceride secretions by cultured rat hepatocytes. *J Clin Invest* 1982;70:63–73.

51. Jackson TK, Salhanic AI, Elovson J, et al: Insulin regulates apolipoprotein B turnover and phosphorylation in rat hepatocytes. *J Clin Invest* 1990;86:1746–1751.

52. Ruotolo G, Micossi P, Galimberti G, et al: Effects of intraperitoneal versus subcutaneous insulin administration on lipoprotein metabolism in type I diabetes. *Metabolism* 1990;39:598–604.

53. Shames DM, Havel RJ: De novo production of low density lipoproteins: Fact or fancy? *J Lipid Res* 1991;32:1099–1112.

54. Curtiss LK, Witztum JL: Plasma apolipoproteins A-I, A-II, B, C-I and E are glucosylated in hyperglycemic diabetics. *Diabetes* 1985;34:452.

55. Howard BV, Abbott WGH, Beltz WF, et al: Integrated study of low density lipoprotein metabolism and very low density lipoprotein metabolism in non-insulin-dependent diabetes. *Metabolism* 1987;36:870–877.

56. Chait A, Bierman EL, Albers JJ: Low-density lipoprotein receptor activity in cultured human skin fibroblasts. Mechanism of insulin-induced stimulation. *J Clin Invest* 1979; 64:1309–1319.

57. Witztum JL, Mahoney EM, Branks MJ, et al: Nonenzymatic glucosylation of low-density lipoprotein alters its biological activity. *Diabetes* 1982;31:283–291.

58. Hiramatsu K, Bierman EL, Chait A: Metabolism of low-density lipoprotein from patients with diabetic hypertriglyceridemia by cultured human skin fibroblasts. *Diabetes* 1985;34:8–14.

59. Rosenstock J, Vega GL, Raskin P: Effect of intensive diabetes treatment on low-density lipoprotein apolipoprotein B kinetics in type I diabetes. *Diabetes* 1988;37:393–397.

60. Rosenstock J, Strowig S, Cercone S, et al: Reduction in cardiovascular risk factors with intensive diabetes treatment in insulin-dependent diabetes mellitus. *Diabetes Care* 1987;10:729–734.

61. Abrams JJ, Ginsberg H, Grundy SM: Metabolism of cholesterol and plasma triglycerides in nonketotic diabetes mellitus. *Diabetes* 1982;31:903–910.

62. Dunn FL, Raskin P, Bilheimer DW, et al: The effect of diabetic control on very low-density lipoprotein-triglyceride metabolism in patients with type II diabetes mellitus and marked hypertriglyceridemia. *Metabolism* 1984;33:117–123.

63. Taskinen MR, Beltz WF, Harper I, et al: Effects of NIDDM on very-low-density lipoprotein triglyceride and apolipoprotein B metabolism. Studies before and after sulfonylurea therapy. *Diabetes* 1986;35:1268–1277.

64. Weisgraber KH, Innerarity TL, Mahley RW: Role of the lysine residues of plasma lipoproteins in high affinity binding to cell surface receptors on human fibroblasts. *J Biol Chem* 1978;253:9053–9062.

65. Steinbrecher UP, Witztum JL, Kesaniemi YA, et al: Comparison of glucosylated LDL with methylated or cyclohexandione-treated LDL in the mesurement of receptor-independent LDL catabolism. *J Clin Invest* 1983;71:960–964.

66. Kesaniemi YA, Witztum JL, Steinbrecher UP: Receptor-mediated clearance of LDL in man—new estimates using glucosylated LDL. *J Clin Invest* 1983;71:950–959.

67. Wiklund O, Witztum JL, Carew TE, et al: Turnover and tissue sites of degradation of glucosylated low density lipoprotein in normal and immunized rabbits. *J Lipid Res* 1987;28:1098–1109.

68. Steinbrecher UP, Witztum JL: Glucosylation of low-density lipoprotein to an extent comparable to that seen in diabetes slows their catabolism. *Diabetes* 1984;33:130–134.

69. Nordestgaard BG, Zilversmit DB: Comparison of arterial intimal clearances of LDL from diabetic and nondiabetic cholesterol-fed rabbits. Differences in intimal clearance explained by size differences. *Arteriosclerosis* 1989;9:176–183.

70. Lopes-Virella MF, Sherer GK, Lees AM: Surface binding, internalization and degradation by cultured human fibroblasts of low density lipoproteins isolated from type 1 (insulin-dependent) diabetic patients: Changes with metabolic control. *Diabetologia* 1982;22:430–436.

71. Witztum JL, Koschinsky T: Metabolic and immunological consequences of glycation of low density lipoproteins, in Baynes JW, Monnier VM (eds): *The Maillard Reaction in Aging, Diabetes, and Nutrition.* New York, Alan R. Liss, 1989, pp 219–234.

72. Aviram M, Lundkatz S, Phillips MC, et al: The influence of the triglyceride content of low density lipoproteins on the interaction of apoprotein B-100 with cells. *J Biol Chem* 1988;263:6842–6848.

73. de Graaf J, Hak-Lemmers HL, Hectors MP, et al: Enhanced susceptibility to in vitro oxidation of the dense low density lipoprotein subfraction in healthy subjects. *Arterioscler Thromb* 1991;11:298–306.

74. Curtiss LK, Witztum JL: A novel method for generating region-specific monoclonal antibodies to modified proteins: Application to the identification of human glucosylated low density lipoproteins. *J Clin Invest* 1983;72:1427–1438.

75. Lyons TJ, Klein RL, Baynes JW, et al: Stimulation of cholesteryl ester synthesis in human monocyte-derived macrophages by low-density lipoproteins from type 1 (insulin-dependent) diabetic patients: The influence of nonenzymatic glycosylation of low-density lipoproteins. *Diabetologia* 1987;30:916–923.

76. Lopes-Virella MF, Klein RL, Lyons TJ, et al: Glucosylation of low density lipoprotein enhances cholesteryl ester synthesis in human monocyte-derived macrophages. *Diabetes* 1988;37:550–557.

77. Khoo JC, Miller E, McLoughlin P, et al. Prevention of low density lipoprotein aggregation by high density lipoproteins or apolipoprotein AI. *J Lipid Res* 1990;31:645–652.

78. Steinberg D, Witztum JL: Lipoproteins and atherogenesis: Current concepts. *JAMA* 1990;264:3047–3052.

79. Witztum JL, Steinberg D: Role of oxidized LDL in atherogenesis. *J Clin Invest* 1991;88:1785–1792.

80. Morel DW, Chisolm GM: Antioxidant treatment of diabetic rats inhibits lipoprotein oxidation and cytotoxicity. *J Lipid Res* 1989;30:1827–1834.

81. Cerami A, Vlassara H, Brownlee M: Role of advanced glycosylation products in complications of diabetes. *Diabetes Care* 1988;11:73–79.

82. Brownlee M, Vlassara H, Cerami A: Nonenzymatic glycosylation products on collagen covalently trap low density lipoprotein. *Diabetes* 1985;34:938–941.

83. Baynes JW: Role of oxidative stress in development of complications in diabetes. *Diabetes* 1991;40:405–412.

84. Ceriello A, Giugliano D, Quatraro A, et al: Vitamin E reduction of protein glycosylation in diabetes. New Prospect for prevention of diabetic complications? *Diabetes Care* 1991;14:68–72.

85. Davie SJ, Gould BJ, Yudkin JS: Effect of vitamin C on glycosylation of proteins. *Diabetes* 1992;41:167–173.

86. Steinbrecher UP, Fisher M, Witztum JL, et al: Immunogenicity of homologous low density lipoprotein after methylation, ethylation, acetylation or carbamylation: Generation of antibodies specific for derivatized lysine. *J Lipid Res* 1984;25:1109–1116.

87. Witztum JL, Steinbrecher UP, Kesaniemi YA, et al: Autoantibodies to glucosylated proteins in the plasma of patients with diabetes mellitus. *Proc Natl Acad Sci USA* 1984;81:3204–3208.

88. Brownlee M, Vlassara H, Kooney A, et al: Aminoguanidine prevents diabetes-induced arterial wall protein cross-linking. *Science* 1986;232:1629–1632.

89. Picard S, Parthasarathy S, Fruebis J, et al: Aminoguanidine inhibits the oxidative modification of low density lipoprotein and the subsequent increase in macrophage uptake via scavenger receptor. *Proc Natl Acad Sci USA* 1992;89:6876–6880.

90. James RW, Pometta D: The distribution profiles of very low density and low density lipoproteins in poorly-controlled male, type 2 (non-insulin-dependent) diabetic patients. *Diabetologia* 1991;34:246–252.

91. Pan SR, Hu SX, Yong G, et al: Lipoprotein and apoprotein A1 levels in diabetics and coronary heart disease patients and controls. *Chin Med J* 1987;100:204–207.

92. Falko JM, Parr JH, Simpson RN, et al: Lipoprotein analyses in varying degrees of glucose tolerance: Comparison between non-insulin-dependent diabetic, impaired glucose tolerant, and control populations. *Am J Med* 1987;83:641–647.

Chapter 3

Triglyceride-Rich Lipoproteins in Diabetes

Gary F. Lewis, MD, FRCP(C), and
George Steiner, MD, FRCP(C)

Hypertriglyceridemia resulting from the accumulation of triglyceride-rich lipoproteins (TRLs) in the circulation is the most common lipid abnormality in diabetes mellitus and is found in up to a third of all diabetic patients.[1–3] Diabetes is characterized by a number of abnormalities in the metabolic pathway of TRLs, reflecting the complex interaction between carbohydrate and lipid metabolism.

Alterations of TRL metabolism in type I diabetes (insulin-dependent diabetes mellitus; IDDM), a state characterized primarily by pancreatic B cell insulin secretory deficiency, are distinct from those of type II diabetes (non-insulin-dependent diabetes mellitus; NIDDM), a state of combined tissue resistance to insulin and a less profound insulin-secretory defect. In fact, in many NIDDM patients the serum immunoreactive insulin (IRI) levels may exceed those in nondiabetics. In both IDDM and NIDDM, the degree of effective insulinization is a critical determinant of TRL metabolism, and any discussion of TRL metabolism in diabetes must consider this.

The metabolism of both principal classes of TRLs—chylomicrons derived from the intestinal absorption of dietary fat, and very-low-density lipoprotein (VLDL) from hepatic synthesis—is affected by the diabetic state. Alterations in the metabolism of the exogenous pathway (ie, chylomicron metabolism) are discussed in this chapter in the section on postprandial TRL metabolism in diabetes.

The relationship between hypertriglyceridemia and atherosclerotic cardiovascular disease (ASCD) in the nondiabetic population has been extensively investigated for many years and no consistent conclusion has been reached.[4,5] In diabetic patients, however, a number of studies have shown that triglycerides are a risk factor for ASCD even when other established risk factors are considered in the analysis.[6–9] In addition, at least two studies have emphasized the importance of hypertriglyceridemia in the etiology of peripheral vascular disease in diabetic patients.[10,11] A detailed discussion of the epidemiology of hypertriglyceridemia as it relates to atherosclerosis in diabetes is beyond the scope of this chapter. Suffice it to say that there is mounting evidence that abnormalities of TRL metabolism play an important role in the pathogenesis of the increased incidence of premature atherosclerosis in diabetic patients.

In this chapter we discuss the relationship between insulin, insulin resistance and VLDL production, VLDL metabolism in NIDDM and IDDM, intermediate-density lipoprotein (IDL) metabolism in NIDDM, VLDL compositional abnormalities in diabetes, the relationship between glycemic control and VLDL metabolism, and some of the more recent work examining postprandial TRL metabolism in diabetes mellitus.

The Role of Insulin in VLDL Production

Insulin plays a key role in coordinating the complex metabolic process responsible for the assembly and secretion of VLDL from dietary and tissue-derived precursors, ensuring plasma lipid balance and an adequate supply of fuel for energy-requiring peripheral tissues.[12,13] Insulin also plays an important direct role at the level of the peripheral tissues in controlling the catabolism of VLDL and other triglyceride-rich particles and determining rates of synthesis and release of stored triglyceride.[14] This peripheral effect of insulin thus controls the release of free fatty acid (FFA), which in turn is an important determinant of hepatic triglyceride and VLDL production rate.[15-17]

Because of the well-described association between chronic hyperinsulinemia and VLDL overproduction,[18-20] it has generally been assumed that insulin stimulates VLDL production in vivo. This may imply that insulin has a direct stimulatory effect on hepatocytes. Although this may be true in certain chronic states of hyperinsulinemia, the evidence for such a direct stimulatory effect of acute hyperinsulinemia is quite controversial, with some studies showing that insulin stimulates and others that insulin actually inhibits VLDL production. At least three in vivo studies demonstrated an acute inhibitory effect of insulin on VLDL production.[21-23] In vivo studies are frequently unable to differentiate primary from secondary effects of insulin, but at least one of these studies,[21] by infusing insulin directly into the portal vein and measuring simultaneous substrate delivery to the liver, claimed that the inhibitory effect of insulin was independent of FFA availability. We demonstrated that VLDL triglyceride production decreases to the same extent in normal-weight and chronically hyperinsulinemic, obese, nondiabetic individuals in response to a 6-hour euglycemic hyperinsulinemic clamp.[23] Whether this was a direct effect of insulin or indirectly related to the dramatic decrease in plasma FFA levels with insulin could not be determined. VLDL apolipoprotein B production decreased in the normal-weight controls but not in the obese subjects, suggesting that obese, chronically hyperinsulinemic individuals may be resistant to this acute effect of insulin.

Studies performed using perfused rat livers have mostly shown a stimulatory effect of insulin on VLDL production rate.[24-29] Recent experiments in perfused rat livers indicate that acutely added insulin stimulates the triglyceride secretion rate in perfused livers taken from normal and chronically hyperinsulinemic rats. However, it did so to a lesser extent in the latter,[28] suggesting that the chronically hyperinsulinemic livers are partly resistant to the acute effects of insulin. Topping et al have drawn attention to the fact that the results of perfused rat liver experiments are dependent on perfusion conditions, with insulin being either stimulatory or inhibitory on triglyceride secretion rates depending on the rate of blood perfusion and hematocrit (ie, oxygen supply).[29]

The majority of in vitro experiments using isolated rat hepatocytes have

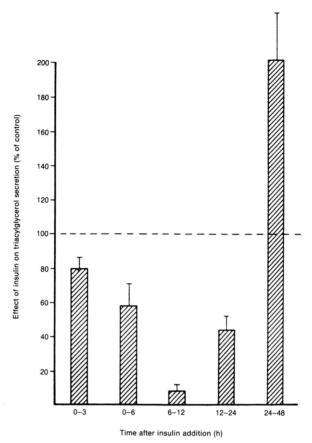

Figure 3.1 Relationship between VLDL triacylglycerol secretion and length of time of exposure of hepatocytes to insulin, illustrating an initial inhibitory effect of insulin followed by stimulation when exposure to insulin continues for longer than 24 hours. (*Reprinted, by permission, from Gibbons GF: Biochem Soc Trans 1989;17:49–51.*)

shown an inhibitory effect of insulin on VLDL triglyceride secretion rates during the initial 24-hour period.[30–35] Of interest is the fact that insulin appeared to block secretion of VLDL into the medium, with an accumulation of intracellular lipid.[30,31,33–35] In addition, the acute inhibitory effect of insulin was diminished and even reversed in some studies with longer exposure time (over 24 or 48 hours) of the hepatocytes to insulin[32–34] (Figure 3.1). At least one study reported a stimulatory effect of insulin on triglyceride and VLDL production and release from cultured rat hepatocytes.[36] Similar experiments using the hepatoma cell line, HepG$_2$ cells, found that insulin inhibited the secretion of VLDL[37,38] and apo B,[38] but did not alter the levels of apo B mRNA. Furthermore, hepatocytes cultured from chronically hyperinsulinemic rats synthesize more apo B than do those from normal rats.[39]

An essential drawback to in vitro experiments of this nature is removal from the influence of multiple factors that may regulate the production of VLDL in vivo. In addition to insulin, the availability of FFA,[37] carbohydrate,[30] glucagon,[40] and glucocorticoids[41] may regulate VLDL production. In fact, the particular type of carbohydrate may be important, with glucose and sucrose having different effects.[42]

Two of the metabolic abnormalities commonly associated with NIDDM, hyperglycemia and elevated plasma FFAs, have been shown to stimulate VLDL secretion directly from cultivated hepatocytes in vitro.[27,30] It has been postulated that in NIDDM, in the presence of an increased flux of these substrates to the liver, chronic hyperinsulinemia facilitates the overproduction of VLDL.[18,43] Reaven and Mondon[44] have provided evidence that the ability of a given FFA concentration to stimulate hepatic VLDL triglyceride secretion is a function of the ambient insulin level. The hypothesis that insulin-facilitated hepatic VLDL overproduction in NIDDM is driven by an increased flux of FFA and glucose delivery to the liver as a result of peripheral tissue insulin resistance presumes differential insulin sensitivity at the level of the liver and the peripheral tissues. An alternate hypothesis,[12] focusing on the in vitro evidence that acute hyperinsulinemia inhibits VLDL secretion, suggests that increased VLDL production in NIDDM results from resistance to the normal insulin-mediated restraint on VLDL production. While such resistance could prevent an insulin-induced inhibition of VLDL production, it would still require an additional factor to stimulate VLDL production above baseline.

In addition to the postulated effects of hyperinsulinemia on VLDL production, insulin resistance per se is closely correlated with hypertriglyceridemia in obese[45] and lean[46,47] nondiabetic individuals (Figure 3.2). Although insulin resistance and hyperinsulinemia are generally accepted as playing an important role in the development of hypertriglyceridemia, it is also important to note that hypertriglyceridemia itself may decrease insulin sensitivity,[48,49] and treatment of the hypertriglyceridemia results in improvement in insulin sensitivity.[50]

The exact role of insulin itself in directly stimulating VLDL production remains a critical but unanswered question. Whereas insulin may play an important direct role in the regulation of VLDL production in certain situations, other factors such as plasma FFA availability may assume a more important regulatory role in certain physiologic situations. The decrease in triglyceride levels and the suppression of VLDL triglyceride production that occur during the euglycemic hyperinsulinemic clamp[23,51] or with short-term improvement in glycemic control in insulin-dependent diabetic subjects[52] may be related to a dramatic decrease in FFA availability rather than a direct inhibitory effect of insulin.

In summary, it appears that the effect of insulin on VLDL production is dependent on a number of additional factors, such as the availability of substrate for VLDL production (FFA), duration of exposure to hyperinsulinemia, degree of insulin resistance, and nutritional state of the individual. Whether the divergent results of experiments using different experimental models are an artifact of the experimental conditions or merely a reflection of these complex interrelated regulatory factors is yet to be determined.

VLDL Metabolism in NIDDM

The majority of studies of VLDL metabolism in NIDDM, using tracer kinetics and mathematical modeling, have shown increased VLDL triglyceride turnover in NIDDM.[53-59] Some studies have also demonstrated a decreased fractional catabolic rate (FCR) of VLDL in some NIDDM subjects but not in others.[53-55,58,59]

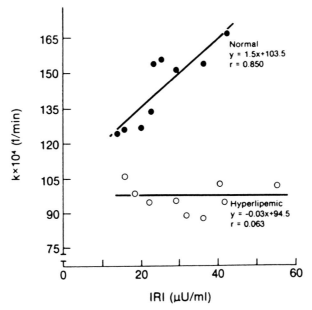

Figure 3.2 Fractional disappearance of glucose in relation to serum before and during glucagon infusion in normolipidemic (●) and lean hypertriglyceridemic (○) subjects. In the normal subjects, the fractional disappearance rate of glucose was positively related to serum levels of insulin, whereas in the hypertriglyceridemic subjects, it was lower than normal and did not change in relation to insulin concentration, demonstrating that lean hypertriglyceridemics are resistant to insulin with respect to glucose utilization. (*Reprinted, by permission, from Steiner G, Morita S, Vranic M: Resistance to insulin but not glucagon in lean human hypertriglyceridemia. Diabetes 1980;29:899–905.*)

This decreased FCR appears to be more marked in hypertriglyceridemic NIDDM,[53,54] reflecting the inability to increase removal capacity in response to increased VLDL mass. In a minority of NIDDM subjects, the degree of hypertriglyceridemia is out of proportion to transport rates, and these individuals appear to have a primary removal defect with or without increased VLDL production.[53,54] Perhaps this is related to a deficiency of adipose tissue lipoprotein lipase, which is known to occur in NIDDM.[60–62] Alternatively, the abnormal composition of VLDL in diabetes and/or its nonenzymatic glycation may decrease the affinity of the particle for lipoprotein lipase or for the receptors involved in removal of VLDL remnants.[55,63]

Greenfield and colleagues have shown that the relationship between plasma triglyceride concentration and VLDL secretion rate in NIDDM subjects follows the pattern in nondiabetic individuals and is qualitatively normal (Figure 3.3). In the majority of NIDDM subjects, the plasma triglyceride concentration–turnover ratio follows the predictable saturation kinetics lines of normal individuals, suggesting a normal removal system in the face of increased production.

Some studies in the Pima Indian NIDDM population indicate that a decreased clearance capacity is an important cause of the mild degree of hypertriglyceridemia in these subjects,[55,64,65] raising the possibility that this genetically homogeneous obese diabetic population is distinct from other diabetic groups studied.

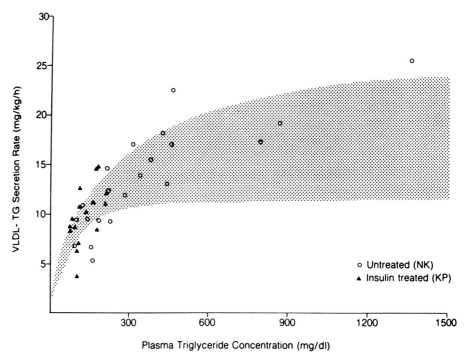

Figure 3.3 Relationship between plasma triglyceride concentration and VLDL triglyceride secretion rate in diabetic patients. The shaded area represents the 95% confidence interval for the relationship between these two variables in 92 patients with normal fasting glucose and creatinine levels. (*Reprinted, by permission, from Greenfield M, Kolterman O, Olefsky J, et al: Diabetologia 1980;18:441–446.*)

There are fewer studies examining the metabolism of apo B in NIDDM. Kissebah and colleagues[53] found an increase in VLDL apo B turnover in NIDDM in both normo- and hypertriglyceridemic individuals. There was a high degree of correlation between VLDL triglyceride and VLDL apo B turnover, resulting in an increased rate of secretion of VLDL of normal composition. In contrast, Howard and colleagues[55,65,66] found that, in Pima Indians with untreated NIDDM, VLDL triglyceride but not VLDL apo B production rate was increased compared to obese nondiabetics, resulting in VLDL particles with abnormal composition, as indicated by a higher triglyceride–apo B ratio. The FCR for both VLDL apo B and VLDL triglyceride were similarly reduced in the diabetics. They concluded from these data that NIDDM does not increase apo B production rate over and above that shown to be associated with obesity.[67,68] Taskinen et al,[69] labeling both large and small VLDL subfractions, concluded that NIDDM patients overproduce VLDL triglyceride but not apo B when compared to weight-matched controls.

IDL Metabolism in NIDDM

The apo B kinetic studies have also enabled investigators to examine the metabolism of IDL and its conversion to low density lipoprotein (LDL) in NIDDM. There appears to be heterogeneity among NIDDM subjects with respect to their ability to convert VLDL efficiently to IDL and LDL. The alternative pathway involves direct removal of IDL via a non-LDL pathway, and this process appears to be influenced by the degree of hyperlipidemia and glycemic control. Kissebah et al[53] found that, in normolipidemic mildly diabetic patients, only a small fraction of VLDL apo B was removed via a non-LDL pathway, whereas, in hyperlipidemic NIDDM, removal of VLDL apo B through the non-LDL pathway was five times greater than normal.

Howard et al[55] found that a higher proportion of VLDL apo B was removed without conversion to LDL in diabetic patients compared to nondiabetics. They suggested that the triglyceride-rich VLDL secreted in NIDDM may be a poor precursor for conversion to LDL. Taskinen et al[69] found that NIDDM patients convert VLDL to IDL and ultimately to LDL at normal rates and that neither IDL mass nor its overall production or clearance rates are affected by insulin therapy, although the proportion of precursor small VLDL relative to large VLDL increased with insulin therapy.

The potential importance to atherogenesis of an increase in the direct removal (VLDL remnant) pathway is underscored by the ability of these smaller cholesteryl ester and apo E–rich IDL particles to cross the capillary endothelial surface[70] and bind to receptors on arterial wall smooth muscle cells,[71] and by the demonstration that early atherosclerosis is associated with high levels of IDL.[72] The quantitative importance in diabetic patients of an accelerated VLDL remnant pathway still needs to be determined.

Association Between Improved Glycemic Control and VLDL Metabolism in NIDDM

The importance of glycemic control and insulinization in determining the above metabolic abnormalities is emphasized by the numerous studies that have shown improvement and in some cases normalization of TRL metabolism with various therapeutic measures aimed at improving glycemia. An energy-restricted diet was found to decrease plasma triglycerides dramatically.[57,73] In one of these studies,[57] VLDL triglyceride transport rate was reduced while the FCR remained constant.

High-carbohydrate, low-saturated-fat diets in individuals with NIDDM[74] and nondiabetic individuals[74,75] have been shown primarily to decrease the rate of conversion of VLDL to LDL, thus decreasing LDL levels while increasing VLDL levels. The effect was qualitatively similar in individuals with NIDDM and nondiabetic individuals. The exact mechanisms responsible for this are not clear but have been postulated to be related either to a decrease in lipolytic enzyme activity, to a change in composition of VLDL particles affecting their affinity for lipoprotein lipase, or to a decrease in the exchange of VLDL and high-density lipoprotein (HDL) core lipids.

The addition of ω-3 fatty acids to the diet of NIDDM patients can in some cases lower plasma triglyceride levels while adversely affecting glycemic control.[76,77]

Studies using oral hypoglycemic agents have generally shown a decrease in plasma VLDL and triglyceride concentrations with improved glycemic control.[59,65,78] Taskinen et al[65] showed an increase in FCR, an increase in adipose tissue lipoprotein lipase activity, a decrease in hepatic lipase activity, and a decrease in the triglyceride–apo B ratio of VLDL particles with 6 weeks of sulfonylurea therapy. Kissebah et al[59] found that 3 to 6 months of phenformin significantly lowered the plasma FFA and triglyceride concentrations, normalized FFA turnover and triglyceride clearance, and reduced triglyceride turnover rate.

Insulin therapy in NIDDM subjects had similar beneficial effects on TRL metabolism.[56,58,69,79] Abrams et al[56] showed that insulin therapy in NIDDM lowered both synthesis and concentration of VLDL triglyceride to near normal. Dunn et al[58] found a decrease in VLDL triglyceride synthesis and an increase in FCR but failed to restore them to normal. Taskinen et al[69] found that insulin therapy decreased large VLDL mass to a greater extent than small VLDL mass. The major effects of insulin were to reduce large VLDL apo B transport and increase the direct input of small VLDL into the plasma.

VLDL Metabolism in IDDM

VLDL metabolism in IDDM is critically dependent on the state of insulinization. Plasma VLDL and triglyceride levels in well-controlled IDDM patients may be entirely normal.[22,80–82] Triglyceride levels correlate with indices of glycemic control[81–83] and may be decreased with short-term improvement in diabetic control.[22,52,83–86]

Although it is well recognized that insulin is an important regulator of lipoprotein lipase (LPL) activity,[87] in the absence of frank diabetic ketoacidosis or extremely poor diabetic control, it appears that it is the production rate of VLDL and not the clearance that is most affected with changes in glycemic control. This is supported by the finding that LPL activity in postheparin plasma in insulin-treated IDDM patients is either normal or increased, regardless of the degree of glycemic control.[88] Ginsberg et al[89] found a combined increase in synthesis and decreased FCR of VLDL triglyceride in insulin-deficient IDDM subjects in extremely poor diabetic control. Others, however, have found that conventionally insulin-treated IDDM subjects have a normal FCR.[52,54,83]

Nikkila and Kekki[54] found that, in uncontrolled but nonketotic IDDM patients, the mean plasma triglyceride turnover rate and concentration were both significantly increased, whereas the FCR was normal in most cases. Pietri et al[84] reported that normotriglyceridemic IDDM subjects can have a normal VLDL triglyceride synthesis rate and FCR while on conventional insulin therapy. Studies that have examined VLDL triglyceride kinetics after improved glycemic control have demonstrated decreased VLDL turnover without change in FCR to be the mechanism responsible for triglyceride reduction,[22,52,54] with triglycerides in some cases decreasing to levels below those found in nondiabetic controls.

Of interest is the fact that VLDL and plasma triglyceride levels begin decreasing by 12 hours after instituting strict diabetic control with the artificial beta cell[90] but are unaffected after 2 weeks of deliberate moderate deterioration in glycemic control without ketosis.[91] The reason for this discrepancy is not readily apparent. The rapid inhibition of VLDL triglyceride production with strict glycemic control may be due to inhibition of hormone-sensitive lipase-mediated lipolysis of adipose tissue triglyceride with a subsequent reduction in FFA flux to the liver or to an acute inhibitory effect of hyperinsulinemia directly at the level of the hepatocyte. The increase in VLDL triglyceride production when glycemic control deteriorates may be regulated by different mechanisms that take longer to manifest.

Absolute insulin deficiency resulting in ketoacidosis has a far more profound effect on LPL activity, and the acute withdrawal of insulin from IDDM subjects results in a rapid decrease in LPL activity and subsequent elevation of plasma triglycerides.[92] Nikkila and Kekki[54] found a marked increase in VLDL triglyceride production in the early stages of diabetic ketoacidosis, in addition to a decrease in FCR. The increased VLDL triglyceride production is presumably related to the marked mobilization and flux of FFA from the peripheral tissues in this insulin-deficient state. Of interest is the demonstration that prolonged insulin deficiency itself may actually decrease VLDL production in vivo in dogs despite continued FFA mobilization from the periphery.[93]

The chylomicronemia syndrome (diabetic lipemia) occurring in some patients is clearly related to a profound acquired deficiency of LPL.[94] However, it is believed by some to represent the coexistence of diabetes with a familial form of hypertriglyceridemia.[95] The marked hypertriglyceridemia is fairly rapidly reversed after instituting insulin therapy and a low-fat diet, but triglyceride levels may take weeks to return to absolutely normal levels. Persistent elevation of triglycerides after 3 to 6 months of good diabetic control usually signifies the coexistence of an additional lipid disorder.

The effects of portal versus subcutaneously administered insulin on lipid and lipoprotein metabolism appear to differ in IDDM. Kazumi et al[96] showed that subcutaneously administered insulin in rats resulted in a higher peripheral serum insulin, a lower serum glucose and FFA, a higher LPL activity with lower serum triglycerides, and a similar rate of triglyceride secretion to portally administered insulin. Ruotolo et al[97] found that continuous intraperitoneal insulin infusion resulted in lower peripheral insulin levels, VLDL triglycerides, and VLDL apo B than did continuous subcutaneous insulin infusion. The decreased VLDL with intraperitoneal infusion appeared to be due to both decreased production and increased clearance of VLDL apo B. More studies are needed to determine whether the more physiologic route of insulin administration (ie, into the portal system) has clear-cut benefits with respect to its effect on plasma lipoproteins.

VLDL Compositional Changes in NIDDM and IDDM

The above discussion has focused on gross changes in lipid and lipoprotein levels in NIDDM and IDDM. Not only can alterations in TRL metabolism also lead to changes in VLDL, IDL, and HDL composition, but more subtle compositional changes in TRL particles can in turn be responsible for abnormalities in receptor recognition, lipoprotein interactions, and clearance of the particles in diabetic individuals.

In NIDDM, several studies have found VLDL particles to be large and triglyceride rich, with a disproportionate increase in the larger VLDL subfraction and the triglyceride–apo B ratio,[55,65,69] and this abnormality reverts toward normal with treatment.[65,69] Ishibashi et al[98] found no differences in the relative composition of VLDL isolated from patients with NIDDM when compared with VLDL from individuals with similarly elevated triglyceride concentration, suggesting that these abnormalities are not specific for diabetes but are a result of hypertriglyceridemia, whatever the etiology. These large triglyceride-rich VLDLs may be less efficiently converted to LDLs,[99] increasing direct removal from the circulation via non-LDL pathways.[53,55] Although the VLDL particles are triglyceride enriched, it is important not to lose sight of the fact that, at least in nondiabetics, approximately 70% of any increase in triglyceride production results in an increase in the number of particles, the remainder being due to an increase in the amount of triglyceride carried per particle.[100]

Abnormalities in the distribution of apolipoproteins in VLDL have been described in NIDDM,[101–103] with increases in the proportion of apo C and apo E being reported. The detailed analysis of Ishibashi et al[98] found that the absolute content of apo C-II, apo C-III, and apo E per VLDL particle increases as the concentration of triglycerides in VLDL increases, both in NIDDM as well as nondiabetic subjects. In addition, the ratio of apo C-III to apo C-II increases in hypertriglyceridemia. Taskinen et al[65] found that the changes in VLDL apo E appeared to reflect those of apo B, with a relative decrease in apo E with respect to triglycerides in these triglyceride-rich VLDL particles. The VLDL of diabetics, however, had a greater proportion of total apo E in the VLDL fraction, and this proportion returned toward that of controls during therapy with sulfonylureas.

An increased apo E2–apo E3 ratio in NIDDM has been reported by some investigators[103] but not by others.[104] The latter investigators,[104] however, found that apo E isoform pattern influences the incidence of hyperlipidemia within the diabetic population, with the highest incidence of hyperlipidemia being associated with inheritance of the apo E3/E2 pattern, followed by the apo E4/E3 and apo E3/E3 groups.

In IDDM with hypertriglyceridemia, similar lipoprotein alterations probably occur. Normolipemic IDDM patients have also been found to have VLDL compositional abnormalities, with a high proportion of apo B and free and esterified cholesterol and lower triglyceride concentrations.[105–107] These compositional abnormalities suggest the presence of smaller and more atherogenic VLDL particles and are not corrected fully by intensive insulin therapy. Bagdade et al[106] found an increase in the free cholesterol–lecithin ratio in VLDL, and this may be a risk factor for the development of atherosclerosis.[108]

Oxidative and glycation modifications of VLDL particles in both IDDM and NIDDM also appear to be extremely important in increasing their atherogenicity and interaction with endothelial cells, smooth muscle cells, and macrophages. This topic is discussed in detail elsewhere in this book.

Postprandial Metabolism of TRL in Diabetes Mellitus

There has been a resurgence of interest in the postprandial metabolism of TRL in diabetic and nondiabetic populations for the following reasons:

1. Humans ingest on average three meals a day with snacks in between. Since chylomicron remnants can be detected in the circulation for up to 14 hours following a high-fat meal in normolipidemic individuals,[109] the importance of studying subjects in the postprandial state becomes evident.
2. The large influx of dietary fat following a meal stresses the common, saturable triglyceride removal mechanism for chylomicrons and VLDL,[110] and may

reveal abnormalities in TRL metabolism that may not be evident in the basal postabsorptive state.

3. The dynamic interaction and exchange of lipids between TRL and higher density lipoproteins, particularly HDL, can be studied in vivo in the postprandial state.[109,111]

4. Chylomicron remnant particles generated by the lipolysis of chylomicrons are believed to be atherogenic,[112,113] and increased levels may be related to a higher incidence of coronary artery disease.[114]

The postprandial studies in IDDM[91,115,116] and NIDDM[111,117,118] reported to date, as well as those in obese hyperinsulinemic nondiabetic subjects,[109] have found a consistent relationship between fasting triglyceride level and postprandial triglyceride response (Figure 3.4). The most likely explanation for this strikingly consistent finding is that there is competition for clearance of chylomicrons and VLDL by the same lipolytic enzymes,[110] and that the fasting VLDL pool size therefore affects the clearance rate of chylomicrons, even in the presence of normal LPL activity. Alternatively, if decreased clearance is responsible for the fasting hypertriglyceridemia, this abnormality in LPL activity will also manifest in the postprandial state, delaying chylomicron clearance.

This concept is supported by the finding of slower removal of chylomicrons in NIDDM subjects with fasting hypertriglyceridemia,[56,111,119] and the reversal of this abnormality with insulin-induced lowering of the fasting triglyceride level.[56] Whether this is related purely to a mass effect or to concurrent changes in LPL activity affecting both VLDL and chylomicron clearance is not entirely

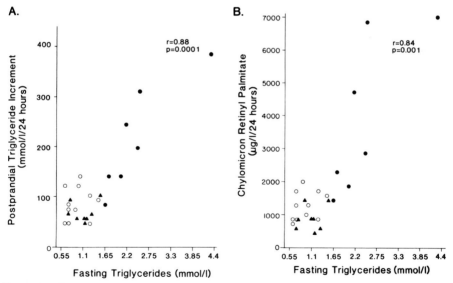

Figure 3.4 Correlations between fasting triglyceride concentration and postprandial triglyceride increment (A) and postprandial chylomicron concentration (labeled with retinyl palmitate) (B) in normotriglyceridemic NIDDM subjects, (○), hypertriglyceridemic NIDDM subjects, (●), and nondiabetic controls (▲). (*Reprinted, by permission, from Lewis GF, O'Meara NM, Soltys PA, et al: Fasting hypertriglyceridemia in noninsulin-dependent diabetes mellitus is an important predictor of postprandial lipid and lipoprotein abnormalities. J Clin Endocrinol Metab 1991;72:934–944.*)

clear. In addition, we cannot rule out the possibility that changes in the composition of the triglyceride-rich lipoprotein particles with increasing triglyceridemia affects their clearance by LPL.

As might be expected from the above findings, NIDDM subjects with fasting hypertriglyceridemia have a markedly increased postprandial triglyceride response, and this is contributed to by an increase in both chylomicron and nonchylomicron fractions.[110] Postprandial response in normotriglyceridemic NIDDM subjects does not differ significantly from that in weight-matched nondiabetic controls (Figure 3.5). There is also evidence that at least some of the postprandial increase in TRL is of endogenous VLDL origin,[109] but the mechanism responsible for this rise in VLDL is not clearly understood.

The postprandial elevation of chylomicron remnant particles in hypertriglyceridemic NIDDM subjects[111] appears to be a function of the overall postprandial TRL excursion that occurs in these individuals and not the result of a specific clearance defect related to the diabetic state per se, although such a defect cannot be ruled out absolutely. This increase in chylomicron remnant concentration in postprandial plasma may have important implications for atherogenesis, as discussed above. Others have found an elevated apo B-48–apo B-100 ratio in the VLDL and IDL fractions of NIDDM subjects postprandially,

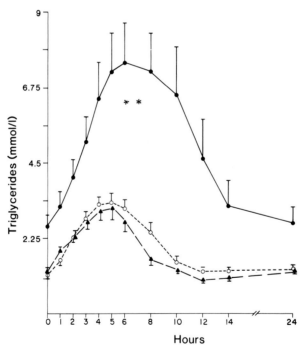

Figure 3.5 Plasma triglyceride concentrations following ingestion of a high-fat mixed meal at zero time in hypertriglyceridemic NIDDM subjects (●), normotriglyceridemic NIDDM subjects (○), and weight-matched normo⁺riglyceridemic controls (▲). There were no significant differences in postprandial triglyceride response between the latter two groups, but the hypertriglyceridemic NIDDM subjects had a greater postprandial triglyceride response (*p* = .001). (*Reprinted, by permission, from Lewis GF, O'Meara NM, Soltys PA, et al: Fasting hypertriglyceridemia in noninsulin-dependent diabetes mellitus is an important predictor of postprandial lipid and lipoprotein abnormalities. J Clin Endocrinol Metab 1991;72:934–944.*)

suggesting that chylomicron remnants may be relatively elevated in NIDDM postprandially.[120]

The major postprandial change in HDL particles in NIDDM subjects—triglyceride enrichment at the expense of cholesteryl ester—was qualitatively similar to that described in nondiabetic subjects.[111] The magnitude of the triglyceride enrichment reflected the magnitude of postprandial lipemia and was inversely correlated with fasting HDL levels, suggesting that triglyceride enrichment of HDL may be related to the lower HDL levels in NIDDM.

One of the most striking findings in hypertriglyceridemic NIDDM subjects is the marked postprandial elevation of FFA levels for up to 14 hours following a high-fat meal,[111] despite normal fasting FFA levels. The timing of this late postprandial surge in FFAs suggests that they are derived from the peripheral lipolysis of chylomicrons, although the exact origin of the postprandial FFAs still needs to be determined. Whether the increased flux of FFA in hypertriglyceridemic NIDDM is merely a reflection of the greater TRL load undergoing lipolysis, or whether this represents a more basic abnormality in FFA uptake and/or mobilization from peripheral tissues in these individuals, is yet to be determined. This increased postprandial FFA flux may play a role in stimulating hepatic triglyceride overproduction in certain individuals with NIDDM.

Postprandial triglyceride elevation in IDDM can be decreased by reducing the fasting triglyceride level,[115,116,121] again demonstrating the close relationship between fasting and postprandial triglyceridemia. There does not appear to be any specific gross abnormality of TRL metabolism in IDDM subjects compared to matched nondiabetic controls,[91] but abnormal fasting TRL composition in IDDM is also reflected in postprandial TRL compositional differences between diabetic and nondiabetic subjects and between males and females.[121]

Alterations in insulinization affecting glycemic control in IDDM, aside from the well-described effects on fasting triglyceride levels, do not appear to independently affect postprandial triglyceride, chylomicron, or chylomicron remnant metabolism.[91] Although the level of insulin replacement at the time of the meal does not influence these parameters, it does have a profound effect on FFA levels postprandially. Adequate insulinization at the time of the meal prevents the marked excursion in postprandial FFA seen when only a low basal level of insulin is provided. Whether insulin acts directly in facilitating FFA uptake by peripheral cells or indirectly via its action on hormone-sensitive lipase, thereby controlling tissue levels of FFA, remains to be determined.

Summary

There are multiple abnormalities in TRL metabolism in both NIDDM and IDDM subjects. Many of these abnormalities result in potentially atherogenic changes to lipid homeostasis. Because of the diversity and heterogeneity of these alterations, it has been difficult to prove a simple, direct relationship between hypertriglyceridemia and premature atherosclerosis.

NIDDM is characterized by increased FFA and glucose availability to the hepatocyte, which, together with insulin, play a pivotal role in the overproduction of VLDL. Abnormalities of lipoprotein lipase leading to decreased clearance of VLDL appear to play a lesser role in most NIDDM subjects. Apo B production is increased in NIDDM but to a lesser extent than triglyceride production, resulting in larger triglyceride-rich VLDLs that may be poorly converted to LDLs via IDLs. Elevated fasting VLDL concentrations are associated with postprandial hypertriglyceridemia and elevated postprandial FFA concentrations, fueling the vicious cycle leading to VLDL overproduction. The exact role that insulin plays in VLDL overproduction is not clear, but improved glycemic control by whatever means generally is associated with reversal of many of the above abnormalities.

IDDM, in contrast, is characterized by normolipidemia when glycemic control is good. With insulin deficiency there is a marked acquired defect in the action of LPL, leading to hypertriglyceridemia. In the moderately controlled IDDM subject, more intensive insulin therapy appears to act by decreasing hepatic VLDL production, and there is a good correlation between plasma triglyceride levels and glycemic control. Despite normal or subnormal VLDL levels in well-controlled IDDM subjects, there may be potentially atherogenic alterations in VLDL composition that are not fully corrected with improved glycemic control. Whereas postprandial triglyceride levels in IDDM generally reflect fasting triglyceride concentrations, FFA levels appear to be a far more sensitive index of insulinization than triglycerides.

References

1. Barrett-Connor E, Grundy SM, Holdbrook MJ: Plasma lipids and diabetes mellitus in an adult community. *Am J Epidemiol* 1982;115:657–663.
2. Laakso M, Voutilainen E, Sarlund H, et al: Serum lipids and lipoproteins in middle-aged non-insulin-dependent diabetics. *Atherosclerosis* 1985;56:271–281.
3. Howard BV, Knowler WC, Vasquez B, et al: Plasma and lipoprotein cholesterol and triglyceride in the Pima Indian population. Comparison of diabetics and nondiabetics. *Arteriosclerosis* 1984;4:462–471.
4. Austin MA: Plasma triglyceride and coronary heart disease. *Arterioscler Thromb* 1991;11:2–14.
5. Assman G, Gotto AM Jr, Paoletti R, et al: The hypertriglyceridemias: Risk and management. *Am J Cardiol* 1991;68:1A–42A.
6. West KM, Ahuja MMS, Bennett PH, et al: The role of circulating glucose and triglyceride concentrations and their interactions with other risk factors as determinants of arterial disease in nine diabetic population samples from the WHO multinational study. *Diabetes Care* 1983;6:361–369.
7. Janka HU: Five-year incidence of major macrovascular complications in diabetes mellitus. *Horm Metab Res Suppl* 1985;15:15–19.
8. Fontbonne A, Eschwege E, Cambien F, et al: Hypertriglyceridemia as a risk factor for coronary heart disease mortality in subjects with impaired glucose tolerance or diabetes. Results from the 11-year follow-up of the Paris Prospective Study. *Diabetologia* 1989;32:300–304.
9. Santen RJ, Willis PW, Fajans SS: Atherosclerosis in diabetes mellitus. Correlations with serum lipid levels, adiposity and serum insulin levels. *Arch Intern Med* 1972; 130:833–843.
10. Laakso M, Pyorala K: Lipid and lipoprotein abnormalities in diabetic patients with peripheral vascular disease. *Atherosclerosis* 1988;74:55–63.
11. Uusitupa MI, Niskanen LK, Siitonen O, et al: 5-year incidence of atherosclerotic vascular disease in relation to general risk factors, insulin level, and abnormalities in lipoprotein composition in non-insulin-dependent diabetic and non-diabetic subjects. *Circulation* 1990;82:27–36.
12. Gibbons GF: Hyperlipidemia of diabetes [review]. *Clin Sci* 1986;71:477–486.

13. Gibbons GF: Assembly and secretion of hepatic very-low-density lipoprotein [review]. *Biochem J* 1990;268:1–13.
14. Howard BV: Lipoprotein metabolism in diabetes mellitus [review]. *J Lipid Res* 1987; 28:613–628.
15. Fukuda N, Ontko JA: Interactions between fatty acid synthesis, oxidation and esterification in the production of triglyceride-rich lipoproteins by the liver. *J Lipid Res* 1984;25:831–842.
16. Kohout M, Kohoutova B, Heimberg M: The regulation of hepatic triglyceride metabolism by free fatty acids. *J Biol Chem* 1971;246:5067–5074.
17. Levinson M, Oswald B, Quarfordt S: Serum factors influencing cultured hepatocyte exogenous and endogenous triglyceride. *Am J Physiol* 1990;259:G15–G20.
18. Reaven GM, Greenfield MS: Diabetic hypertriglyceridemia. Evidence for three clinical syndromes. *Diabetes* 1981;30(suppl 2):66–75.
19. Tobey TA, Greenfield M, Kraemer F, et al: Relationship between insulin resistance, insulin secretion, very-low-density lipoprotein kinetics and plasma triglyceride levels in normotriglyceridemic man. *Metabolism* 1981;30:165–171.
20. Steiner G, Haynes FJ, Yoshino G, et al: Hyperinsulinemia and in vivo very-low-density lipoprotein-triglyceride kinetics. *Am J Physiol* 1982;246:E187–E192.
21. Vogelberg KH, Gries FA, Moschinski D: Hepatic production of VLDL-triglycerides. Dependence of portal substrate and insulin concentration. *Horm Metab Res* 1980; 12:688–694.
22. Pietri AO, Dunn FL, Grundy SM, et al: The effect of continuous subcutaneous insulin infusion and very-low-density lipoprotein triglyceride metabolism in type 1 diabetes mellitus. *Diabetes* 1983;32:75–81.
23. Lewis G, Uffelman K, Steiner G: Acute hyperinsulinemia decreases VLDL triglyceride and VLDL apolipoprotein B production *in vivo* in humans. *Diabetes* 1992;41(suppl 1):25A.
24. Topping DL, Mayes PA: The immediate effects of insulin and fructose on the metabolism of the perfused liver. Changes in the lipoprotein secretion, fatty acid oxidation and esterification, lipogenesis and carbohydrate metabolism. *Biochem J* 1972;126:295–311.
25. Woodside WF, Heimberg M: Effects of antiinsulin serum, insulin and glucose on output of triglycerides and on ketogenesis by the perfused rat liver. *J Biol Chem* 1976;251:13–23.
26. Laker ME, Mayes PA: Investigations into the direct effects of insulin on hepatic ketogenesis, lipoprotein secretion and pyruvate dehydrogenase activity. *Biochim Biophys Acta* 1984;795:427–430.
27. Topping DL, Mayes PA: Insulin and non-esterified fatty acids. Acute regulators of lipogenesis in perfused rat liver. *Biochem J* 1982;204:433–439.
28. Raman M, Steiner G: Effect of insulin on VLDL-triglyceride secretion and glucose production in the perfused rat liver [abstract]. *Diabetes* 1990;39(suppl 1):45A.
29. Topping DL, Storer GB, Trimble RP: Effects of flow rate and insulin on triacylglycerol secretion by perfused rat liver. *Am J Physiol* 1988;255:E306–E313.
30. Durrington PN, Newton RS, Weinstein DB, et al: Effects of insulin and glucose on very-low-density lipoprotein triglyceride secretion by cultured rat hepatocytes. *J Clin Invest* 1982;70:63–73.
31. Patsch W, Franz S, Schonfeld G: Role of insulin in lipoprotein secretion by cultured rat hepatocytes. *J Clin Invest* 1983;71:1161–1174.
32. Bartlett SM, Gibbons GF: Short- and longer-term regulation of very-low-density lipoprotein secretion by insulin, dexamethasone and lipogenic subsrates in cultured hepatocytes. A biphasic effect of insulin. *Biochem J* 1988;249:37–43.
33. Duerden JM, Bartlett SM, Gibbons GF: Long term maintenance of high rates of very-low-density lipoprotein secretion in hepatocyte cultures. A model for studying the direct effects of insulin and insulin deficiency in vitro. *Biochem J* 1989;263:937–943.

34. Duerden JM, Bartlett SM, Gibbons GF: Regulation of very-low-density lipoprotein lipid secretion in hepatocyte cultures derived from diabetic animals. *Biochem J* 1989; 262:313–319.

35. Sparks CE, Sparks JD, Bolognino M, et al: Insulin effects on apolipoprotein B lipoprotein synthesis and secretion by primary cultures of rat hepatocytes. *Metabolism* 1986;35:1128–1136.

36. Beynen AC, Haagsman HP, Van Golde LMG, et al: The effects of insulin and glucagon on the release of triacylglycerols by isolated rat hepatocytes are mere reflections of the hormonal effects on the rate of triacylglycerol synthesis. *Biochim Biophys Acta* 1981;665:1–7.

37. Dashti N, Wolfbauer G: Secretion of lipids, apolipoproteins, and lipoproteins by human hepatoma cell line, HepG2: Effects of oleic acid and insulin. *J Lipid Res* 1987; 28:423–436.

38. Pullinger CR, North JD, Teng B-B, et al: The apolipoprotein B gene is constitutively expressed in HepG2 cells: Regulation of secretion by oleic acid, albumin, and insulin, and measurement of the mRNA half-life. *J Lipid Res* 1989;30:1065–1077.

39. Salhanick AI, Deichman ML, Anatruda JM: Chronic in vivo and acute in vitro effects of insulin on apolipoprotein B synthesis and secretion in rat hepatocytes. *Diabetes* 1992;41:(suppl 1):17A.

40. Eaton RP, Schade DS, Conway M: Decreased glucagon activity. A mechanism for genetic and acquired endogenous hyperlipidaemia. *Lancet* 1974;2:1545–1547.

41. Martin-Sanz P, Vance JE, Brindley DN: Stimulation of apolipoprotein secretion in very-low-density and high-density lipoproteins from cultured rat hepatocytes by descamethasone. *Biochem J* 1990;271:575–583.

42. Kazumi T, Vranic M, Steiner G: Triglyceride kinetics: Effects of dietary glucose, sucrose, or fructose alone or with hyperinsulinemia. *Am J Physiol* 1986;250:E325–E330.

43. Reaven GM: Abnormal lipoprotein metabolism in non-insulin-dependent diabetes mellitus. Pathogenesis and treatment. *Am J Med* 1987;83(suppl 3A):31–40.

44. Reaven GM, Mondon CE: Effect of in vivo plasma insulin levels on the relationship between perfusate free fatty acid concentration and triglyceride secretion by perfused rat livers. *Horm Metab Res* 1984;16:230–232.

45. Abbott WGH, Lillioja S, Young AA, et al: Relationships between plasma lipoprotein concentrations and insulin action in an obese hyperinsulinemic population. *Diabetes* 1987;36:897–904.

46. Zuniga-Guarjardo S, Steiner G, Shumak S, et al: Insulin resistance and action in hypertriglyceridemia. *Diabetes Res Clin Pract* 1991;14:55–62.

47. Steiner G, Morita S, Vranic M: Resistance to insulin but not to glucagon in lean human hypertriglyceridemia. *Diabetes* 1980;29:899–905.

48. Thiebaud D, DeFronzo RA, Jacot E, et al: Effect of long chain triglyceride infusion on glucose metabolism in man. *Metabolism* 1982;31:1128–1136.

49. Ferrannini E, Barrett E, Bevilacqua S, et al: Some interactions of free fatty acids on glucose metabolism in man. *Diabetologia* 1981;21:270–275.

50. Steiner G: Altering triglyceride concentrations changes insulin-glucose relationships in hypertriglyceridemic patients. *Diabetes Care* 1991;14:1077–1081.

51. Shumak SL, Zinman B, Zuniga-Guarjardo S, et al: Triglyceride-rich lipoprotein metabolism during acute hyperinsulinemia in hypertriglyceridemic humans. *Metabolism* 1988;37:461–466.

52. Dunn FL, Carroll PB, Beltz WF: Treatment with artificial B cell decreases very-low-density lipoprotein triglyceride synthesis in type I diabetes. *Diabetes* 1987;36:661–666.

53. Kissebah AH, Alfarsi S, Evans DJ, et al: Integrated regulation of very low density lipoprotein triglyceride and apolipoprotein B kinetics in non-insulin-dependent diabetes mellitus. *Diabetes* 1982;31:217–225.

54. Nikkila EA, Kekki M: Plasma triglyceride transport kinetics in diabetes mellitus. *Metabolism* 1973;22:1–22.
55. Howard BV, Abbott WGH, Beltz WF, et al: Integrated study of low density lipoprotein metabolism and very-low density lipoprotein metabolism in non-insulin-dependent diabetes. *Metabolism* 1987;36:870–877.
56. Abrams JJ, Ginsberg H, Grundy SM: Metabolism of cholesterol and plasma triglycerides in nonketotic diabetes mellitus. *Diabetes* 1982;31:903–910.
57. Ginsberg H, Grundy SM: Very low density lipoprotein metabolism in non-ketotic diabetes mellitus: Effect of dietary restriction. *Diabetologia* 1982;23:421–425.
58. Dunn FL, Raskin P, Bilheimer DW, et al: The effect of diabetic control on very-low-density lipoprotein-triglyceride metabolism in patients with type II diabetes mellitus and marked hypertriglyceridemia. *Metabolism* 1984;33:117–123.
59. Kissebah AH, Adams PW, Wynn V: Inter-relationship between insulin secretion and plasma free fatty acid and triglyceride transport kinetics in maturity onset diabetes and the effect of phenethylbiguanide (phenformin). *Diabetologia* 1974;10:119–130.
60. Taskinen M-R, Nikkila EA, Kuusi T, et al: Lipoprotein lipase activity and serum lipoproteins in untreated type 2 (insulin-independent) diabetes associated with obesity. *Diabetologia* 1982;22:46–50.
61. Nikkila EA, Huttunen JK, Ehnholm C: Postheparin plasma lipoprotein lipase and hepatic lipase in diabetes mellitus. Relationship to plasma triglyceride metabolism. *Diabetes* 1977;26:11–21.
62. Taylor KG, Galton DJ, Holdsworth G: Insulin-independent diabetes: A defect in the activity of lipoprotein lipase in adipose tissue. *Diabetologia* 1979;16:313–317.
63. Mamo JCL, Szeto L, Steiner G: Glycation of very low density lipoprotein from rat plasma impairs its catabolism. *Diabetologia* 1990;33:339–345.
64. Howard BV, Reitman JS, Vasquez B, et al: Very-low-density lipoprotein triglyceride metabolism in non-insulin-dependent diabetes mellitus. Relationship to plasma insulin and free fatty acids. *Diabetes* 1983;32:271–276.
65. Taskinen MR, Beltz WF, Harper I, et al: Effects of NIDDM on very-low-density lipoprotein triglyceride and apolipoprotein B metabolism. Studies before and after sulphonylurea therapy. *Diabetes* 1986;35:1268–1277.
66. Howard BV, Abbott WGH, Egusa G, et al: Coordination of very low-density lipoprotein triglyceride and apolipoprotein B metabolism in humans: Effects of obesity and non-insulin-dependent diabetes mellitus. *Am Heart J* 1987;113:522–526.
67. Egusa G, Biltz WF, Grundy SM, et al: Influence of obesity on the metabolism of apolipoprotein B in humans. *J Clin Invest* 1985;76:596–603.
68. Kissebah AH, Alfarsi S, Adams PW: Integrated regulation of very low density lipoprotein triglyceride and apolipoprotein B kinetics in man: Normolipemic subjects, familial hypertriglyceridemia and familial combined hyperlipidemia. *Metabolism* 1981;30:856–868.
69. Taskinen M-R, Packard CJ, Shepherd J: Effect of insulin therapy on metabolic fate of apolipoprotein B-containing lipoproteins in NIDDM. *Diabetes* 1990;39:1017–1027.
70. Reichl D, Myant NB, Pflug JJ, et al: The passage of apoproteins from plasma lipoproteins into the lipoproteins of peripheral lymph in man. *Clin Sci Mol Med* 1977; 53:221–226.
71. Bierman EL, Eisenberg S, Stein O, et al: Very low density lipoprotein "remnant" particles: Uptake by aortic smooth muscle cells in culture. *Biochim Biophys Acta* 1973;329:163–169.
72. Steiner G, Schwartz L, Shumak S, et al: The association of increased levels of intermediate density lipoproteins with smoking and with coronary artery disease. *Circulation* 1987;75:124–130.
73. Vessby B, Selinus I, Lithell H: Serum lipoprotein and lipoprotein lipase in overweight, type II diabetics during and after supplemented fasting. *Arteriosclerosis* 1985;5:93–100.

74. Abbott WGH, Swinburn B, Ruotolo G, et al: Effect of a high-carbohydrate, low-saturated-fat diet on apolipoprotein B and triglyceride metabolism in Pima Indians. *J Clin Invest* 1990;86:642–650.

75. Ginsberg HN, Le N-A, Melish J, et al: Effect of a high carbohydrate diet on apolipoprotein-B catabolism in man. *Metabolism* 1981;30:347–353.

76. Friday KE, Childs MT, Tsunehara CH, et al: Elevated plasma glucose and lowered triglyceride levels from omega-3 fatty acid supplementation in type II diabetes. *Diabetes Care* 1989;12:276–281.

77. Borkman M, Chisholm DJ, Furler SM, et al: Effects of fish oil supplementation on glucose and lipid metabolism in NIDDM. *Diabetes* 1989;38:1314–1319.

78. Schneider J, Erren T, Zofel P, et al: Metformin-induced changes in serum lipids, lipoproteins and aploproteins in non-insulin-dependent diabetes mellitus. *Atherosclerosis* 1990;82:97–103.

79. Hughes TA, Clements RS, Fairclough PK, et al: Effect of insulin therapy on lipoproteins in non-insulin dependent diabetes mellitus (NIDDM). *Atherosclerosis* 1987;67: 105–114.

80. Nikkila EA, Hormila P: Serum lipids and lipoproteins in insulin-treated diabetes. Demonstration of increased high density lipoprotein concentrations. *Diabetes* 1978; 27:1078–1086.

81. Lopes-Virella MF, Wohltmann HJ, Loadholt CB, et al: Plasma lipids and lipoproteins in young insulin-dependent diabetic patients. Relationship with control. *Diabetologia* 1981;21:216–223.

82. Sosenko JM, Breslow JL, Miettinen OS, et al: Hyperglycemia and plasma lipid levels. A prospective study of young insulin-dependent diabetic patients. *N Engl J Med* 1980;302:650–654.

83. Gonen B, White N, Schonfeld G, et al: Plasma levels of apoprotein B in patients with diabetes mellitus: The effect of glycemic control. *Metabolism* 1985;34:675–679.

84. Pietri A, Dunn FL, Raskin P: The effect of improved diabetic control on plasma lipid and lipoprotein levels. A comparison of conventional therapy and continuous subcutaneous insulin infusion. *Diabetes* 1980;29:1001–1005.

85. Hershcopf R, Plotnick LP, Kaya K, et al: Short term improvement in glycemic control utilizing continuous subcutaneous insulin infusion: The effect on 24-hour integrated concentrations of counterregulatory hormones and plasma lipids in insulin-dependent diabetes mellitus. *J Clin Endocrinol Metab* 1982;54:504–509.

86. Tamborlane WV, Genel M, Sherwin RS, et al: Restoration of normal lipid and aminoacid metabolism in diabetic patients treated with a portable insulin-infusion pump. *Lancet* 1979;1:1258–1261.

87. Taskinen M-R: Lipoprotein lipase in diabetes [review]. *Diabetes Metab Rev* 1987;3: 551–570.

88. Nikkila EA, Huttunen JK, Ehnholm C: Postheparin plasma lipoprotein lipase and hepatic lipase in diabetes mellitus. Relationship to plasma triglyceride metabolism. *Diabetes* 1977;26:11–21.

89. Ginsberg H, Mok H, Grundy S, et al: Increased production of very low density lipoprotein triglyceride in insulin-deficient diabetics [abstract]. *Diabetes* 1977;26(suppl 1):399.

90. Vlachokosta FV, Asmal AC, Ganda OP, et al: The effect of strict control with the artifical beta-cell on plasma lipid levels in insulin-dependent diabetes. *Diabetes Care* 1983;6:351–355.

91. Lewis GF, O'Meara NM, Cabana VG, et al: Postprandial triglyceride response in type I (insulin-dependent) diabetes mellitus is not altered by short-term deterioration in glycaemic control or level of postprandial insulin replacement. *Diabetologia* 1991; 34:253–259.

92. Bagdade JD, Porte D Jr, Bierman EL: Acute insulin withdrawal and the regulation of plasma triglyceride removal in diabetic subjects. *Diabetes* 1968;17:127–132.

93. Steiner G, Poapst ME, Davidson JK: Production of chylomycron-like lipoproteins from endogenous lipid by the intestine and liver of dogs. *Diabetes* 1975;24:263–271.

94. Bagdade JD, Porte D Jr, Bierman EL: Diabetic lipemia: A form of acquired fat-induced lipemia. *N Engl J Med* 1967;276:427–433.

95. Chait A, Robertson HT, Brunzell JD: Chylomicronemia syndrome in diabetes mellitus. *Diabetes Care* 1981;4:343–348.

96. Kazumi T, Vranic M, Bar-On H, et al: Portal v. peripheral hyperinsulinemia in very low density lipoprotein triglyceride kinetics. *Metabolism* 1986;35:1024–1028.

97. Ruotolo G, Micossi P, Galimberti G, et al: Effects of intraperitoneal versus subcutaneous insulin administration on lipoprotein metabolism in type I diabetes. *Metabolism* 1990;39:598–604.

98. Ishibashi S, Yamada N, Shimano H, et al: Composition of very-low-density lipoproteins in non-insulin-dependent diabetes mellitus. *Clin Chem* 1989;35:808–812.

99. Packard CJ, Munro A, Lorimer AR, et al: Metabolism of apolipoprotein B in large triglyceride-rich very low density lipoproteins of normal and hypertriglyceridemic subjects. *J Clin Invest* 1984;74:2178–2192.

100. Poapst M, Reardon M, Steiner G: Relative contribution of triglyceride-rich lipoprotein particle size and number to plasma triglyceride concentration. *Arteriosclerosis* 1985;5:381–390.

101. Gabor J, Spain M, Kalant N: Composition of serum very-low density and high-density lipoproteins in diabetes. *Clin Chem* 1980;26:1261–1265.

102. Stalenhoef AF, Demacker PNM, Lutterman JA, et al: Apolipoprotein C in type 2 (non-insulin-dependent) diabetic patients with hypertriglyceridemia. *Diabetologia* 1982;22:489–491.

103. Weiswueiler P, Jungst D, Schwandt P: Quantitation of apolipoprotein E-isoforms in diabetes mellitus. *Horm Metab Res* 1983;15:201.

104. Eto M, Watanabe K, Iwashima Y, et al: Apolipoprotein E polymorphism and hyperlipemia in type II diabetics. *Diabetes* 1986;35:1374–1382.

105. James RW, Pometta D: Differences in lipoprotein subfraction composition and distribution between type I diabetic men and control subjects. *Diabetes* 1980;39:1158–1164.

106. Bagdade JD, Helve E, Taskinen M-R: Effects of continuous insulin infusion therapy on lipoprotein surface and core lipid composition in insulin-dependent diabetes mellitus. *Metabolism* 1991;40:445–449.

107. Rivellese A, Riccardi G, Romano G, et al: Presence of very low density lipoprotein compositional abnormalities in type I (insulin-dependent) diabetic patients; effects of blood glucose optimisation. *Diabetologia* 1988;31:884–888.

108. Kuksis A, Myher JJ, Geher K, et al: Decreased plasma phosphatidylcholine/free cholesterol ratio as an indicator of risk for ischemic vascular disease. *Arteriosclerosis* 1982;2:296–302.

109. Lewis GF, O'Meara NM, Soltys PA, et al: Postprandial lipoprotein metabolism in normal and obese subjects: Comparison after the vitamin A fat-loading test. *J Clin Endocrinol Metab* 1990;71:1041–1050.

110. Brunzell JD, Hazzard WR, Port D Jr, et al: Evidence for a common, saturable, triglyceride removal mechanism for chylomicrons and very low density lipoproteins in man. *J Clin Invest* 1973;52:1578–1585.

111. Lewis GF, O'Meara NM, Soltys PA, et al: Fasting hypertriglyceridemia in noninsulin-dependent diabetes mellitus is an important predictor of postprandial lipid and lipoprotein abnormalities. *J Clin Endocrinol Metab* 1991;72:934–944.

112. Zilversmit DB: Atherogenesis: A postprandial phenomenon. *Circulation* 1979;60:473–485.

113. Floren CH, Albers JJ, Bierman EL: Uptake of chylomicron remnants causes cholesterol accumulation in cultured human arterial smooth muscle cells. *Biochim Biophys Acta* 1981;663:336–349.

114. Simons LA, Dwyer T, Simons J, et al: Chylomicrons and chylomicron remnants in coronary artery disease: A case-control study. *Atherosclerosis* 1987;65:181–189.
115. Georgopoulos A, Margolis S, Bachorik P, et al: Effect of improved glycemic control on the response of plasma triglycerides to ingestion of a saturated fat load in normotriglyceridemic and hypertriglyceridemic diabetic subjects. *Metabolism* 1988;37: 866–871.
116. Georgopoulos A, Applebaum-Bowden D, Margolis S: Improved glycemic control lowers plasma apolipoprotein E and triglyceride levels following ingestion of a fat load in insulin-dependent diabetic subjects. *Metabolism* 1988;37:837–843.
117. Williams CM, Moore F, Wright J: Fasting and postprandial triacylglycerol responses to a standard test meal in subjects taking dietary supplements of n-3 fatty acids. *Biochem Soc Trans* 1990;18:909–910.
118. Lerman I, Ahumada AM, Cardoso SG, et al: Postprandial lipids and lipoproteins in NIDDM patients with hypoalphalipoproteinemia and patients with primary hypoalphalipoproteinemia [abstract]. *Diabetes* 1991;40(suppl 1):391A.
119. Haffner SM, Foster DM, Kushwaha RS, et al: Retarded chylomicron apolipoprotein-B catabolism in type 2 (non-insulin-dependent) diabetic subjects with lipaemia. *Diabetologia* 1984;26:349–354.
120. Onuma T, Boku A, Yanada A, et al: Postprandial changes of chylomicron remnant in non-insulin-dependent diabetes mellitus [abstract]. *Diabetes* 1991;40(suppl 1): 390A.
121. Georgopoulos A, Rosengard AM: Abnormalities in the metabolism of postprandial and fasting triglyceride-rich lipoprotein subfractions in normal and insulin-dependent diabetic subjects: Effects of sex. *Metabolism* 1989;38:781–789.

Chapter 4

High-Density Lipoprotein Transport in Diabetes Mellitus

John D. Bagdade, MD

The results of early studies employing ultracentrifugation to separate the major plasma lipoprotein classes led Gofman to first suggest almost 30 years ago that high-density lipoproteins (HDLs) may protect against the development of coronary heart disease (CHD).[1] This notion received scant attention until three important epidemiologic studies—the Honolulu Heart Study, the Tromso Heart Study, and the Framingham Heart Study—all showed that HDL was an independent predictor of CHD.[2] A negative correlation between plasma HDL cholesterol concentration and the risk of CHD has subsequently been documented in angiographic and autopsy studies, the characterization of kindreds with familial disorders in which HDL is either increased or decreased, and recent clinical trials with drugs and hormones that increase HDLs.[3]

These antiatherogenic associations of HDL appear to reflect its central role in reverse cholesterol transport (RCT), the series of metabolic steps involved in the transport of cholesterol from peripheral cells, through the plasma lipoproteins, and to ultimate clearance by the liver (see Figure 4.1). Even in the presence of an intact and normally functioning low-density lipoprotein (LDL) receptor mechanism, arterial wall cells appear to take up cholesterol continuously by receptor-independent pathways. Since peripheral tissues lack a system to catabolize cholesterol, a RCT system is essential to homeostatically control its intracellular concentration. RCT in humans is believed to have four basic steps:

1. The efflux of cell membrane free (unesterified) cholesterol to HDL.
2. Esterification of diffusible free cholesterol by lecithin : cholesterol acyltransferase (LCAT), which converts it into insoluble cholesteryl ester.
3. Transfer of esterified cholesterol to the apolipoprotein B–containing lipoproteins, very-low-density lipoprotein (VLDL) and LDL.
4. Hepatic uptake of lipoprotein cholesterol.

The rate of RCT is the balance between efflux and influx. Many patients with non-insulin-dependent diabetes mellitus (NIDDM) have reduced HDL levels (with or without an associated increase in plasma triglyceride), which are believed to compromise RCT and contribute to their three- to fourfold increase in CHD risk.[4] Unexplained, however, is the fact that treated patients with insulin-dependent diabetes mellitus (IDDM) who have normal or even increased HDL cholesterol levels experience the same acceleration of atherogenesis as NIDDM patients with low HDL levels. This seemingly paradoxical finding suggests that, in the presence of IDDM, HDL loses its antiatherogenic properties. In this chapter an attempt is made to demonstrate how the altered physiology of lipoproteins in IDDM and NIDDM adversely affects the metabolism and function of HDL, and how these disturbances may contribute to the macrovascular complications of diabetes. Several excellent recent reviews provide relevant background on this subject.[5-9]

Overview of HDL Metabolism

Among the various lipoprotein classes, the transport of lipids and lipoproteins within HDL is probably the most complex. The number of functions ascribed to HDL continues to grow. Foremost among these is the capacity to act as a reservoir in plasma for several apoproteins that serve as ligands for specific cell surface receptors and modulators of enzymes involved in the metabolism of lipoprotein. Indeed, HDL appears to interact with most enzymes and lipid transfer proteins present either in plasma or in close proximity to the plasma compartment. These include the two lipases (lipoprotein lipase and hepatic lipase), the LCAT system, and lipid transfer proteins (neutral lipid or cholesteryl ester–triglyceride transfer protein and phospholipid transfer protein). Because of their intimate involvement in the regulation of key processes in lipid transport,[10] HDLs exert an important influence on lipid accumulation in arterial tissues. HDL delivers cholesterol sequestered in plasma to the liver and steroidogenic tissues and thereby plays an important role in bile acid formation and steroidogenesis. New information suggests that, in addition, HDL may also function in immunoregulation, detoxification, and cell proliferation.[11]

Characteristics of HDL

Mature HDL particles in plasma are small, spherical, dense lipid–protein complexes of which about 50% is protein and 50% is lipid. The overall structure of HDL resembles that of all other lipoproteins in that it has a hydrophobic neutral lipid core consisting mainly of cholesteryl esters and variable amounts of triglyceride (depending on the plasma triglyceride level) that is surrounded by a surface monolayer of unesterified (free) cholesterol, phospholipids, and apoproteins. Phospholipids play a key role in lipoprotein metabolism in plasma by complexing to apoproteins, free cholesterol, and the neutral lipids triglyceride and cholesteryl ester. Apoproteins do not bind to free cholesterol, and instead associate with phospholipids, which can then sequester free cholesterol. The small amount of core cholesteryl ester and triglyceride present on the surface of HDLs makes them accessible to the action of lipolytic enzymes and lipid transfer proteins. Subclasses of HDL vary considerably in size, density, and apoprotein and core and surface lipid composition (Table 4.1). The major apoproteins of HDL are apo A-I (molecular weight 28,000) and apo A-II (molecular weight 17,000), but others, such as apo A-IV, apo E, and the apo Cs (C-I, C-II, and C-III), which are present in small concentrations, may be metabolically important (Table 4.2).

Because of their small size, surface components constitute the majority of

Table 4.1 Composition of High-Density Lipoprotein Subclasses[a]

	HDL$_3$	HDL$_2$
	(moles/mole lipoprotein)	
Molecular weight	200,000	200,000
Apolipoproteins		
Apo A-I	3	4
Apo A-II	1	1
Apo C	±	1
Phospholipids	93	189
Free cholesterol	11	52
Cholesteryl ester	44	109
Triglycerides	9	18

(Adapted from Eisenberg.[10])

[a] Data are number of protein and lipid molecules in average particles.

the HDL mass; core lipids represent about only 20%. Although HDLs are heterogeneous, they have been conventionally separated by ultracentrifugation according to density into two major subclasses: the larger (95 to 120 Å), less dense HDL$_2$ and the smaller (55 to 95 Å), more dense HDL$_3$. Alaupovic's more physiologic approach to the separation of HDL and other lipoprotein subpopulations, based on their immunochemical characteristics and apoprotein composition,[12] has revealed that HDL has two major lipoprotein subfractions, one containing apo A-I only (LpA-I) and another containing both apo A-I and apo A-II (LpA-I/A-II). The intestine only produces LpA-I particles, whereas the liver synthesizes and secretes both LpA-I and LpA-I/A-II. Particles containing these apoproteins are polydisperse, however, and may differ in density, size, and lipid content. Therefore, LpA-I and LpA-I/A-II particles can be found in both HDL$_2$ and HDL$_3$, although LpA-I particles are more abundant in HDL$_2$. In vitro studies with most cultured cell systems have shown that LpA-I and LpA-I/A-II are equally effective promoters of cholesterol efflux. Indeed, as a ligand for specific HDL binding, apo A-I mediates a dose-related efflux of cholesterol from cells.[11] The antiatherogenic properties of apo A-I also may include its capacity to inhibit complement, since the complement system has been implicated in endothelial cell damage and components of complement have been identified in human atherosclerotic lesions.[13]

Falcone and Fielding have shown that a minor small, low-molecular-weight, pre-β–migrating subfraction of HDL$_3$ containing apo A-I only is a particularly effective promoter of cholesterol efflux from cells.[14] Pre-β HDL may be derived in part from the surface of triglyceride-rich lipoproteins during lipoprotein lipase (LPL)-mediated lipolysis that normally occurs in the postprandial state.[10] Consequently, a precursor–product relationship exists between the delipidation and remodeling of the apo B–containing lipoproteins of hepatic and intestinal origin and HDL. This particular subpopulation of HDL particles, which appear to be the primary acceptor of cellular cholesterol in plasma, also are the dominant site of LCAT action and occupy a central role early in RCT (Figure 4.1). The apo A-I associated with these particles activates LCAT, which catalyzes the transfer of *sn*-2-acyl groups from lecithin to cholesterol, forming cholesteryl ester and

Table 4.2 Site of Synthesis, Principal Functions, and Properties of HDL-Associated Proteins

Protein	Molecular Mass (kD)	Site of Synthesis	Functions and Properties
Apo A-I	28	Intestine, liver	Promotes cholesterol efflux; ligand for specific HDL binding; LCAT activator; may regulate hydrolysis of cholesteryl ester in lipoproteins; involved in membrane complement inhibition (??)
Apo A-II	17	Liver, intestine	Phospholipid binding; modulates LCAT activity; activates lipoprotein and hepatic lipase
Apo A-IV	46	Intestine, liver	Transports lipids; activates LCAT; modulates LPL and apo C-II release from VLDL and HDL; participates in HDL interconversion
LCAT	63	Liver	Reverse cholesterol transport; esterifies cholesterol of cell membranes and lipoproteins; participates in lipoprotein interconversion processes; facilitates apo A-IV enrichments of HDL
CETP	74	Liver, skeletal	Reverse cholesterol transport; facilitates muscle, adipose tissue, adrenal glands lipid transfer (TG, CE) between lipoproteins and between lipoproteins and cells; participates in lipoprotein interconversion processes
LTIP[a]	29	?	Inhibits CETP-mediated lipid transfer
Apo-E	34	Liver, brain, spleen, adrenal glands; appears to be ubiquitous	Reverse cholesterol transport; intratissue lipid transport; regulates cell transport; regulates cell growth by binding to heparin-like structures; exhibits immunoregulatory properties; inhibits phospholipid turnover in T-lymphocytes
Apo C-I	6.6	Liver	Activates LPL; activates LCAT
Apo C-II	8.9	Liver	Activates LPL
Apo C-III	8.8	Liver	Inhibits LPL; inhibits hepatic uptake of TG-rich lipoproteins
Apo D	19.0	Liver, intestine brain adrenals, pancreas, spleen	Potential radical scavenger

(Reprinted, by permission, from Schmitz G, Williamson E: High density lipoprotein metabolism reverse cholesterol transport and membrane. *Curr Opin Lipidol* 1991;12:177–189.)

[a] LTIP = lipid transfer inhibitory protein.

lysolecithin. As a result of the LCAT reaction, the pre-β HDLs are transformed into more complex HDL species. Because of its very low solubility, cholesteryl ester does not readily transfer back to cells, although special conditions may be present in the liver to facilitate this process. Cell membranes or lipoproteins in the HDL$_3$ density range provide cholesterol for the LCAT reaction. Alimentary lipemia has a significant effect on HDL. Serving as a reservoir for apoproteins, HDL can transfer apo C and apo E to triglyceride-rich apo B–containing lipoproteins, where they facilitate the metabolism of these lipoproteins. Through the process of transferring of lipolytic products—especially phospholipid—from dietary particles to apo A-I during the postprandial state, pre-β HDL particles are produced and RCT stimulated. In the basal state, HDLs function as a circulating repository for cholesterol and phospholipid that are transferred from other lipoproteins, erythrocytes, and endothelial cells, and to a lesser degree are by-products of lipolysis.

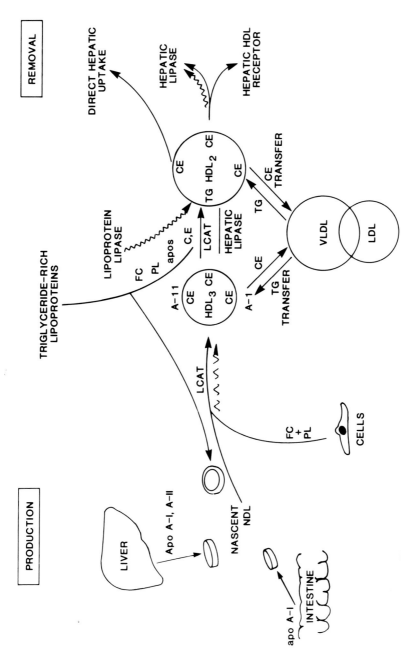

Figure 4.1. High-density lipoprotein metabolism in humans. Heavily shaded continuous arrows indicate steps regulated by insulin. Discontinuous arrow indicates possible regulation by insulin. FC = free cholesterol; PL = phospholipid; CE = cholesteryl ester; TG = triglyceride.

Secretion and Remodeling in Plasma.

HDL particles are derived from three principal sources: (1) the coalescence in plasma of surface coat constituents of triglyceride-rich lipoproteins generated by LPL, consisting of cholesterol-poor phospholipid discs associated with apoproteins (A-I, A-II, A-IV, E and the Cs); (2) direct secretion from the liver and small intestine; and (3) the direct interaction in plasma of phospholipids from cellular origin and apolipoproteins, as mentioned in the paragraph above describing pre-β HDL. Eisenberg has presented data[10] that strongly suggest that the first of these—the products generated by LPL—are a major source of HDL precursors (Figure 4.1). Because of their density and small size, these particles are present in the HDL$_3$ subfraction. When secreted as nascent particles by the intestine and liver, HDLs appear to be disc-shaped bilayers containing mainly phospholipids and cholesterol with apoproteins surrounding the perimeter. Not all HDL precursor particles that are devoid of neutral lipids, however, are necessarily discoidal.

During the postprandial state, the delipidating action of LPL in plasma is closely linked temporally with the activity of lipid transfer proteins,[15] which interact with HDL and other lipoproteins in plasma (Figures 4.1 and 4.2). One such protein that facilitates the net transfer of phospholipid to HDL is specific for phospholipid transfer; another, which also has some phospholipid transfer capability, has as its major function the exchange of core neutral lipids among the lipoproteins in plasma. This hydrophobic 74-kDa glycoprotein, known as cholesteryl ester transfer protein (CETP), simultaneously shuttles cholesteryl ester from HDL to VLDL and LDL and triglyceride from VLDL to HDL. The transfer of cholesteryl ester appears to involve the binding of CETP to lipoproteins. Although CETP can bind to all lipoproteins with high affinity, it has particular avidity for HDL.[16] The CETP-mediated heteroexchange of core lipids serves to redistribute cholesteryl ester synthesized by LCAT on HDL to the apo B–containing lipoproteins, which can deliver it either to the liver, where it can be

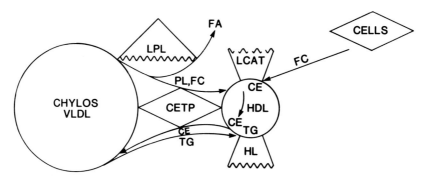

Figure 4.2. Enzymatic modifications of HDL in plasma. The delipidation of chylomicrons and VLDLs by lipoprotein lipase (LPL) in tissue and muscle results in fatty acid (FA) uptake by these tissues and transfer of phospholipid (PL) and free cholesterol (FC) into HDLs, which are utilized as substrates by LCAT to form cholesteryl esters (CE). Cholesteryl ester transfer protein (CETP) facilitates the transfer of PE, CE, and triglyceride (TG). Hepatic lipase (HL) hydrolyzes HDL, PL, and TG in the liver. Heavy wavy lines indicate steps regulated by insulin; discontinuous wavy line indicates possible regulation by insulin. (*After Tall AR: Plasma high density lipoproteins: Metabolism and relationship to atherogenesis. J Clin Invest 1990*); 86: 379.)

reutilized or excreted as bile acids, or to steroidogenic tissues, where it can be used for hormone synthesis. Transfer proteins are major modifiers of lipoprotein composition, and as such exert a strong influence on both the core and surface lipid composition and, as a result, the function of HDL and other lipoproteins. It is still unclear precisely how much of the cholesteryl ester derived from the LCAT reaction is actually transferred to other lipoproteins, although it is likely that the major is. Nevertheless, once a mature HDL particle is formed, it appears to undergo continuous remodeling in the circulation. Equilibria that affect the directional flux of HDL constituents are continually changing as a result of the actions of the lipases, lipid transfer proteins, and LCAT and the production and removal of lipoproteins from plasma (Figure 4.2). The transfer rates for cholesterol are so rapid that the equilibrium distribution is completed more rapidly than other processes of cholesterol and lipoprotein metabolism.[17]

Role of HDL in Cholesterol Trafficking

There is now evidence indicating that the first step in RCT may involve the interaction of HDL with a cell-surface receptor, although the nature of the HDL binding site remains to be resolved.[18] It seems clear that the movement of cholesterol from the plasma membrane to HDL, however, does not require specific HDL binding.[19] Like the better characterized LDL receptor, activity of the putative HDL receptor also is affected by an intracellular cholesterol pool. In contrast to the LDL receptor, however, activity of the HDL receptor is down-regulated by mitogens such as platelet-derived growth factor and insulin and up-regulated when the cell is cholesterol loaded and cell proliferation is inhibited.[20] Both LpA-I and LpA-I/A-II particles appear equally capable of interacting with the candidate HDL receptor protein. When the putative HDL receptor is activated by the protein moieties of HDL (apo A-I, apo A-II), it transduces an intracellular signal involving the generation of protein kinase C that stimulates the translocation of excess intracellular sterol to the plasma membrane. The efflux of this sterol from the cell surface is mediated by the lipid constituents of HDL or another lipid-rich acceptor particle. The smallest HDLs, which are cholesterol poor and contain primarily phospholipid and apo A-I, have a built-in gradient that makes them well suited to accept free cholesterol from cells by diffusion. The action of LCAT, which utilizes both free cholesterol and lecithin, maintains a gradient for free cholesterol between cell membranes and acceptor lipoproteins and thereby sustains the influx of both phospholipid and free cholesterol into HDL. For this reason LCAT is considered to be the "driving force of RCT." To some extent LCAT also can esterify cholesterol on VLDLs, intermediate-density lipoproteins (IDLs), and LDLs, and its activity on these lipoproteins is designated β-LCAT activity, whereas that involving HDL (the dominant component) is called α-LCAT activity. When hydrophobic cholesteryl ester is formed by LCAT on HDL, it partitions into the inner core region, progressively transforming a disclike nascent particle into a sphere (Figure 4.1). The maturation of small HDL_3 into larger HDL_2 particles is analogous to inflating a balloon and involves a two- to threefold increase in the number of cholesteryl ester molecules in the lipid core (from 40 to 50 to 100 to 120 molecules) (Table 4.1). To accommodate this expansion of core volume, HDL_3 acquires an additional apo A-I molecule and requisite amounts of surface constituents (phospholipid, free cholesterol, and apo C-II, apo C-III, and apo E) generated by the lipolytic actions of LPL.

HDL and Cholesteryl Ester Transfer Protein

The normal LPL-mediated postprandial delipidation of triglyceride-rich lipoproteins stimulates the action of CETP.[21] It is generally believed that, during lipid transfer, most of the cholesteryl ester formed within HDL by LCAT appears in chylomicron and VLDL remnants, IDL, and LDL particles that may be cleared by either the apo B, E, remnant, or other receptor-mediated pathways. At first glance an enhancement of cholesteryl ester transfer might seem advantageous because it could increase the flux of cholesterol from tissues and facilitate its hepatic excretion. This does not, however, appear to be true because the activity of CETP has been found to correlate directly with atherosclerosis. Animals such as the rat, dog, and swine that are resistant to dietary-induced atherosclerosis have very low levels of CETP activity, whereas CETP activity is high in atherosclerosis-prone species such as the rabbit and human.[15]

It is now recognized that facilitated cholesteryl ester transfer may be atherogenic because it pathologically modifies the core and likely the surface lipid composition of subpopulations of apo B–containing lipoproteins. These changes appear to adversely affect the behavior and metabolism of these particles and may result in their being selectively cleared from the circulation by arterial wall cells. Clinical evidence supports the position that accelerated cholesteryl ester transfer is pathogenetic. An abnormal increase in cholesteryl ester transfer has been reported in patients predisposed to accelerated atherosclerosis with dyslipidemia,[22] hypercholesterolemia,[23] and hypertriglyceridemia,[24] and in both IDDM[25,26] and NIDDM.[27]

Pathways of Hepatic Cholesteryl Ester Excretion

The cholesteryl ester that is retained in HDL (about 30% of the cholesterol esterified on HDL) and not transferred from HDL to the apo B–containing lipoproteins may be taken up selectively by different tissues[28] via the interaction of apo E–free HDL particles with the surface of membranes, without actual internalization of the whole particle. In contrast, those HDLs formed normally from HDL$_3$ during the intravascular phase of RCT that contain apo E can be taken up intact by hepatic receptors that recognize apo E.[29] Animals lacking CETP tend to have low LDL levels and transport the bulk of cholesteryl ester in plasma in HDL. These species (rat, dog, swine) typically demonstrate large numbers of apo E–containing HDLs[15] which are cleared from plasma by this pathway primarily. In humans this route of cholesterol transport is probably quantitatively less important than in species lacking CETP. However, apo E–containing HDLs may become more prominent not only when the intake of dietary cholesterol and saturated fat is high and tissue delivery of cholesterol is increased but also when cholesteryl ester cannot be efficiently transported out of HDL, as occurs in patients who lack either CETP[30] or acceptor lipoproteins (i.e., those with abetalipoproteinemia).

Like the apo B–containing lipoproteins, HDL can, however, also deliver cholesteryl ester from plasma to the liver directly via a liver cell plasma membrane receptor-mediated pathway involving the recognition of apo A-I and apo A-IV, which may mediate the endocytosis of intact HDL particles.[31] Studies in rats showing that the hepatic uptake of HDL cholesteryl ester is several times greater than that of HDL apo A-I[32] suggest that cholesteryl ester dissociates from HDL particles that bind at the surfaces of hepatic cells. Evidence indicating that HDL can be taken up by endocytosis into a nonlysosomal pathway in macrophages[33] and hepatic sinusoidal cells[34] suggests that, once internalized, cholesteryl ester dissociates from HDL. The mechanism of transfer of free cholesterol from lipoproteins to the liver is unclear. Since it is likely that the gradient for free cholesterol between lipoproteins and hepatic cells determines its directional flux, the phospholipase activity of hepatic endothelial lipase may facilitate this process by raising the free cholesterol–phospholipid ratio at the surface of HDL.[35] This gradient may also be promoted by the continuous conversion of cholesterol to bile acids and the secretion of free cholesterol into bile by lowering the free cholesterol–phospholipid ratio in hepatocytes.

The removal and catabolism of HDL apoproteins also is not straightforward. Removal of apoproteins C-II, C-III, and E, which normally cycle between HDL and VLDL and chylomicrons, may take place when the remnants of VLDL and chylomicrons are internalized by cells. When HDL particles are internalized by hepatocytes, some catabolism of these same apoproteins may occur. The mechanism for the removal of apo A-I from plasma is not well understood, although it appears that the liver may degrade apo A-I when it internalizes HDL particles containing apo E. The kidney also appears to play an important role in apo A-I catabolism. Little is known about the sites of apo A-II and apo A-IV degradation.

Impact of Diabetes Mellitus on HDL Transport

Insulin's pervasive effects on lipoprotein transport include important influences on a number of steps in the metabolism of HDL (Figures 4.1 and 4.2). The nature and extent of the perturbation in HDL will vary considerably among patients depending on the type of diabetes present and the adequacy of glycemic control. Insulin modulates not only the activities of both LPL and hepatic lipase[6] and the LDL receptor, but probably also that of the putative HDL receptor. There is no consistent evidence as yet, however, that the synthesis and secretion of nascent HDL particles from either the intestine (LpA-I) or the liver (LpA-I, LpA-I/A-II) are adversely affected by diabetes mellitus.

HDL Transport in IDDM

Taskinen et al's[36] finding that, in IDDM patients receiving conventional subcutaneous insulin treatment (CIT), the concentration of cholesterol and phospholipids in HDL_2 correlated with postheparin lipolytic activity, an indirect measure of LPL, indicates that this enzyme is an important determinant of HDL mass in IDDM. As mentioned above in the section describing the role of HDL in cholesterol trafficking, the conversion of HDL_3 into HDL_2 and achieving maximal concentrations of HDL_2 depend on the availability of surface constituents derived from the delipidating actions of LPL. The fact that HDL_2 and LPL activity in skeletal muscle and postheparin plasma are increased in treated IDDM patients

Table 4.3 Parameters of HDL Surface Lipid Composition (Expressed as mol/mol Ratios) in Patients with Diabetes Mellitus Receiving Conventional Treatment

	NIDDM[a]	IDDM[b]	Ref. Group
HDL$_2$			
Sphingomyelin–lecithin	0.44 ± 0.15	0.23 ± 0.12	0.29 ± 0.20
Free cholesterol–lecithin	0.52 ± 0.24	0.89 ± 0.49	0.66 ± 0.15
HDL$_3$			
Sphingomyelin–lecithin	0.25 ± 0.12	0.13 ± 0.02	0.15 ± 0.05
Free cholesterol–lecithin	0.38 ± 0.15	0.66 ± 0.31	0.43 ± 0.07

[a] Data from Bagdade et al.[38]

[b] Data from Bagdade and Subbaiah[41] and Bagdade et al.[52]

has suggested that these changes might result from the hyperinsulinism associated with CIT stimulating LPL.

The strong influence of LPL on plasma VLDL (triglyceride) and HDL concentrations is manifested in contrasting profiles in IDDM and NIDDM. In IDDM patients with iatrogenic hyperinsulinism in whom glycemic control is excellent and LPL levels are increased, a decidedly benign and antiatherogenic lipid profile is present, characterized by low triglyceride levels and often increased HDL. In contrast, in NIDDM patients with insulin resistance, increased VLDL production, relatively lower insulin levels, and normal or reduced LPL levels, plasma triglyceride is frequently increased. As in hypertriglyceridemic nondiabetics in whom VLDL production exceeds LPL-mediated removal capacity, HDL estimated as HDL-cholesterol is reduced in NIDDM.

Although no consistent abnormality has been noted in either IDDM or NIDDM in HDL$_3$ cholesterol concentrations, changes in HDL$_3$ surface phospholipids and/ or free cholesterol have been described[37,38] (Table 4.3). These alterations in surface composition assume potential pathophysiologic significance in light of Oram's recent finding that the actual desorption of free cholesterol by HDL$_3$ or other acceptor particles is affected by their lipid rather than their apoprotein content.[19] Glycation of HDL$_3$ apoproteins may impair HDL's interaction with its receptor. Duell et al have observed that HDL$_3$ from IDDM patients and HDL$_3$ from controls that has been glycated in vitro has a reduced capacity to promote the receptor-mediated efflux of radiolabeled cholesterol from cholesterol-loaded cells in culture.[39] These findings raise the possibility that glycemic control may influence the signal transduction step in RCT, which affects the movement of intracellular cholesterol to the plasma membrane. Further studies are required to determine the extent to which the changes observed in HDL composition in diabetes compromise its interactions with (1) circulating cells and tissues, and (2) the proteins in plasma (LCAT, CETP, hepatic lipase) that contribute continuously to HDL remodeling.

Lipoprotein Composition in IDDM

Perhaps the most significant abnormality among those present in lipoprotein surface and core lipid composition in IDDM patients treated conventionally with CIT[40] is an enrichment of lipoproteins in unesterified or free cholesterol that is manifested by an increase in the ratio of free cholesterol to lecithin in plasma.[37,41] This specific marker of altered lipoprotein surface composition is of interest because Kuksis et al[42] found it to be a strong predictor of risk for CHD in a Lipid Research Clinic study of nondiabetic patients with hypercholesterolemia. This abnormality has been found in other nondiabetic patients with premature coronary artery disease.[43] A disturbance in the free cholesterol content may have adverse functional consequences because free cholesterol gradients among lipoproteins[44] are required to maintain the normal directional fluxes of cholesterol in plasma. For this reason, alterations in free cholesterol content may compromise the normal movement of free cholesterol among lipoproteins and between lipoproteins and cells. In IDDM, the free cholesterol enrichment appears to involve both HDL_2 and HDL_3 (Table 4.2). The increase observed in the HDL_2 free cholesterol–lecithin ratio may facilitate receptor-independent hepatic cholesterol delivery and increase intracellular pools of cholesterol available for VLDL synthesis, leading to a potential enrichment of VLDL with free cholesterol. This pathway constitutes another example of how changes in lipoprotein composition in IDDM that affect the retrograde movement of cholesterol can have a deleterious outcome. Further study is required to assess these possibilities.

Core lipid alterations also are present in the lipoproteins of IDDM patients. These changes are inapparent in the routinely performed measurement of plasma lipids and are expressed as triglyceride–cholesteryl ester ratios. These disturbances involve reciprocal changes in the normal proportions of cholesteryl ester and triglyceride in $VLDL_1$[25] and in HDL_2 and HDL_3 (Table 4.4). A recently recognized consequence of this alteration is that IDDM VLDL causes increased cholesteryl ester accumulation in cultured human monocyte-derived macrophages.[45] Although it is possible that this abnormality in VLDL core lipid composition could result from de novo synthesis, it also could be a consequence of increased cholesteryl ester transfer. Studies to assess this possibility have in fact demonstrated that cholesteryl ester transfer from HDL to VLDL, estimated by both the mass[25] and isotopic assays,[26] is accelerated in IDDM (Figure 4.3). Recombination experiments with lipoprotein fractions isolated from IDDM sub-

Table 4.4 HDL Core Lipid Composition in Patients With Diabetes Mellitus Receiving Conventional Treatment

	NIDDM[a]	IDDM[b]	Ref. Group
HDL_2			
Triglycerides (mg/dL)	7.4 ± 1.5	6.5 ± 2.8	4.6 ± 1.9
Total cholesterol (mg/dL)	6.4 ± 4.0	18.1 ± 6.3	17.5 ± 4.0
Cholesteryl ester (mg/dL)	3.6 ± 2.7	8.7 ± 4.4	9.6 ± 3.9
Triglyceride–cholesteryl ester ratio (mg/mg)	2.65 ± 1.76	0.83 ± 0.3	0.78 ± 0.27
HDL_3			
Triglycerides (mg/dL)	30.9 ± 7.3	19.1 ± 3.2	17.2 ± 3.2
Total cholesterol (mg/dL)	29.1 ± 6.5	37.7 ± 11.1	37.7 ± 6.7
Cholesteryl ester (mg/dL)	22.9 ± 6.6	25.8 ± 10.6	28.4 ± 6.4
Triglyceride–cholesteryl ester ratio (mg/mg)	1.41 ± 0.62	0.85 ± 0.4	0.68 ± 0.15

[a] Data from Bagdade et al.[38]

[b] Data from Bagdade and Subbaiah[41] and Bagdade et al.[52]

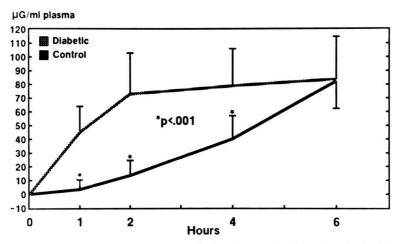

Figure 4.3. Cholesteryl ester mass transfer in plasma of IDDM and control subjects.

jects have shown that this abnormality results from dysfunction of the $VLDL_1$ subfraction rather than from the small increase found in the mass of CETP.[25] The cause for this disturbance in cholesteryl ester transfer is unclear. A number of observations together suggest the intriguing possibility that accelerated cholesteryl ester transfer in IDDM might be in part a consequence of peripheral hyperinsulinism resulting from conventional insulin treatment. One important finding is that basal activity of the insulin-sensitive enzyme LPL in IDDM is increased (I. D. Bagdade and R. H. Eckel, unpublished observations); another is that exposure of VLDL to LPL has been shown earlier to enhance its interaction with CETP.[21] If elevated insulin levels do in fact tonically stimulate LPL, this could explain why assiduous management of IDDM with additional subcutaneous insulin, which exacerbates the hyperinsulinism, fails to correct this particular parameter of lipoprotein function.

Preliminary studies in IDDM patients indicate that, when insulin is delivered into the portal circulation from an intraperitoneal catheter connected to an implanted radioprogrammable infusion pump, which reduces peripheral insulin concentrations by one half, these disturbances in LPL and cholesteryl ester transfer, as well as those in lipoprotein composition, are normalized. These observations support the long-held suspicion that high insulin levels resulting from the unphysiologic route of subcutaneous insulin administration might cause proatherogenic changes in lipoprotein composition and function that contribute to the accelerated development of macrovascular complications in normolipidemic IDDM patients.

HDL Transport in NIDDM

In contrast to IDDM patients, HDL and apo A-I[46] levels are reduced in about 25% to 30% of NIDDM patients who (not coincidentally) have the same frequency of triglyceride elevation. As described above, the close association that the delipidation of triglyceride-rich lipoproteins has with the generation and maturation of HDL probably accounts for the fact that these abnormalities in HDL and plasma triglyceride frequently coexist in the same patient. Since the concentration of

HDL depends on the normal catabolism of VLDL, a reduction in LPL activity in NIDDM will tend to lower HDL levels.[6] The metabolic basis for this profile of changes in triglyceride and HDL-cholesterol concentrations in NIDDM is complicated and is related to a combination of obesity, insulin resistance, and often the presence of coexisting familial dyslipidemias, which are usually exacerbated in the presence of diabetes. The varying degrees of insulin deficiency and insulin resistance that accompany NIDDM increase the flux and hepatic delivery of free fatty acids, which promote the synthesis and secretion of VLDL, IDL, and/or LDL particles without necessarily causing an obvious increase in plasma triglyceride concentrations. If HDLs lack surface constituents, their susceptibility to degradation appears to be increased and their residence time in plasma shortened. LPL activity may be reduced in some NIDDM patients because of insulin deficiency. Consequently, the generation of surface constituents during the delipidation of VLDL and chylomicrons may impair the maturation of HDL_3 into larger HDL_2 particles. In addition to HDL production being reduced in this way, the catabolism of apo A-I also may be accelerated,[47] although the fractional catabolic rate of apo A-I in NIDDM patients does not appear to be any greater than that of nondiabetic subjects with compromised LPL systems and similarly reduced HDL levels. This increase in HDL catabolism in NIDDM may be selective and involve only certain subpopulations of HDL and the simultaneous enhancement of hepatic lipase activity.[48] This possibility is suggested by the inverse correlation between HDL cholesterol and hepatic lipase activity shown earlier in NIDDM by Taskinen.[6] Although there is some evidence suggesting that low HDL cholesterol levels in NIDDM might result in part from defective LCAT activity,[49] there is so far none to indicate that the HDL_3-mediated efflux of free cholesterol from cells is impaired, or that HDL cholesterol is reduced because the hepatic extraction of HDL_2 cholesteryl ester or apo E–containing HDL is enhanced. Witztum et al[50] have shown that glycosylation of HDL accelerates its catabolism in guinea pigs, but no comparable effect has been demonstrated in humans.

Lipoprotein Composition in NIDDM

Abnormalities in lipoprotein lipid composition are present in NIDDM that resemble those found in IDDM. Certain lipoproteins in NIDDM, including HDL, demonstrate abnormal amounts of free cholesterol and alterations in the proportions of the two principal surface phospholipids, sphingomyelin and lecithin, and in core triglyceride and cholesteryl ester (Tables 4.3 and 4.4). The distribution of this disturbance in free cholesterol among the lipoproteins differs in IDDM and NIDDM. It is interesting that the magnitude of these compositional changes, including the previously described enrichment of VLDL with free cholesterol,[51] does not correlate with glycemic control, and some of these changes persist even after normal hemoglobin A_1 levels have been achieved for 6 months with chronic subcutaneous insulin infusion therapy.[38,52] Because of differences in glycemic control and the high frequency of dyslipidemia in NIDDM, it has not yet been possible to clearly discern the relative contribution made to these compositional abnormalities in lipoprotein composition by NIDDM itself, unrelated inherited dyslipidemia, and possibly treatment. A number of observers have shown that intensively treating NIDDM patients with insulin results in favorable directional changes in plasma lipid and lipoprotein levels.[9] However, as was observed in studies in IDDM,[52] near-normalization of glycemic control failed to restore these disturbances in surface lipoprotein lipid composition to normal, raising the possibility that insulin itself may in some way contribute to these changes. The free cholesterol–lecithin ratio in plasma remained abnormally increased and was little changed by insulin treatment; whereas the amount of triglyceride in HDL decreased, the triglyceride–cholesteryl ester ratios of HDL_2 and HDL_3 remained high. Because of this directional change in HDL core lipid composition following insulin, the reduction in HDL cholesterol and in HDL_2 cholesterol in NIDDM may be disproportionate to that of the apo A-I concentration, with the result that the HDL cholesterol measurement may give the mistaken impression that HDL particle number is reduced to a greater extent than it in fact is.

It should be remembered that both the number of cholesterol molecules (especially cholesteryl ester) in each HDL particle and the number of HDL particles determine the HDL cholesterol level in plasma. It may be that those apo A-I–containing HDL particles whose cores are triglyceride enriched are the ones that are rapidly catabolized by hepatic lipase and account for the increased fractional catabolic rate of apo A-I in NIDDM. Although most lipoproteins in diabetes tend to be free cholesterol enriched, a slight decrease in free cholesterol of uncertain physiologic significance was found in HDL_3 in a heterogeneous population of NIDDM patients.[38] If real, this small change could alter the gradient for free cholesterol and actually promote the efflux of cholesterol from cells, as Brinton et al[53] have shown in in vitro studies. Other specific compositional modifications involving the two principal lipoprotein phospholipids, spingomyelin (S) and lecithin (L), expressed as the S/L ratio, also are present in both HDL subfractions in NIDDM but not in IDDM. NIDDM patients treated with oral hypoglycemic agents who are normolipidemic have less marked alterations in lipoprotein composition than insulin-treated NIDDM patients with the typical spectrum and frequency of hyperlipidemia. Even in the absence of hyperlipidemia, however, women with NIDDM demonstrate increases in the triglyceride–cholesteryl ester ratio of both HDL subfractions and a reduction in the HDL_2 free cholesterol–lecithin ratio.[54]

HDL Function in NIDDM

Theoretically, glycation of apo A-I could impair its capacity to activate LCAT and reduce cholesterol esterification in NIDDM. There is no evidence, however, that LCAT activity is reduced in either NIDDM or IDDM. When HDL_3 from nondiabetic control subjects is nonenzymatically glycated in vitro to achieve a 40% to 50% reduction in free lysine residues, it has been shown that its capacity to interact with the HDL receptor of human skin fibroblasts and to promote cholesterol efflux declines.[39] This type of in vitro modification results in a loss of protein relative to lipid and actually enhances the capacity of HDL_3 to act as an acceptor for the HDL receptor–dependent efflux of free cholesterol from cells. Since interaction of HDL_3 with the putative HDL receptor is the first step in RCT, an in vivo impairment in the capacity of glycated HDL to engage its receptor would promote cholesterol accumulation in arterial cells. It is as yet unclear, however, whether a sufficient degree of glycation occurs in vivo to adversely affect these functions of HDL.

The increase in HDL subfraction triglyceride–cholesteryl ester ratios (Table 4.4) suggests that the flux of HDL core lipids also may be increased in NIDDM because of increased lipid transfer protein activity.[27] Indeed, measurements with both mass and isotopic assays in non-insulin-treated NIDDM patients indicate the cholesteryl ester transfer is increased.[27] Preliminary studies show, as in IDDM, that accelerated cholesteryl ester transfer in NIDDM results from abnormal behavior and composition of VLDL$_1$ and not from altered functions of HDL or CETP. Preliminary studies in IDDM suggest that this same defect in transfer results from peripheral hyperinsulinism associated with conventional insulin treatment and pathologic activation of LPL. It is uncertain whether systemic insulin levels in NIDDM are sufficiently elevated to stimulate basal LPL activity, as has been observed in IDDM (J. D. Bagdade and R. H. Eckel, unpublished observations).

Ginsberg[5] has suggested that the turnover of certain HDL subpopulations in NIDDM may be increased because accelerated cholesteryl ester transfer leads to the cholesterol depletion and triglyceride enrichment of their lipid cores. Hence alterations in the remodeling of HDL that lead to changes in the conformation of apo A-I may make it more susceptible to premature removal.

Summary

It is apparent from the complex relationships that HDLs have with other lipoproteins in plasma and with cells in a variety of different tissues that there is no simple explanation for why increased HDL cholesterol and apo A-I levels are antiatherogenic in nondiabetic populations. It is likely that these measurements are markers of other critical steps in lipoprotein transport that influence the flux of cholesterol between tissues, plasma lipoproteins, and the liver. The cholesteryl ester content of HDL, which is reflected in the HDL cholesterol level, is affected significantly by the activity of CETP.[30] In most (but not necessarily all) common disorders in which VLDL, IDL, and LDL lipoprotein lipids and apoproteins are abnormal, cholesteryl ester transfer is accelerated, HDL cholesterol is reduced, and HDL-derived cholesteryl esters may be directed back to peripheral tissues. These events appear to occur in NIDDM. In this setting, elevated plasma VLDL and IDL levels may provide not only particles that serve as acceptors of cholesteryl esters from HDL but particles that can both contribute to and expand the LDL pool. In addition to the qualitative changes present in HDL particles that could theoretically compromise RCT, accelerated catabolism of apo A-I can lead to an absolute reduction in HDL particle number. Thus the changes in HDL in NIDDM are only one component of a pervasive disturbance in lipoprotein transport manifested by changes in both lipoprotein concentration and quality.

The situation differs in IDDM, in which quantitative disturbances in plasma lipids and lipoprotein usually are absent. Since CET also is accelerated in IDDM, however, many of the same qualitative changes in core lipids of the apo B–containing lipoproteins (VLDL, IDL, LDL) and HDL are present. This defect in CET appears to contribute to the accelerated development of macrovascular disease in both NIDDM and IDDM by promoting the formation of cholesteryl ester–enriched, atherogenic, apo B–containing lipoprotein particles and likely simultaneously compromising the functional capacity of HDL. Therefore, in both IDM and NIDDM, HDL may be rendered dysfunctional by a combination of diabetes-induced disturbances in lipoprotein transport and possibly by hypergly-cemia and hyperinsulinism as well.

Acknowledgment

Supported by grant DK 43227 from the National Institutes of Health.

References

1. Gofman JW, Delalla O, Glazier F, et al: Serum lipoprotein transport system in health metabolic disorders, atherosclerosis and coronary heart disease. *Plasma* 1954;2:413–484.
2. Gordon DJ, Rifkind BM: High density lipoprotein—the clinical implications of recent studies. *N Engl J Med* 1989;21:1311–1316.
3. Reichl D, Miller NE: Pathophysiology of reverse cholesterol transport. Insights from inherited disorders of lipoprotein metabolism. *Arteriosclerosis* 1989;9:785–797.
4. Kannel WB, McGee DL: Diabetes and glucose intolerance as risk factors for cardio-vascular disease: The Framingham Study. *Diabetes Care* 1979;2:120–126.
5. Ginsburg HN: Lipoprotein physiology in nondiabetic and diabetic states. Relationship to atherogenesis. *Diabetes Care* 1991;14:839–855.
6. Taskinen MR: Hyperlipidemia in diabetes. *Bailliere's Clin Endocrinol Metab* 1990;4: 743–775.
7. Betteridge DJ: Diabetes, lipoprotein metabolism and atherosclerosis. *Br Med Bull* 1989;45:285–311.
8. Orchard TJ: Dyslipoproteinemia and diabetes. *Endocrinol Metab Clin North Am* 1954; 19:361–380.
9. Dunn FL: Hyperlipidemia in diabetes mellitus. *Diabetes Metab Rev* 1990;6:47–61.
10. Eisenberg S: High density lipoprotein metabolism. *J Lipid Res* 1984;25:1017–1058.
11. Schmitz G, Williamson E: High density lipoprotein metabolism, reverse cholesterol transport and membrane. *Curr Opin Lipidol* 1991;2:177–189.
12. Alaupovic P: The concepts, classification systems and nomenclature of human plasma lipoproteins, in Lewis LA, Opplt JJ (eds): *Lipoproteins: Basic Principles and Concepts.* Boca Raton, FL, CRC Press Inc, 1980, vol 1, pp 27–46.
13. Hansson GK: Complement receptors and regulatory proteins in human atheroscle-rotic lesions. *Arteriosclerosis* 1989;9:802–811.
14. Falcone OL, Fielding CJ: Initial steps in reverse cholesterol transport: The role of short-lived cholesterol acceptors. *Eur Heart J* 1990;11:218–224.
15. Tall AR: Plasma lipid transfer proteins. *J Lipid Res* 1986;27:359–365.
16. Morton RE: Binding of plasma-derived lipid transfer protein to lipoprotein substrates. *J Biol Chem* 1985;260:12593–12599.
17. Patsch JR, Gotto AM Jr: Metabolism of high density lipoproteins, in Gotto AM Jr (ed): *Plasma Lipoproteins.* Amsterdam, Elsevier Science Publishers BV (Biomedical Divi-sion), 1987, pp 260–325.
18. Karlin JB, Johnson WJ, Benedict CR, et al: Cholesterol flux between cells and high density lipoprotein: Lack of relationship to specific binding of the lipoprotein to the cell surface. *J Biol Chem* 1987;262:12557–12564.
19. Oram JR: Cholesterol trafficking in cells. *Curr Opin Lipidol* 1990;1:416–421.
20. Oram JF, Brinton EA, Bierman EL: Regulation of high density lipoprotein receptor activity in cultured human skin fibroblasts and human arterial smooth muscle cells. *J Clin Invest* 1983;72:1611–1621.

21. Hesler CB, Swenson TL, Tall AR: Purification and characterization of a human plasma cholesteryl ester transfer protein. *J Biol Chem* 1987;262:2275–2282.
22. Tall AR, Granot R, Brocia R, et al: Accelerated transfer of cholesteryl esters in dyslipidemic plasma. Role of cholesterol ester transfer protein. *J Clin Invest* 1987;79:1217–1225.
23. Bagdade JD, Subbaiah PV, Ritter MC: Accelerated cholesteryl ester transfer in plasma of patients with hypercholesterolemia. *J Clin Invest* 1991;87:1259–1265.
24. Mann CJ, Yen FT, Grant AM, et al: Mechanisms of plasma cholesteryl ester transfer in hypertriglyceridemia. *J Clin Invest* 1991;88:2059–2066.
25. Bagdade JD, Ritter MC, Subbaiah PV: Accelerated cholesteryl ester transfer in patients with insulin dependent diabetic mellitus. *Eur J Clin Invest* 1991;21:161–167.
26. Dullaart RPF, Groener JEM, Dikkeschei LD, et al: Increased cholesteryl ester transfer activity in complicated type I (insulin-dependent) diabetes mellitus–its relationship with serum lipids. *Diabetologia* 1989;32:14–19.
27. Bagdade JD, Lane JT, Subbaiah PV, et al: Accelerated cholesteryl ester transfer in noninsulin-dependent diabetes: Effect of probucol treatment. *Diabetes,* to be published.
28. Pittman RC, Knecht TP, Rosenbaum MS, et al: A non-endocytotic mechanism for the selective uptake of high density lipoprotein-associated cholesterol esters. *J Biol Chem* 1987;262:2443–2451.
29. Mahley RW: Apolipoprotein E: Cholesterol transport protein with expanding role in cell biology. *Science* 1988;240:622–630.
30. Brown ML, Inazu A, Hesler CB, et al: Molecular basis of lipid transfer protein deficiency in a family with increased high-density lipoprotein. *Nature* 1989;342:448–451.
31. Mendel CM, Kunitake ST, Hong K, et al: Radiation inactivation of binding sites for high density lipoproteins in human liver membranes. *Biochim Biophys Acta* 1988;961:188–193.
32. Glass C, Pittman RC, Weinstein D, et al: Dissociation of tissue uptake of cholesterol ester from that of apoprotein A-I of rat plasma high density lipoprotein. Selective delivery of cholesterol ester to liver, adrenal and gonad. *Proc Natl Acad Sci USA* 1983;80:5435–5439.
33. Schmitz G, Robenek H, Lottman V, et al: Interaction of HDL with cholesterol ester-laden macrophages: Biochemical and morphological characterization of cell surface receptor binding, endocytosis and resecretion of HDL by macrophages. *EMBO J* 1985;4:613–622.
34. Takata K, Huriuchi S, Rahim A, et al: Receptor-mediated internalization of HDL by rat sinusoidal liver cells: Identification of a non-lysosomal endocytotic pathway by fluorescent-labeled ligand. *J Lipid Res* 1988;29:1117–1126.
35. Bamburger M, Glick JM, Rothblat GH: Hepatic lipase stimulates the uptake of high density lipoprotein cholesterol by hepatoma cells. *J Lipid Res* 1983;24:869–876.
36. Taskinen MR, Kuusi T, Nikkila E: Regulation of HDL and its subfractions in chronically insulin treated patients with type I diabetes, in Crepaldi G, Tiengo A, Baggio G (eds): *Diabetes, Obesity and Hyperlipidemias 111*, Amsterdam, Elsevier Science Publishers, 1985, pp 251–259.
37. Bagdade JD, Subbaiah PV: Abnormal high-density lipoprotein composition in insulin-dependent diabetic women. *J Lab Clin Med* 1988;113:235–240.
38. Bagdade JD, Buchanan WF, Kuusi T, et al: Persistent abnormalities in lipoprotein composition in noninsulin-dependent diabetes following intensive insulin therapy. *Arteriosclerosis* 1990;10:232–239.
39. Duell PB, Oram JF, Bierman EL: Nonenzymatic glycosylation of HDL and impaired HDL-receptor-mediated cholesterol efflux. *Diabetes* 1991;40:377–384.
40. Rivellese A, Riccardi G, Romano G, et al: Presence of very low density lipoprotein compositional abnormalities in type I (insulin-dependent) diabetes patients: Effects of blood glucose optimization. *Diabetologia* 1988;31:884–888.

41. Bagdade JD, Subbaiah PV: Whole plasma and high density lipoprotein subfraction surface lipid composition in insulin-dependent diabetic males. *Diabetes* 1989;38: 1226–1230.
42. Kuksis A, Myher JJ, Geher K: Decreased plasma phosphatidylcholine/free cholesterol ratio as an indicator of risk for ischemic vascular disease. *Arteriosclerosis* 1982;2: 296–302.
43. Paucillo P, Rubba P, Marotta G, et al: Abnormalities in serum lipoprotein composition in patients with premature coronary heart disease compared to serum lipid matched controls. *Atherosclerosis* 1988;73:241–246.
44. Fielding CJ: The origin and properties of free cholesterol potential gradients in plasma and their relationship to atherogenesis. *J Lipid Res* 1984;25:1624–1628.
45. Klein RL, Lyons TJ, Lopes-Virella MF: Interaction of very-low-density lipoprotein isolated from type I (insulin-dependent) diabetes subjects with human monocyte-derived macrophages. *Metabolism* 1989;38:1108–1114.
46. Howard BV: Lipoprotein metabolism in diabetes mellitus. *J Lipid Res* 1987;28:613–628.
47. Golay A, Zech L, Shim Z: High density lipoprotein (HDL) metabolism in noninsulin-dependent diabetes mellitus: Measurement of HDL turn-over using tritiated HDL. *J Clin Endocrinol Metab* 1987;65:512–518.
48. Kasim SE, Tseng K, Jen K-LC, et al: Significance of hepatic triglyceride lipase in the regulation of serum high density lipoproteins in type II diabetes mellitus. *J Clin Endocrinol Metab* 1987;65:183–187.
49. Schernthaner G, Kostner GM, Dieplinger H, et al: Apolipoproteins (A-I, A-II, B) Lp(a) lipoprotein and lecithin : cholesterol acyltransferase activities in diabetes mellitus. *Atherosclerosis* 1983;49:277–293.
50. Witztum JL, Fisher M, Pietro T, et al: Nonenzymatic glycosylation of high-density lipoprotein accelerates its catabolism in guinea pigs. *Diabetes* 1982;31:1029–1032.
51. Fielding CJ, Reaven GM, Liv G, et al: Increased free cholesterol in plasma low and very low density lipoproteins in noninsulin-dependent diabetes mellitus: Its role in the inhibition of cholesteryl ester transfer. *Proc Natl Acad Sci USA* 1984;81:2512–2516.
52. Bagdade JD, Helve E, Taskinen M-R: Effects of continuous insulin infusion on lipoprotein surface and core lipid composition in insulin-dependent diabetes mellitus. *Metabolism* 1991;40:445–449.
53. Brinton EA, Oram JF, Bierman EL: The effect of variations in lipid composition of high-density lipoproteins on its interaction with receptors on human fibroblasts. *Biochim Biophys Acta* 1987;920:68–75.
54. Lane JT, Subbaiah PV, Otto ME, et al: Lipoprotein composition and HDL particle size distribution in women with non-insulin-dependent diabetes mellitus and the effects of probucol treatment. *J Lab Clin Med* 1991;118:120–128.

Chapter 5

Lipoprotein Lipases and Diabetes Mellitus

Robert H. Eckel, MD

As detailed elsewhere in this text, diabetes mellitus is often associated with alterations in lipid and lipoprotein levels and/or lipoprotein composition. Most common is hypertriglyceridemia, which in part could be attributable to alterations in one or both of the lipoprotein lipases. In this chapter, both lipoprotein lipase (LPL) and hepatic triglyceride lipase (HTGL) are reviewed, with emphasis on the regulation of the lipases by glucose and insulin, and how hyperglycemia caused by insulin deficiency and/or insulin resistance impacts lipase-dependent lipoprotein metabolism. First, a background of the biochemistry and physiology of LPL and HTGL is provided.

Biochemistry and Physiology of the Lipases

LPL and HTGL are both members of the lipase gene family, which also includes pancreatic lipase.[1] The three-dimensional structure of pancreatic lipase provided by x-ray crystallography[2] reveals two structural domains connected by a relatively short spanning region. Based on the high degree of sequence homology of the three lipases, the location and number of disulfide bonds, and similar substrate preferences, a similar three-dimensional structure for LPL and HTGL is presumed. A triad of serine, histidine, and aspartic acid in the catalytic region of the lipases is shared by all three enzymes.[1,2] Comparative biochemical properties of LPL and HTGL are portrayed in Table 5.1.

LPL

More than 40 years ago, Hahn noticed that the intravenous injection of heparin totally cleared diet-induced lipemia in dogs.[3] The addition of heparin to plasma in vitro did not reproduce this effect, suggesting that the substance(s) responsible for lipid clearing was(were) activated and/or released into plasma by heparin in vivo. Ultimately, the discovery that one of the factors was activated by lipoproteins (apolipoprotein C-II)[4] resulted in the designation of the lipase as lipoprotein lipase (LPL).

LPL resides on the capillary walls of many tissues, where it is activated by

Table 5.1 Biochemical Properties of Lipoprotein Lipase and Hepatic Triglyceride Lipase

	Gene	mRNAs	Protein	Activation	Inhibition	Predominant Substrates	Optimum pH
LPL	10 exons 9 introns	3.6 ± 3.4 kbp	448 aa (55 kD)	Apo C-II n-linked glycosylation	Protamine SO_4 1M NaCl Apo C-III	Triacylglycerol	8–9
HTGL	9 exons 8 introns	1.7 kbp	476 aa (59 kD)	Protamine SO_4 SDS		Triacylglycerol Phosphatidyl- ethanolamine Phosphatidyl- choline Monoacylglycerol	8–8.5

apolipoprotein C-II to hydrolyze triacylglycerol (triglycerides) in triglyceride-rich lipoproteins (ie, chylomicrons, produced in the intestinal epithelium, and very-low-density lipoproteins [VLDLs], formed in the liver). Free fatty acids (FFAs), monoglycerides, and remnant lipoproteins are the products of this reaction[5] (Figure 5.1). Further metabolism of LPL-derived smaller VLDL remnants results in low-density lipoproteins (LDLs), whereas larger VLDL remnants and chylomicron remnants return to the liver, where they are further hydrolyzed by HTGL and taken up and degraded.[6] LPL also hydrolyzes monoglycerides and phospholipids but at a rate that is much slower.

LPL is synthesized in the parenchymal cells of many tissues, including ad-

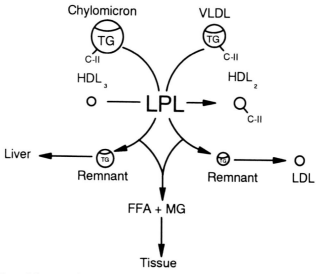

Figure 5.1 LPL and lipoprotein metabolism. LPL is activated by apolipoprotein C-II on the triglyceride (TG)–rich lipoproteins (chylomicrons and VLDL) to produce FFA and monoacylglycerol (MG). FFA and MG are delivered to the tissues wherein LPL is produced. As a part of this reaction, HDL_3 is converted to HDL_2 and apolipoprotein C-II is transferred from the TG-rich lipoproteins to HDL_2. Also generated are chylomicron remnants, which return to the liver for further processing, and VLDL remnants, which in part are converted to LDL.

ipose tissue, muscle, lung, lactating mammary gland, breast, kidney, and adrenal gland,[5] but the in vivo function of the lipase requires binding to the vascular endothelium. Glycosaminoglycans (eg, heparin) can displace LPL from vascular binding sites and increase the concentration in plasma up to 2,000-fold.[7] This effect of glycosaminoglycans appears to be due to competitive binding.[8] An effect of heparin to slow the metabolic clearance rate of LPL from plasma has also been demonstrated.[9]

In adipose cells, LPL is synthesized in the endoplasmic reticulum and proximal Golgi apparatus, where progressive trimming of high-mannose-containing lipase units results in a higher percentage of complex n-linked glycosylated LPL, the active form of the lipase[10,11] (Figure 5.2). This active form of LPL is a homodimer.[12,13] After transit through the Golgi apparatus, the enzyme is packaged into secretory vesicles in preparation for release from cells. After release, the lipase either moves to the glycocalyx of the endothelium or reassociates with the cell surface, where it can be taken up by the cell of origin and degraded.[10]

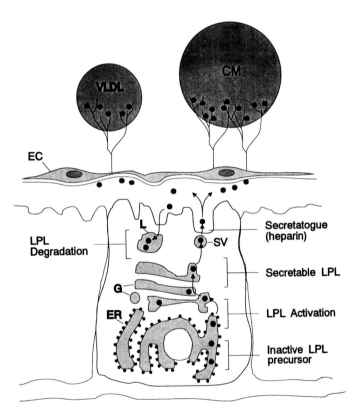

Figure 5.2 Cell biology of LPL. LPL (●) is synthesized as an inactive process in the endoplasmic reticulum (ER). Activation of the lipase relates to glucose trimming and n-linked glycosylation in terminal phases of the ER and Golgi apparatus (G) processing. The active lipase is then packaged into secretory vesicles (SV), where it is available for secretion. Following secretion, LPL is transported and bound to the glycocalyx on endothelial cells (EC) where the lipase has access to triglycerides in triglyceride-rich lipoproteins, chylomicrons (CM), and VLDL. Uptake of LPL by the cell of synthesis occurs by binding of the secreted lipase to glycosaminoglycans on the cell surface. Following uptake, a pathway of degradation in lysosomes (L) has been demonstrated.

Because W/W^v mice, which are deficient in heparin, have reductions in postheparin LPL,[14] heparin is implicated in the normal transit of LPL to the glycocalyx. At this site, multiple lipase units bind and hydrolyze triglyceride-rich lipoproteins.[15] The lipolysis products appear to displace LPL from the glycocalyx,[16] and some lipase can be found bound to circulating lipoproteins, including chylomicron and VLDL remnants.[17] The relationship between the activity of LPL spontaneously displaced from the endothelium into plasma and LDL[18] suggests that these LPL-containing remnants may be targeted for further processing to LDL. Once released into plasma, LPL is rapidly removed, mostly by the liver.[9] However, the presence of abundant LPL in regions of the brain wherein no LPL mRNA is present[19] suggests that LPL is transported and functional in sites wherein it is not synthesized. Such a biology exists for HTGL in the gonads and adrenal gland.[20,21]

HTGL

HTGL is synthesized by the periportal hepatocyte.[22] Unlike LPL, apo C-II and *n*-linked glycosylation of HTGL are not necessary for HTGL activation; however, *n*-linked glycosylation is important for secretion.[23] Although triacylglycerol is the preferential substrate, HTGL is also an effective phospholipase with a preference for phosphatidylethanolamine.[24] Like LPL, HTGL is bound to the vascular endothelium, where it can be displaced by glycosaminoglycans.[25] In the liver, its hydrolytic properties against triglycerides and phospholipids enable the catabolism of chylomicron and VLDL remnants and HDL$_2$.[26,27] In the ovary, HTGL is concentrated within thin-walled vessels of corpus lutea[20]; as yet, the function and relative importance of HTGL at distant sites have not been clarified.

Glucose and Insulin Regulation of the Lipases

The altered regulation of LPL, and to a lesser extent HTGL, in diabetes relates to both direct and indirect effects of hyperglycemia and/or insulin deficiency. This statement implies that the euglycemic/insulin-replete state is important to the physiologic control of the lipases. For LPL this is particularly true, yet this regulation is not the same for the two major tissues that synthesize the lipase, adipose tissue and muscle.

LPL

In adipose tissue, LPL is rate limiting for the uptake and storage of fatty acids for triglyceride storage.[28] However, in patients deficient in the enzyme, the storage of triglycerides in adipose tissue still occurs,[29] presumably an indication that other processes can compensate for the absence of LPL, such as the biosynthesis of fatty acids from glucose; the re-esterification of the products of hormone-sensitive, lipase-mediated lipolysis in adipose tissue; and/or the uptake and esterification of FFA from plasma. In the heart and skeletal muscle (predominantly red fiber), LPL provides triglyceride fatty acids for fuel.[30] The relative contribution of LPL to energy needs of muscle during fasting, feeding, and exercise is unknown.

Although LPL produced in adipose tissue is identical to LPL in muscle, its activity depends on the metabolic state of the tissue. During a fast, plasma insulin levels fall, levels of counterregulatory hormones increase, and the hormone-sensitive, lipase-mediated lipolysis of triglycerides stored in adipose tissue accelerates. These changes are accompanied by decreases in adipose tissue LPL (ATLPL)[28] and stable or even increasing LPL activities in muscle (cardiac, skeletal, or both).[30] These tissue-specific changes in LPL during fasting may be due to increases in levels of cyclic adenosine monophosphate (cAMP) in LPL-producing cells. cAMP has been shown to decrease ATLPL but increase muscle LPL in other systems.[31]

Increases in ATLPL during feeding of mixed nutrients have been repeatedly documented in a number of species.[28] In muscle, LPL either falls or fails to change.[30] Because high-carbohydrate diets are particularly effective in increasing ATLPL, insulin has been considered to be a major regulator of the feeding response. When infused intravenously under conditions of euglycemia (the euglycemic clamp), insulin stimulates ATLPL in a dose- and tissue-dependent manner.[32] Levels of the enzyme in skeletal muscle, however, fall even at identical intervals.[33] Of interest, the magnitude of the insulin-mediated decline of LPL in vastus lateralis was inversely related to the amount of insulin-mediated glucose uptake across the limb.[34] This suggests an important role of the lipase in the provision of fatty acids for muscle. Additional evidence suggests that the regulation of LPL in adipose tissue and skeletal muscle by nutrients is different. Following the ingestion of corn oil at the beginning of a euglycemic clamp, the insulin-stimulated ATLPL response is markedly blunted.[35] This inhibitory effect of fat on the insulin/glucose stimulation of ATLPL may partially explain why the ATLPL response to mixed meals is less than that to high-carbohydrate meals. Unlike this effect of fat ingestion on ATLPL, diets high in fat actually increase skeletal muscle LPL (SMLPL).[30]

The mechanism by which insulin stimulates ATLPL has been investigated in vitro. In adipose tissue pieces, isolated adipocytes, or 3T3-L1 cells, the predominant effect of insulin is to increase the rate of synthesis of the enzyme.[36] The increase in synthetic rate has been associated with or occurs subsequent to increases in LPL mRNA.[36,37] By nuclear run-on transcription assays, it appears that the effect of insulin on LPL mRNA is due not to changes in LPL gene transcription but to increases in LPL mRNA stability.[37] Such an effect of insulin on mRNA stability has been demonstrated for other adipocyte mRNAs (eg, glycerophosphate dehydrogenase).[38] In 3T3-L1 cells, insulin has also been shown to elicit a rapid release of LPL activity into the culture medium,[39,40] an effect mediated in part by the activation of a specific phospholipase that hydrolyzes membrane-associated glucosyl phosphatidylinositol molecules.[40]

It has been known for some time that glucose increases ATLPL activity in vitro, an effect not dependent on protein synthesis.[28] More recently, in adipocytes cultured in the absence of glucose, a lower molecular weight form of LPL (49,000) has been identified that is neither active nor secreted.[41] Following the addition of glucose, increases in LPL synthetic rate and potentiation of the stimulatory effects of insulin were seen; however, there was no effect on LPL mRNA. Thus, the effect of glucose was to enhance LPL translation and post-translational processing, whereas insulin stimulated LPL activity by increasing LPL mRNA.

The regulation of muscle LPL by insulin ex vivo or in vitro is consistent with the in vivo data. In general, when normal hearts were perfused with insulin, no effect was seen.[42] Although cardiomyocytes from insulin-injected control rats demonstrated decreases in heparin-releasable LPL compared to untreated controls,[43] the addition of insulin to cardiomyocytes in vitro failed to change cellular or heparin-releasable LPL.[44] This absence of an in vitro effect of insulin on LPL in cardiomyocytes suggests that insulin does not stimulate cardiac muscle LPL directly and that the reductions in muscle LPL in diabetes must be secondary to an unidentified metabolic factor(s) associated with insulin deficiency. Although a skeletal muscle cell line is now available for study,[45] the effect of insulin has not yet been examined.

HTGL

Studies to examine the effect of glucose/insulin on HTGL are less abundant. In one study, injections of nondiabetic rats with insulin failed to alter HTGL in postheparin plasma.[46] However, in another study a 40% increase was seen after 10 U of protamine zinc insulin every 16 hours for 4 days.[47] In vitro, HTGL is synthesized by both HepG2 cells[48] and rat hepatocytes.[49] In rat hepatocytes, a small stimulatory effect of insulin (20%) on HTGL was seen.[49] In general, HTGL is not viewed as an insulin-responsive lipase.

Lipases in Diabetes Mellitus

When evaluating the impact of hyperglycemia/insulin deficiency on the lipases, particularly LPL, it is important to realize that LPL is synthesized and secreted from many tissues wherein the regulation of the lipase by glucose/insulin may be different. Thus, when measurements are carried out in postheparin plasma, some assumptions can be made about the potential ability of the organism to hydrolyze triglycerides from circulating chylomicrons and VLDLs;[50] however, the site of a defect in triglyceride-rich lipoprotein triglyceride lipolysis (eg, adipose tissue versus muscle) cannot be adequately assessed from the postheparin plasma activities. Moreover, although biopsies of tissues may be helpful in detecting tissue-specific defects in LPL related to diabetes mellitus, activities of ATLPL vary between regions,[51] and SMLPL is variable based on fiber type and conditioning.[30] Assumptions must also be made about organ blood flow. Finally, many abundant sources of LPL (ie, heart and lung) are not accessible in humans for study. Nevertheless, because alterations in triglyceride-rich lipoprotein catabolism and reductions in postheparin and/or tissue LPL activities are associated with diabetes mellitus,[52] measurement of the lipases is relevant to the understanding of the altered biology of lipids and lipoproteins in insulin deficiency/resistance.

The pathophysiology of the lipases in diabetes mellitus is approached first by a discussion of animals with pharmacologic- or pancreatectomy-induced diabetes. Human diabetes is then covered with a further breakdown related to type I, or insulin-dependent, diabetes mellitus (IDDM) and type 2, or non-insulin-dependent, diabetes mellitus (NIDDM). In most areas and where appropriate, the published literature is summarized using a meta-analytic approach.

Animals and Diabetes Mellitus

Postheparin Lipases

Catabolic defects in triglyceride-rich lipoprotein or artificial triglyceride-rich lipoprotein metabolism have been repeatedly demonstrated in animals with alloxan- or streptozotocin-induced diabetes, or following pancreatectomy.[42,53-63] This presumes a defect in the lipases, predominantely LPL, which should be reflected by decrements in postheparin LPL. However, this has rarely been the case. Despite periods of insulin deficiency from 2 days to up to 17 months, postheparin plasma LPL was not less than that measured in nondiabetic controls, but 123 ± 15% ($\bar{x}$ ± SEM) of controls[46,53,64-68] (Table 5.2). This was despite a mean blood or serum glucose of 408 ± 39 mg/dL or greater. Insulin treatment from 2 to 10 days, however, improved blood (serum) glucose from 444 ± 106 to 140 ± 11 mg/dL and increased postheparin plasma LPL by 21 ± 5%.[46,64,67] Although in one study 2 days of insulin treatment reduced triglycerides from about 350 to about 25 mg/dL, LPL levels in postheparin plasma increased by only 15%.[67] These data suggest that the hypertriglyceridemia in diabetic animals is not simply a consequence of LPL deficiency.

A somewhat different story exists for postheparin HTGL. Again, in animals diabetic from 2 days to 17 months, postheparin HTGL has ranged from 36%[67] to 104%[68] of normal. The overall mean was 77 ± 9% that of nondiabetic controls.[46,66-68] Similarly to postheparin LPL, improved glycemic control increased postheparin HTGL, but variably, with one study demonstrating a 22% increase[46] and another a 255% increase.[67] Although glycemia improved in these studies,[46,67,68] triglycerides were only measured in one.[67] Here there was an apparent relationship between the magnitude of change in triglycerides and the change in postheparin HTGL. Although HDL was not measured in any of these studies,

Table 5.2 Postheparin Lipolytic Activites in Diabetic Animals

Species	Duration (Days)	Glucose (mg/dL)	Triglycerides (mg/dL)	LPL (% Control)	HTGL (% Control)	Comments	Ref
Dogs	≥7	206	168	29	—	Total lipase	53
Rats	≥2	250	—	77	—	Total lipase	64
		120		**101**		**INS (? d)**	
Rats	2	475	248	135		Total lipase	65
Rats	7	>300	—	145	60		66
Rats	3	464	—	168	69		67
	5	466	—	147	88		
	7	403	—	137	88		
	9	613	≈350	93	36		
	2	**142**	**≈25**	**107**	**92**	**INS (2 d)**	
Dogs	17 mo	434	128	157	104		68
Rats	10	470	228	108	93		46
	10	**159**	**—**	**128**	**113**	**INS (10 d)**	
All studies		≥408 ± 39	224 ± 38	123 ± 15	77 ± 9	No INS	
		140 ± 11	**—**	**—**	**112 ± 8**	**103 ± 11**	**INS**

Abbreviation: INS = insulin.

Table 5.3 HTGL in Homegenates of Liver from Diabetic Rats

Duration (Days)	Nutritional State	Glucose (mg/dL)	Triglycerides (mg/dL)	HTGL (% Control)	Comments	Ref
5–8	Fast	—	—	76		69
2 h	Fed	326	118	100		47
8 h		93	109	102		
1		425	108	36		
3		430	434	42		
5		458	392	49		
5		**170**	**103**	**155**	**INS (5 d)**	
7		514	517	45		
3	Fed	619	—	41		70
3–4	Fed	508	88	79		71
	Fed	**110**	**37**	**103**	**INS (4 d)**	
	Fast	373	146	86		
	Fed	431	753	59		
4–5	Fed	740	160	53		72
All studies		447 ± 49	283 ± 72	64 ± 7	No INS	
		140 ± 50	**70 ± 53**	**129 ± 26**	**INS**	

Abbreviation: INS = insulin.

the small reduction in postheparin HTGL in diabetic animals would predict, if anything, higher levels of HDL, a metabolic response ordinarily not seen in humans when hypertriglyceridemia is also present.

In some studies the activity of HTGL was directly measured (ie, in liver homogenates of rats but not postheparin plasma)[47,69–72] (Table 5.3). As for HTGL in postheparin plasma, HTGL in liver homogenates was reduced (64 ± 7% of controls), and more consistently. In two studies wherein insulin was utilized to reduce glycemia, HTGL in homogenates increased minimally (23%)[71] or substantially (316%).[47] However, in the study by Knauer et al,[47] insulin had no effect at 90 minutes and had an effect only after days of administration. Unlike HTGL in postheparin plasma, HTGL in liver homogenates was inversely related to blood (serum) glucose ($r = -.669, n = 13, p < .02$). In two studies, the concentration of FFA in plasma was also inversely related to HTGL in homogenates.[47,71] Together, these experiments suggest that hyperglycemia/insulin deficiency in rats decreases levels of HTGL in the liver. Although HTGL in postheparin plasma is somewhat less reduced by diabetes than HTGL in the liver, the impact of insulin deficiency in animals proves to be greater on postheparin plasma HTGL than LPL.

ATLPL in Animals with Diabetes

The important regulatory roles of glucose and insulin on ATLPL in vivo and in vitro would predict reductions in ATLPL in diabetics. The data in animals bear this out (Table 5.4). With the exception of a single study wherein ATLPL was measured in acetone–ether extracts of parametrial and retroperitoneal adipose tissue 10 days after the induction of diabetes,[57] and one study wherein ATLPL was measured in homogenates 1 day after streptozotocin,[56] ATLPL has been

Table 5.4 ATLPL in Diabetic Animals

Species	Duration (Days)	Nutritional State	Glucose (mg/dL)	Triglycerides (mg/dL)	AT depot	Assay	ATLPL (% Control)	Comments	Ref
Rats	30	Fed	≈400	≈450	Epid	HG	≈50	1 d w/o INS	73
							≈33	3 d w/o INS	
Rats	5	Fed	411	372	Epid	HG	39	4 d w/o INS	55
			170	**20**			**199**	**INS**	
Rats	3 h	Fed	441	—	—	HG	28		74
			392				**76**	**INS (3 h)**	
Rats	2	Fed	311	172	Epid	HG	6		65
Rats	1	Fast	—	—	Param	HG	168		56
Rats	10	?	428	713	Param	HG	117		57
					Retrop		159		
Rats	5–8	Fast	—	—	Epid	HG	9		69
Rats	7–10	Fast	≈250	≈170	Retrop	HG	76		75
			≈375	≈190			64		
		Fed	—	—			27		
			—	—			26		
Rats	2	Fed	362	—	Epid	HG	21		76
	4		414	—			10		
Rats	7–10	Fed	326	158	Epid	HG	52		77
						HR	54		
		Fast	282	105		HG	64		
						HR	45		
Rats	3	Fast	>300	—	Epid	HR	41		78
	10						15		
	34						25		
Rats	70	Fast	170	71	Epid	HG	57		79
Rats	21	Fast	370	128	Epid	HG	42		80
Rats	14	Fed	>360	275	Epid	HG	33		81
	15–22		>360	284			100		
			—	**363**			**367**	**INS (2 U/d)**	
			—	**133**			**250**	**INS (3 U/d)**	
			—	**124**			**200**	**INS (4 U/d)**	
Rats	7–8	Fast	373	146			21		71
		Fed	431	753			13		
		Fed	**508**	**88**	**Epid**	**HG**	**36**	**INS (3 d)**	
		Fed	**110**	**37**			**236**	**INS (4 d)**	
Rats	3	Fed	450	160	Epid	HR	92		82
			130	**86**			**222**	**INS (3 d)**	
	3		421	—			12		
			315	—			**98**	**INS (½ d)**	
			150	—			**102**	**INS (1½ d)**	
			99	—			**100**	**INS (3 d)**	
Rats	4–5	Fed	≈750	≈150	Epid	HR	25		72
					Perir		15		
Rats	18	Fast	393		Epid	HR	40		28
			—			HG	67		
Rats	10	Fed	490	425	Epid	HR	25		83
			208	**79**			**139**	**INS (4 d)**	
Mice	7	Fed	380	204	Epid	HG	33		84
			65	**177**			**93**	**INS (7 d)**	
Rats	10–14	Fed	460	75	Param	HR	7		85
Rats	14	Fast	351	378	Epid	HG	50		86
			329	**272**			**177**	**INS (1 d)**	
			187	**199**			**232**	**INS (4 d)**	
All studies			≥388 ± 2	269 ± 43		HR	33 ± 7	No INS	
						HG	52 ± 8		
			222 ± 39	**143 ± 31**			**539 ± 108**	**INS**	

Abbreviations: Epid = epididymal; HG = homogenates; HR = heparin releasable; INS = insulin; Param = parametrial; Perir = perirenal; Retrop = retroperitoneal.

reduced in diabetic animals.[28,55,65,69,71-86] Durations of glucose intolerance without insulin have ranged from 3 hours after mannoheptulose[74] to 10 weeks after streptozotocin.[79] Reductions in both the heparin-releasable enzyme[28,72,77,78,82,83,85] and ATLPL measured in acetone–ether extracts or homogenates[28,55,65,69,71,73-77,79-81,84,86] have been found. For the heparin-releasable lipase, the mean reduction in LPL was to levels 33 ± 7% of nondiabetic controls; for ATLPL in homogenates, the mean reduction was to 52 ± 8% of nondiabetic controls. When comparisons are made between measurements of ATLPL in the fasting versus fed condition, diabetes-related reductions in ATLPL were less in fasted rats (52 ± 10% of nondiabetic controls)[28,56,69,71,75,77-80,86] than fed rats (35 ± 6% of nondiabetic controls).[55,65,71-77,81,83-85] Because in most studies the diabetic animals were severely hyperglycemic (ie, blood [serum] glucose level over 350 mg/dL), the extent of glycemia did not relate to the reduction in ATLPL. There also was no relationship between the extent of hypertriglyceridemia and the level of ATLPL in diabetic animals. Triglyceride concentrations, however, varied widely, from 71 to 713 mg/dL.

In the studies in which insulin was administered to diabetic animals, decreases in blood (serum) glucose and triglycerides were seen in most, and increases in ATLPL in all, animals (mean increase 5.4 ± 1.1-fold above non-insulin-treated diabetic animals).[55,71,74,81-84,86] In general, the increases in the heparin-releasable lipase (mean 6.6 ± 1.2-fold)[82,83] were similar to those for ATLPL in adipose tissue homogenates (5.0 ± 1.5).[55,71,74,81,84,86] There was no relationship between the duration of insulin treatment and the increase in ATLPL; however, treatment periods were all less than 7 days. Nor was there a relationship between the duration of diabetes and the response to insulin, yet the maximum duration of diabetes was brief (2 weeks). Overall, these data support the importance of insulin in the physiologic regulation of ATLPL.

SMLPL in Animals with Diabetes

Unlike the effects of diabetes in animals on ATLPL, diabetes in animals (rats only) has been less consistently associated with decreases in SMLPL (mean 83 ± 9% of nondiabetic controls)[56,71,72,75-77,79,86] (Table 5.5). However, variability in the types of muscle utilized, methods of LPL assay, and duration of diabetes all may have contributed to the experimental differences. When red or oxidative muscle alone is considered, SMLPL was similarly reduced (84 ± 9% of nondiabetic controls.[56,71,72,75,77,79,86] In white or glycolytic muscle, the mean activity was 67 ± 11% of nondiabetic controls.[56,71,72] Because the muscles utilized were different between studies, comparisons are of limited value. However, the soleus muscle was examined in six of the eight reports and overall was not altered by the diabetic state (85 ± 12% of nondiabetic controls). Combining all studies, there was no relationship between the duration of diabetes (from 1 to 70 days) and SMLPL. In addition, fasting versus feeding had no impact on the amount of SMLPL in diabetic rats compared to nondiabetic controls. The extent of glycemia and hypertriglyceridemia also failed to relate to the diabetes-dependent alteration in SMLPL.

Several studies examined the effect of improved glycemia on SMLPL. Following 1 and 4 days of insulin therapy, SMLPL in the vastus lateralis was increased by 30% and 90%, respectively.[86] Triglycerides also fell by 28% and 47%, respectively. In another study, SMLPL in psoas muscle increased 2.2-fold and

Table 5.5 SMLPL in Diabetic Rats

Duration (Days)	Nutri-tional State	Glucose (mg/dL)	Tri-glycerides (mg/dL)	SM Depot	Assay	SMLPL (% Control)	Comments	Ref
1	Fast	—	—	Psoas	HG	40		56
				Soleus		26		
				Diaph		25		
7–10	Fast	≈250	≈170	Soleus	HG	96		75
		≈375	≈190			103		
2	Fed	362	—	Soleus	HG	87		76
4		414	—			167		
7–10	Fed	326	158	Soleus	HG	89		77
				Gastroc		86		
	Fast	282	105	Soleus		105		
				Gastroc		87		
70	Fast	170	71	Soleus	HG	100		79
				Gastroc		120		
7–8	Fast	373	146	Psoas		70		71
				Diaph		43		
	Fed	431	753	Psoas		31		
				Diaph		41		
	Fed	**508**	**88**	**Psoas**	**HG**	**72**	**INS (3 d)**	
				Diaph		**72**		
	Fed	**110**	**37**	**Psoas**		**63**	**INS (4 d)**	
				Diaph		**36**		
4–5	Fed	≈750	≈150	Masseter	HR	213		72
				Pectoralis		115		
				Soleus		47		
				Deep quads		151		
				Superf. quads		68		
14	Fast	351	378	Vastus	HG	56		86
		329	**272**			**72**	**INS (1 d)**	
		187	**199**			**101**	**INS (4 d)**	
All studies		371 ± 44	380 ± 150			83 ± 9	No INS	
		284 ± 88	**149 ± 53**			**168 ± 21**	**INS**	

Abbreviations: Diaph = diaphragm; Gastroc = gastrocnemius; HG = homogenates; HR = heparin releasable; INS = insulin; Vastus = vastus lateralis.

that in the diaphragm by 1.3-fold.[71] Together the mean increase in SMLPL by insulin was 1.7-fold above untreated rats. Importantly, the mean glucose concentration was still substantially elevated in insulin-treated rats (284 ± 58 mg/dL). Overall, data from animals indicate that the predominant effect of hyperglycemia/insulin deficiency on LPL in peripheral tissues is on ATLPL, not SMLPL.

Cardiac Muscle LPL (CMLPL) in Animals with Diabetes

The impact of diabetes in animals on CMLPL is easier to interpret, predominantly because of the uniformity of the muscle examined. Presently, data are only available for rats, but both in vivo and in vitro measurements of CMLPL have been made (Table 5.6). When all experiments are considered, diabetes mellitus has no effect on CMLPL (mean = 89 ± 16% of nondiabetic controls).[42–44,56,64, 65,67,70–72,74,76,79,83,84,86,87] However, as for adipose tissue and skeletal muscle,

Table 5.6 CMLPL in Diabetic Animals

Species	Duration (Days)	Nutri-tional State	Glucose (mg/dL)	Tri-glycerides (mg/dL)	Heart Muscle Preparation	Assay	CMLPL (% Control)	Comments	Ref
Rats	>2	Fast	>250	—	Slices	HR	57		64
			<120				**103**	**INS (? d)**	
					Heart	HG	76		
							94	**INS (? d)**	
Rats	2	Fed	311	172	Heart	HG	67		65
Rats	1	Fast	—	—	Heart	HG	116		56
Rats	2	Fed	362	—	Heart	HG	197		76
	4		414				234		
Rats	3h	Fed	441	—	Heart	HG	168		74
			392	—		**HG**	**145**	**INS (3 h)**	
Rats	70	Fast	170	71	Heart	HG	82		79
Rats	2	Fed	320	71	Perfusion	HR	79		42
						HG	63		
						HR	**100**	**INS (2 h)**	
						HG	108		
Rats	3	Fed	619	—	Perfusion	HR	408		70
Rats	3	Fast	625	260	Heart	HG	13		67
	28		610	140			38		
Rats	7–8	Fast	373	146			64		71
		Fed	431	753			76		
		Fed	**508**	**88**	**Heart**	**HG**	**240**	**INS (3 d)**	
		Fed	**110**	**37**			**135**	**INS (4 d)**	
Rats	3–4				Myo cells	HR	36		87
						HG	53		
						Sonicates	43		
Rats	10	Fed	490	425	Heart	HR	211		83
			208	**79**			**107**	**INS (4 d)**	
Rats	4–5	Fed	≈750	≈150	Heart	HR	89		72
Mice	7	Fed	380	204	Heart	HG	88		84
Rats	14	Fast	351	378	Heart	HG	30		86
			329	**272**			**32**	**INS (1 d)**	
			187	**199**			**44**	**INS (4 d)**	
Rats	3–4	Fed	486	—	Myo cells	HR	41		43
						Sonicates	65		
			108	—		**HR**	**55**	**INS (1 h)**	
						Sonicates	**95**		
Rats	4–5	Fed	486	—	Myo cells	HR	23		44
			151	—			**73**	**INS (1 h)**	
Rats	3–5	Fed	432	523	Perfusion	HR	20		88
					Myo cells	HR	35		
						Sonicates	30		
All studies			441 ± 36	293 ± 62			89 ± 16	No INS	
			235 ± 48	**135 ± 43**			**159 ± 24**	**INS**	

Abbreviations: HG = homogenates; HR = heparin releasable; INS = insulin; Myo = myocardial.

the duration of diabetes, degree of hyperglycemia/hypertriglyceridemia, nutritional state of the animal, and assays utilized have varied substantially.

CMLPL measured from heart slices or in perfusates of hearts as the heparin-releasable enzyme was found to vary from 20% to 408% of nondiabetic controls.[42,64,70,72,83,88] The nutritional state of the rats prior to sacrifice (ie, fasted versus fed) did not predict whether or not alterations in CMLPL were seen. When CMLPL was measured in homogenates or extracts of heart, the activity was unchanged compared to nondiabetic controls (95 $\pm$ 18%).[56,64,65,67,71,74,76,79,84,86] Although CMLPL measured in homogenates or extracts of hearts from diabetic rats appeared relatively higher in the fed (127 $\pm$ 29% of nondiabetic controls) than the fasted (49 $\pm$ 22% of controls) state, this difference was not statistically significant.

The amount of CMLPL releasable by heparin failed to correlate with the degree of glycemia as did the CMLPL measured in homogenates or extracts of cardiac tissue. Following the injection of insulin into diabetic rats, CMLPL was variably affected (ie, a 1.59 $\pm$ 0.24-fold increase was seen).[42,64,71,74,83,86] In two studies, insulin treatment reduced the lipase activity from 226% of nondiabetic controls to 121.[74,83] In the other studies, however, minimal to moderate increases were demonstrated.[64,74,86] No apparent explanation for these differences can be provided. Triglyceride levels at sacrifice (37 to 753 mg/dL) also did not relate to CMLPL. In addition, the duration of hyperglycemia from 1 day after pancreatectomy to 10 weeks after streptozotocin had no influence on CMLPL measured at sacrifice.

Using an alternative approach, Severson et al have concluded that diabetes does reduce CMLPL. Using myocardial cells prepared from diabetic and nondiabetic control rats, early[87] and subsequent[43,44,88] experiments demonstrated diabetes-related reductions in CMLPL measured following heparin treatment of cells or in homogenates of cells. In one report, insulin treatment of diabetic rats prior to sacrifice restored heparin-releasable CMLPL to normal, and partially restored the lipase activity measured in homogenates of cells.[43] The diabetes-related decrease in phospholipase C–mediated release of LPL from myocardial cells suggested that LPL was bound ionically to heparan sulfate proteoglycans that are covalently linked to the cell surface by a phosphatidylinositol–glycan membrane anchor.[44] This reduction in cell surface LPL in vitro was corrected by insulin administration in vivo before sacrifice. A similar mechanism for the effect of insulin on LPL has been suggested in 3T3-L1 cells.[40] Yet, when myocardial cells were incubated in vitro with insulin, no increase in cellular or heparin-releasable LPL was found.[44] This absence of a direct effect of insulin on LPL in myocardial cells suggests that the decrease in CMLPL related to diabetes is not directly attributable to insulin deficiency. Subsequent experiments have suggested that this reduction in LPL in myocardial cells from diabetic rats may be due to an inhibitory effect of FFA, derived either from lipoproteins or from hormone-sensitive, lipase-mediated triglyceride lipolysis in adipose tissue.[88] Despite the reproducibility of the findings from the Severson laboratory,[43,44,87,88] the data from animal experiments as a whole suggest that diabetes has no consistent effect on CMLPL.

Diabetes Mellitus in Humans

As in diabetic animals, reductions in triglyceride-rich lipoprotein removal rate from plasma are commonplace in human diabetics.[89–96] To some extent, this relates to defects in LPL and in part provides an explanation for both the hy-

Table 5.7 Lipases in IDDM

n	Age (Yr)	Duration (Yr)	Mean Glucose (mg/dL)	Glyco-hemoglobin (%)	Tri-glycerides (mg/dL)	LPL (μmol/mL/h)	LPL (% Control)	HT (μmol/mL/h)
7	19–27	2–21	362	—	108	236		
			124	—	51	440		
13	16–47	New	239	—	234	15.6	66	23.8
13	18–31	1–18	164	—	128	25.8	110	26.6
25	45	21	>250	—	169	26.6	131	
15			<100		74	32.9	162	
16	31	New	221	—	203			
					102			
12	21	0.25–11	238	—	73			
			198		60			
12	35	3–31	306	—				
			178					
10	17–42	6–30	225	12.9	87	36.1		18.5
			178	11.2	82	30.3		17.7
			160	11.0	84			
15	7–23	New	222		196	0.5	38	
			162		80	1.3	92	
All studies			258 ± 18		153 ± 24		78 ± 28	
			158 ± 11		**83 ± 8**		**177 ± 35**	

Abbreviations: CHO = cholesterol; Gastroc = gastrocnemius; Glut = gluteus; HR = heparin releasable; INS = insulin; Vastus = vastus lateralis.

pertriglyceridemia and less frequent hypoalphalipoproteinemia seen in human diabetes. For discussion, diabetes is separated into insulin-dependent and non-insulin-dependent types.

Insulin-Dependent Diabetes Mellitus (Table 5.7)

Postheparin Lipases

In the early experiments of the lipoprotein lipases in human diabetes, a distinction between HTGL and LPL in postheparin plasma was not made. The first report of abnormalities in postheparin lipolytic activity in diabetes mellitus examined the effect of 48 hours of insulin withdrawal on total lipolytic capacity and found an approximately 50% reduction.[90] This decrease was accompanied by an increase in plasma triglycerides from 51 ± 8 to 108 ± 45 mg/dL. In two subjects, a delay in the disappearance of ^{14}C-labeled triglycerides accompanied insulin withdrawal.

The first report wherein HTGL and LPL were measured separately in insulin-dependent diabetics demonstrated decreases in postheparin LPL in untreated ketotic diabetics but normal levels in chronically insulin-treated diabetics.[96] A significant negative correlation existed between the LPL activity in postheparin plasma and the log of plasma triglycerides, and a positive correlation was found between postheparin LPL and the fractional turnover of VLDL triglycerides. No changes in HTGL were seen, nor was there a relationship between HTGL and triglyceride-rich lipoprotein levels or metabolism. In a subsequent report,[97] Nikkila and Hormila found higher postheparin LPL activities in the postheparin plasma of subjects with diabetes of 10 or more years' duration than age- and

Postheparin Lipases

GL (% Control)	ATLPL				SMLPL				Comments	Ref
	Site	Assay	(μmol/g/h)	(% Control)	Site	Assay	(μmol/g/h)	(% Control)		
									Total lipase	90
88										96
93										
										97
	Glut	HR	1.1	34	Vastus	HR	0.4	46		98
			1.8	56			0.7	78	INS (14 d)	
					Gastroc	HG	0.9	99		99
							1.3	135	Exercise	
	Glut	HR	2.6	—	Vastus	HR	1.0			100
			3.7				0.9		INS (10 h)	
	Glut	HR	1.7	—						101
			1.5	—					CHO (2 wk)	
			1.9	—					CHO (4 wk)	
										102
				34				73 ± 27	No INS	
				56				78	INS	

sex-matched controls. This in part explained the higher levels of HDL cholesterol found in the diabetics versus the controls. In general, there was no relationship between glycemic control and postheparin LPL. The only exceptions were men who had blood glucose concentrations greater than 250 mg/dL. In these subjects, LPL activities were slightly lower (26.6 μmol/mL/h) than in men with good control (32.9 μmol/mL/h) ($p < .05$). Similar relationships between more severe hyperglycemia, triglycerides, and postheparin LPL have also been shown by Rubba et al.[98] In their study, plasma VLDL triglycerides were inversely correlated with postheparin plasma LPL.

Recently, sensitive bioassays have been developed for the measurements of LPL and HTGL in plasma prior to the injection of heparin.[99] Normally, the proportions of HTGL (approximately 60%) and LPL (approximately 40%) in preheparin plasma are similar to those measured in postheparin plasma.[18,99] In insulin-dependent diabetics who were treated with subcutaneous insulin, however, preheparin LPL represented 52% of the total postheparin activity.[100] Following the delivery of insulin through an intraperitoneal catheter, the postheparin LPL fell from 16.9 to 9.6 nmol/mL/h, an activity that then represented 29% of the total lipase. Of interest, this insulin delivery port–dependent change in postheparin LPL was associated with changes in cholesteryl ester transfer protein (CETP) and lipoprotein composition (cholesterol enrichment of VLDL).[101] Presumably, the higher levels of postheparin LPL in diabetics treated with subcutaneous insulin[97] relate to higher systemic levels of insulin achieved using this route of delivery, and the relatively higher level of stimulation of ATLPL in this setting. Displacement of LPL in other insulin-responsive tissues (ie, muscle) by a phospholipase C–dependent effect could also be contributory.[40,43]

ATLPL and SMLPL

Taskinen and Nikkila were the first to biopsy tissues in insulin-dependent diabetics and measure LPL.[102] Before treatment, diabetics had substantial reductions of heparin-releasable ATLPL (34% of control mean) and SMLPL (45% of control mean). After insulin treatment, LPL increased in both adipose tissue and skeletal muscle ($p < .01$) but was still not normal by 2 weeks. Although plasma triglycerides returned to normal, HDL cholesterol also remained low. With shorter periods of insulin deprivation, ATLPL and SMLPL were largely unchanged. However, during subsequent insulin administration, ATLPL increased by 36% whereas SMLPL failed to change.[103] These data are more consistent with the tissue-dependent differences of the effect of diabetes on LPL in animals.

The responsiveness of tissue LPL to perturbations (ie, diet and exercise) has been tested in several laboratories. To determine if diets high in carbohydrate and fiber altered glycemia, serum lipids, or ATLPL in insulin-dependent diabetes, subjects were studied over 6 weeks of intervention.[104] High-carbohydrate (and high-fiber) diets improved glycemia and LDL cholesterol, decreased HDL cholesterol, but failed to alter triglycerides, postheparin plasma LPL and HTGL, or ATLPL measured in fasting subjects. However, consistent with an impact of the diet on insulin sensitivity, the ATLPL response to a meal was enhanced ($p < .05$). Although no control group was examined, previous studies have suggested a similar impact of high-carbohydrate feeding on ATLPL.[105] In a separate report, the impact of training on SMLPL in diabetics was tested.[106] Here, despite moderately poor glycemic control, the increase in SMLPL with training (44%) was similar to that in nondiabetics.

Overall, in IDDM in humans, alterations in LPL predominate. HTGL measured in pre- or postheparin plasma is not affected. When glycemic control is poor and ketosis is present, decreases in postheparin plasma LPL, ATLPL, and SMLPL are all present. With treatment, recovery of ATLPL and SMLPL is slow, but ultimately levels of pre- and postheparin LPL may be increased by subcutaneous insulin. Although levels of LPL in plasma or tissue often relate to plasma triglyceride and HDL cholesterol levels, the subcutaneous route of insulin delivery may have adverse effects on CETP and lipoprotein composition that relate to higher levels of LPL.

Non-Insulin-Dependent Diabetes (Table 5.8)

Postheparin Lipases

Studies in non-insulin-dependent diabetics have been more extensive than those in insulin-dependent diabetics.[75,89,93,107–121] However, as for insulin-dependent diabetics, early studies examined the effect of diabetes on total postheparin lipolytic activity, not LPL nor HTGL. In diabetics with severe hypertriglyceridemia (greater than 1,000 mg/dL), reductions in postheparin lipolytic activity following a single bolus[89,96,107] or infusion[110] of heparin were found. The abnormality in the late phase of the heparin infusion proved greater than the reduction in postheparin lipolytic activity attained during the early phases of the infusion.[110] Treatment of diabetes with sulfonylureas or insulin corrected the late-phase lipolytic defect by 6 months, with associated decreases in triglycerides.

When assays to distinguish LPL and HTGL became available, it was suggested that the lipase responsible for decreases in total lipolytic activity after heparin in non-insulin-dependent diabetics was LPL, not HTGL.[75,114,117] However, the study of Pollare et al[119] failed to show differences for either of the postheparin lipases in non-insulin-dependent diabetics. Nevertheless, postheparin LPL was still inversely correlated with serum triglyceride and VLDL triglycerides. With the exception of one report wherein HTGL was increased in hypertriglyceridemic diabetics,[121] levels of postheparin HTGL typically have been normal. However, when non-insulin-dependent diabetics are separated on the basis of HDL cholesterol levels, Kasim et al[118] and Agardh et al[115] have found differences. In these reports, diabetics with high levels of HDL cholesterol had decreases in HTGL. As for insulin-dependent diabetics, a greater percentage of the preheparin lipase is represented by LPL (49%) (R. H. Eckel and T. J. Yost, unpublished data). However, this percentage is similar to that in obese male nondiabetic controls (52%). Again, systemic hyperinsulinemia may help explain the similarities in preheparin LPL between diabetic and nondiabetic obese subjects, but not the differences in the preheparin lipase between lean insulin-dependent diabetics and lean controls. Treatment of diabetics with sulfonylureas or insulin has resulted in minimal to moderate increases in postheparin LPL, but no change in HTGL.[114,117]

ATLPL and SMLPL

Decreases in both ATLPL and SMLPL have been identified in non-insulin-dependent diabetics. In the study of Pykalisto et al,[111] diabetics with severe hypertriglyceridemia and mean fasting plasma glucose levels of 248 mg/dL had reductions in both heparin-releasable ATLPL (37% of nondiabetic controls) and that measured in extracts of adipose tissue (67% of nondiabetic controls). Unpublished data from this laboratory suggest that hypertriglyceridemia in non-insulin-dependent diabetics (815 ± 255 mg/dL; $n = 11$) does not alter ATLPL (2.3 ± 0.6 nmol/10^6 cells/min) compared to normotriglyceridemic (136 ± 9 mg/dL; $n = 15$) diabetics (2.9 ± 0.8 nmol/10^6 cells/min) (R. H. Eckel and T. J. Yost, unpublished data). These ATLPL activities, however, are substantially reduced in comparison to those measured in normotriglyceridemic nondiabetic obese subjects (11.9 ± 1.6 nmol/10^6 cells/min; $n = 26$). In the Pykalisto et al study,[111] following 10 to 12 weeks of hypoglycemic therapy, heparin-releasable activity increased 3.5-fold whereas the extractable activity increased nearly twofold. These changes were accompanied by reductions of fasting plasma triglycerides from a mean of 1,849 to 684 mg/dL and glucose from 248 to 140 mg/dL. In addition, the changes in both heparin-releasable and extractable ATLPL were correlated with the percentage increases in plasma insulin concentration. Similar reductions in heparin-releasable and ATLPL activities in tissue homogenates and correction by sulfonylureas or insulin were seen in non-insulin-dependent diabetics in other studies.[93,112,120] In the study of Simsolo et al,[120] the change in ATLPL activity with improved control was related to changes in ATLPL synthetic rate, but not ATLPL mRNA.

Three studies have examined the effect of non-insulin-dependent diabetes on both ATLPL and SMLPL.[93,113,119] In the study of Taskinen et al,[113] heparin-releasable ATLPL was reduced by 44% in diabetic men but not significantly in diabetic women. SMLPL was similar to that measured in nondiabetic controls for both genders. Vessby et al[93] studied non-insulin-dependent diabetics before, during, and 3 months after weight reduction. No control group was included.

Table 5.8 Lipases in NIDDM

n	Age (Yr)	Duration (Yr)	Rx	Glucose (mg/dL)	Glyco-hemoglobin (%)	Triglycerides (mg/dL)	LPL (μmol/mL/h)	LPL (% Control)	HT (μmol/mL/h)	HT (% Control)
8						356	32.4			
6			**INS**			**440**	**29.4**			
4	54		Diet, Sulf			2—5,115	9.6	107		
						2—265	4.8	34		
21			Diet, Sulf or INS	>150						
13			**Ins—8**							
12	41			234		3,156	23.2	78		
12			**INS or Sulf**	**151**		**886**	**20.7**	**70**		
8			**INS or Sulf**	**154**			**35.3**	**119**		
12	45		Diet—8	256		1,412				
5			**INS**	**140**		**684**				
14	16–30			160		116	18.7	80	28.2	104
9	32–56		Diet, Sulf	169		112	19.0	95	23.5	104
11	34–55			211		1,240	14.8	74	31.1	138
11	54			149		301				
9						771				
						487				
25 M	43			160		343				
11 F	46			160		336				
26	17–18	0–21	Diet, Sulf or Met	275	14.3	248	≈5.4		≈15.8	
7			**INS**	**149**	**9.4**	**151**	**≈6.9**		**≈13.8**	
6	**42**	**11**	**INS**	**203**		**71**	**9.1**		**12.2**	
6	**37**	**16**	**INS**	**166**		**213**	**6.6**		**13.8**	
9			—	297						
			Sulf	99						
8	54	4.25			13.8	260	6.4	70	13.3	113
			INS or Sul		11.3	151	8.5	93	13.2	**112**
					10.6	128	8.9	98	12.1	103
	54	4.25			13.8	260	4.1	67	11.1	113
			INS or Sul		11.3	151	4.1	68	11.6	119
					10.6	128	5.4	88	12.2	125
20	53		Diet, Sulf or Met	203		434				
20			Fast	85		151				
17			3 mo outpatient	153		230				
11	68	12	Diet, Sulf or INS	187	11.4	100	≈7.7		≈20.7	
10	96	19		212	11.0	165	≈8.4		≈19.5	
9	69	17		152	9.7	164	≈9.0		≈11.4	
7				173	6.9	268	3.9	108	5.8	95
8	49	New		237	14.1	205				
3			**INS or Sulf**	**141**	**9.7**	**145**				
15	41		Diet, Sulf	171		136				
11	41			198		815				
12	54		Diet, Sulf	275		103	13.6	97	13.3	88
7	48			220		232	12.9	92	20.4	136
All studies				>202 ± 10		694 ± 235	12.1 ± 2.0	82 ± 1	18.4 ± 2.4	111 ± 6
				158 ± 8		**336 ± 88**	**13.5 ± 3.5**	**89 ± 7**	**12.8 ± 0.4**	**115 ± 5**

Abbreviations: Abd = abdominals; Fem = femoralis; Glut = gluteus; HG = homogenates; HR = heparin releasable; INS = insulin; Met = metformin; Sulf = sulfonylureas; Vastus = vastus lateralis.

Postheparin Lipases

	ATLPL				SMLPL				
Site	Assay	(μmol/g/h)	(% Control)	Site	Assay	(μmol/g/h)	(% Control)	Comments	Ref
								Total lipase	89
								Total lipase	107
—	HR	4.5	70						108
—	**HR**	**4.3**	**45**					**HR/106 cells**	**109**
								Total lipase **Rx (2 mo)** **Rx (6 mo)**	110
Glut	HR	1.0	37					HR/106 cells	111
	HG	0.8	67						
	HR	**3.5**	**130**					**INS (10–12 wk)**	
	HG	1.6	133						
									75
Abd	HR	90	47						112
	HG	105	61						
	HG	50	28					Before INS	
	HG	**140**	**80**					**After INS**	
Glut	HR	114	56	Vastus	HR	0.6	71		113
	HR	33.4	70		HR	0.5	80		
									114
									115
Fem	HR	6.6	50						116
		9	68						
								Early phase **Rx (1 mo)** **Rx (3 mo)** Late phase **Rx (1 mo)** **Rx (3 mo)**	117
Abd	HR	9.5		vastus	HR	2.3			93
		6.1				1.1			
		11.9				2.5			
								Increased HDL Normal HDL Decreased HDL	118
Abd	HR	5.8	95	Vastus	HR	1.9	135		119
	HR	5.7							**120**
	HG	12							
	HR	**96**							
	HG	**63**							
	HR	**2.9**	**24**						
	HR	**2.3**	**19**						
									121
	HR		54 ± 7				95 ± 20	No INS	
	HG		**52 ± 12**					**INS**	

Table 5.9 Lipases in Diabetes Mellitus

	Postheparin Lipases		Homogenates			
	LPL	HTGL	HTGL	ATLPL	SMLPL	CMLPL
Animals	NC	↓	—	↓	± ↓	± ↓
Humans						
IDDM	NC	NC	—	± ↓	± ↓	—
NIDDM	± ↓	NC	—	↓	NC	—

ATLPL and SMLPL fell during weight loss but, after maintenance of the reduced-obese state, SMLPL increased to baseline but ATLPL increased to levels above baseline. Although there were no significant correlations between ATLPL and plasma triglycerides or intravenous fat tolerance, SMLPL and intravenous fat tolerance related to triglyceride concentrations. For adipose tissue, these data are very similar to those reported for nondiabetic obese subjects before, during, and after weight reduction.[122] In the study of Pollare et al,[119] however, neither ATLPL nor SMLPL was lower in untreated non-insulin-dependent diabetics than in nondiabetic obese controls.

Overall, NIDDM most often, but not always, is associated with decreases in postheparin LPL and ATLPL, with minimal reductions in postheparin LPL and normal SMLPL. Both postheparin LPL and ATLPL increase with improved glycemia. When non-insulin-dependent diabetes is well managed, and other conditions known to alter the lipases are absent, the entire lipolytic system appears to function normally.

Summary

Uncontrolled diabetes mellitus in animals and humans can variably reduce LPL in postheparin plasma, adipose tissue, skeletal muscle, and cardiac muscle. However, the predominant effect is in the adipose tissue (Table 5.9). The response to the treatment of hyperglycemia is predictable but may be slower in humans than animals. Ultimately, normal or even elevated levels of ATLPL and postheparin LPL result. Elevated levels could be a consequence of systemic hyperinsulinemia. In animals but not humans, HTGL is reduced, a modest metabolic abnormality corrected by insulin administration. Although reduction in the lipases may contribute to the hypertriglyceridemia of diabetes, overproduction of VLDL probably occurs earlier and is a more consistent pathophysiologic mechanism.

References

1. Wion KL, Kirchgessner TG, Lusis AJ, et al: Human lipoprotein lipase complementary DNA sequence. *Science* 1987;235:1638–1641.
2. Winkler FK, D'Arcy A, Hunziker W: Structure of human pancreatic lipase. *Nature* 1990;343:771–774.

3. Hahn PF: Abolishment of alimentary lipemia following injection of heparin. *Science* 1943;98:19–20.

4. Korn ED, Quigley TW, Quigley N Jr: Studies of lipoprotein lipase of rat heart and adipose tissue. *Biochim Biophys Acta* 1955;18:143–145.

5. Eckel RH: Lipoprotein lipase. A multifunctional enzyme relevant to common metabolic diseases. *N Engl J Med* 1989;320:1060–1068.

6. Goldberg IJ, Le N-A, Ginsberg HN, et al: Lipoprotein metabolism during the acute inhibition of lipoprotein lipase in the cynomolgus monkey. *J Clin Invest* 1988;81: 561–568.

7. Quinn DK, Shirai K, Jackson RL: Lipoprotein lipase: Mechanism of action and role in lipoprotein metabolism. *Prog Lipid Res* 1983;22:35–78.

8. Bengtsson G, Olivecrona T, Hook M, et al: Interaction of lipoprotein lipase with native and modified heparin-like polysaccharides. *Biochem J* 1980;189:625–633.

9. Wallinder L, Bengtsson T, Olivecrona T: Rapid removal to the liver of intravenously injected lipoprotein lipase. *Biochim Biophys Acta* 1977;575:166–173.

10. Bensadoun A: Lipoprotein lipase. *Annu Rev Nutr* 1991;11:217–237.

11. Ben-Zeev O, Doolittle MH, Davis RC, et al: Maturation of lipoprotein lipase: Expression of full catalytic activity requires glucose trimming but not translocation to the *cis*-Golgi compartment. *J Biol Chem* 1992;267:6219–6227.

12. Garfinkel AS, Kempner ES, Ben-Zeev O, et al: Lipoprotein lipase: Size of the functional unit determined by radiation inactivation. *J Lipid Res* 1983;24:775–780.

13. Osborne JC Jr, Bengtsson-Olivecrona G, Lee NS, et al: Studies on inactivation of lipoprotein lipase. Role of the dimer to monomer dissociation. *Biochemistry* 1985; 24:5606–5611.

14. Hatanaka A, Tanishita H, Ishibashi-Ueda H, et al: Hyperlipidemia in mast cell-deficient W/W^v mice. *Biochim Biophys Acta* 1986;878:440–445.

15. Blanchette-Mackie EJ, Masuno H, Dwyer NK, et al: Lipoprotein lipase in myocytes and capillary endothelium of heart: Immunocytochemical study. *Am J Physiol* 1989; 256:E818–E828.

16. Saxena V, Witte LD, Goldberg IJ: Release of endothelial cell lipoprotein lipase by plasma lipoproteins and free fatty acids. *J Biol Chem* 1989;264:4349–4355.

17. Goldberg IJ, Kandel JJ, Blum CB, et al: Association of plasma lipoproteins with postheparin lipase activities. *J Clin Invest* 1986;78:1523–1528.

18. Glaser DS, Yost TJ, Eckel RH: Preheparin lipoprotein lipolytic activities: Relationship to plasma lipoproteins and postheparin lipolytic activities. *J Lipid Res* 1992;33:209–214.

19. Vilaro S, Camps L, Reina M, et al: Localization of lipoprotein lipase to discrete areas of the guinea pig brain. *Brain Res* 1990;506:249–253.

20. Hixenbaugh EA, Sullivan TR, Strauss JF, et al: Hepatic lipase in the rat ovary. Ovaries cannot synthesize hepatic lipase but accumulate it from the circulation. *J Biol Chem* 1989;264:4222–4230.

21. Jansen H, De Greef WJ: Heparin-releasable lipase activity of rat adrenals, ovaries and testes. *Biochem J* 1981;196:739–745.

22. Verhoeven AJN, Jansen H: Secretion of liver lipase activity by periportal and perivenous hepatocytes. *Biochim Biophys Acta* 1989;1001:239–242.

23. Stahnke G, Sprengel R, Augustin J, et al: Human hepatic triglyceride lipase: cDNA cloning, amino acid sequence and expression in a cultured cell line. *Differentiation* 1987;35:45–52.

24. Jackson RL, McLean LR: Human postheparin plasma lipoprotein lipase and hepatic triglyceride lipase. *Methods Enzymol* 1991;197:339–345.

25. Kuusi T, Nikkila EA, Virtanen I, et al: Localization of the heparin-releasable lipase *in situ* in the rat liver. *Biochem J* 1979;181:245–246.

26. Sultan F, Lagrange D, Jansen H, et al: Inhibition of hepatic lipase activity impairs chylomicron-remnant removal. *Biochim Biophys Acta* 1989;1042:150–152.

27. Rubinstein A, Gibson JC, Paterniti JR, et al: Effect of heparin-induced lipolysis on the distribution of apolipoprotein E and hepatic triglyceride lipase. *J Clin Invest* 1985;75:710–721.

28. Eckel RH: Adipose tissue lipoprotein lipase, in Borensztajn J (ed): *Lipoprotein Lipase*. Chicago, Evener, 1987, pp 79–132.

29. Brun L-D, Gagne C, Julien P, et al: Familial lipoprotein lipase activity deficiency: Study of total body fatness and subcutaneous fat tissue distribution. *Metabolism* 1989;38:1005–1009.

30. Borensztajn J: Heart and skeletal muscle lipoprotein lipase, in Borensztajn J (ed): *Lipoprotein Lipase*. Chicago, Evener, 1987, pp 133–148.

31. Cryer A. Comparative biochemistry and physiology of lipoprotein lipase, in Borensztajn J (ed): *Lipoprotein Lipase*. Chicago, Evener, 1987, pp 277–328.

32. Sadur CN, Eckel RH: Insulin stimulation of adipose tissue lipoprotein lipase: Use of the euglycemic clamp technique. *J Clin Invest* 1982;69:1119–1125.

33. Farese RV Jr, Yost TJ, Eckel RH: Tissue-specific regulation of lipoprotein lipase activity by insulin in normal weight subjects. *Metabolism* 1991;40:214–216.

34. Kiens V, Lithell H, Mikines KJ, et al: Effects of insulin and exercise on muscle lipoprotein lipase activity in man and its relation to insulin action. *J Clin Invest* 1989; 84:1124–1129.

35. Sadur CN, Yost TJ, Eckel RH: Fat feeding decreases insulin responsiveness of adipose tissue lipoprotein lipase. *Metabolism* 1984;33:1043–1047.

36. Ong JM, Kirchgessner TG, Schotz MC, et al: Insulin increases the synthetic rate and mRNA level of lipoprotein lipase in isolated rat adipocytes. *J Biol Chem* 1988;2623: 12933–12938.

37. Raynolds MV, Awald PD, Gordon DF, et al: Lipoprotein lipase gene expression in rat adipocytes is regulated by isoproterenol and insulin through different mechanisms. *Mol Endocrinol* 1990;4:1416–1422.

38. Dani C, Bertrand B, Bardon S, et al: Regulation of gene expression by insulin in adipose cells: Opposite effects on adipsin and glycerophosphate dehydrogenase genes. *Mol Cell Endocrinol* 1989;63:199–208.

39. Eckel RH, Fujimoto WY, Brunzell JD: Insulin regulation of lipoprotein lipase in cultured 3T3-L1 cells. *Biochem Biophys Res Commun* 1978;84:1069–1075.

40. Chan BL, Lisanti MP, Rodriguez-Boulan E, et al: Insulin-stimulated release of lipoprotein lipase by metabolism of its phosphatidylinositol anchor. *Science* 1988;241: 1670–1672.

41. Ong JA, Kern PA: The role of glucose and glycosylation in the regulation of lipoprotein lipase synthesis and secretion in rat adipocytes. *J Biol Chem* 1989;264:3177–3182.

42. O'Looney P, Maten MV, Vahouny GV: Insulin-mediated modifications of myocardial lipoprotein lipase and lipoprotein metabolism. *J Biol Chem* 1983;258:12994–13002.

43. Braun JEA, Severson DL: Diabetes reduces heparin- and phopholipase C-releasable lipoprotein lipase from cardiomyocytes. *Am J Physiol* 1991;260:E477–E485.

44. Braun JEA, Severson DL: Lipoprotein lipase release from cardiac myocytes is increased by decavanadate but not insulin. *Am J Physiol* 1992;262:E663–E670.

45. Raynolds MV, Jensen DR, Eckel RH: C2 skeletal myoblasts: A new model for studying regulation of muscle-specific lipoprotein lipase gene expression [abstract #1777]. The Endocrine Society Program and Abstracts, 1991, p 475.

46. Murase T, Inoue S: Hepatic triglyceride lipase is not an insulin-dependent enzyme in rats. *Metabolism* 1985;34:531–534.

47. Knauer TE, Woods JA, Lamb RG, et al: Hepatic triacylglycerol lipase activities after induction of diabetes and administration of insulin or glucagon. *J Lipid Res* 1982; 23:631–637.

48. Busch SJ, Barnhart RL, Martin GA, et al: Differential regulation of hepatic triglyceride lipase and 3-hydroxy-3-methylglutaryl-CoA reductase gene expression in a human hepatoma cell line, Hep G2. *J Biol Chem* 1990;265:22474–22479.

49. Yoon TH, Yamada N, Ishibashi S, et al: The release of hepatic triglyceride lipase from rat monolayered hepatocytes in primary culture. *Endocrinol Jpn* 1990;37:437–442.

50. Reardon MF, Sakai H, Steiner G: Roles of lipoprotein lipase and hepatic triglyceride lipase in the catabolism *in vivo* of triglyceride-rich lipoproteins. *Arteriosclerosis* 1982;2:396–402.

51. Rebuffe-Scrive M, Andersson B, Olbe L, et al: Metabolism of adipose tissue in intraabdominal depots of non-obese men and women. *Metabolism* 1989;38:453–458.

52. O'Looney PA, Vahouny GV: Diabetes and lipoprotein lipase activity, in Borensztajn J (ed): *Lipoprotein Lipase.* Chicago, Evener, 1987, pp 229–246.

53. Kessler JI: Effect of insulin on release of plasma lipolytic activity and clearing of emulsified fat intravenously administered to pancreatectomized and alloxanized dogs. *J Lab Clin Med* 1962;60:747–755.

54. Brown DF, Olivecrona T: The effect of glucose availability and utilization on chylomicron metabolism in the rat. *Acta Physiol Scand* 1966;66:9–18.

55. Brown DF, Daudiss K, Durrant J: Triglyceride metabolism in the alloxan-diabetic rat. *Diabetes* 1967;16:90–95.

56. Linder C, Chernick SS, Fleck TR, et al: Lipoprotein lipase and uptake of chylomicron triglyceride by skeletal muscle of rats. *Am J Physiol* 1976;231:860–864.

57. Redgrave TG, Snibson DA: Clearance of chylomicron triacylglycerol and cholesteryl ester from the plasma of streptozotocin-induced diabetic and hypercholesterolemic hypothyroid rats. *Metabolism* 1977;26:493–500.

58. Van Tol A: Hyprtriglyceridemia in the diabetic rat. Defective removal of serum very-low-density lipoprotein. *Atherosclerosis* 1977;26:117–128.

59. Bar-On H, Chen Y-DI, Reaven GM: Evidence for a new cause of defective plasma removal of very-low-density lipoproteins in insulin-deficient rats. *Diabetes* 1981;30:496–499.

60. Bar-On H, Levy E, Oschry Y, et al: Removal of defective very-low-density lipoproteins from diabetic rats. *Biochim Biophys Acta* 1984;793:115–118.

61. Minnich A, Zilversmit DB: Impaired triacylglycerol catabolism in hypertriglyceridemia of the diabetic, cholesterol-fed rabbit: A possible mechanism for protection from atherosclerosis. *Biochim Biophys Acta* 1989;1002:324–332.

62. Basso LV, Havel RJ: Hepatic metabolism of free fatty acids in normal and diabetic dogs. *J Clin Invest* 1970;49:537–547.

63. Redgrave TG, Callow MJ: The effect of insulin deficiency on the metabolism of lipid emulsion models of triacylglycerol-rich lipoproteins in rats. *Metabolism* 1990;39:1–10.

64. Aktin E, Meng HC: Release of clearing factor lipase (lipoprotein lipase) *in vivo* and from isolated perfused heart of alloxan diabetic rats. *Diabetes* 1972;21:149–156.

65. Elkeles RS, Williams E: Post-heparin lipolytic activity and tissue lipoprotein lipase activity in the alloxan-diabetic rat. *Clin Sci Mol Med* 1974;46:661–664.

66. Jansen H, Hulsmann WC: On hepatic and extra hepatic postheparin serum lipase activities and the influence of experimental hypercortisolism, and diabetes on these activities. *Biochim Biophys Acta* 1975;398:337–346.

67. Nakai P, Yamada S, Tamai T, et al: The effects of streptozotocin diabetes on hepatic triglyceride lipase activity in the rat. *Metabolism* 1979;28:30–40.

68. Muller DL, Saudek CD, Applebaum-Bowden D: Hepatic triglyceride lipase in diabetic dogs. *Metabolism* 1985;34:251–254.

69. Elkeles RS, Hambley J: The effects of fasting and streptozotocin diabetes on hepatic triglyceride lipase activity in the rat. *Diabetes* 1977;26:58–60.

70. Stam H, Schoonderwoerd K, Breeman W, et al: Effects of hormones, fasting and diabetes on triglyceride lipase activities in rat heart and liver. *Horm Metab Res* 1984;16:293–297.

71. Nomur T, Hagino Y, Gotoh M, et al: The effects of streptozotocin diabetes on tissue-specific lipase activities of the rat. *Lipids* 1984;19:594–599.

72. Wilson DE, Zeikus R, Chan I-F: Relationship of organ lipoprotein lipase activity and ketonuria to hypertriglyceridemia in starved and streptozotocin-induced diabetic rats. *Diabetes* 1987;36:485–490.

73. Schnatz JD, Williams RH: The effect of acute insulin deficiency in the rat on adipose tissue lipolytic activity and plasma lipids. *Diabetes* 1963;12:174–178.

74. Borensztajn J, Samols DR, Rubenstein AH: Effects of insulin on lipoprotein lipase activity in the rat heart and adipose tissue. *Am J Physiol* 1972;223:1271–1275.

75. Chen Y-DI, Risser TR, Cully M, et al: Is the hypertriglyceridemia associated with insulin deficiency caused by decreased lipoprotein lipase activity? *Diabetes* 1979; 28:893–898.

76. Rauramaa R, Kuusela P, Hietanen E: Adipose, muscle and lung tissue lipoprotein lipase activities in young streptozotocin treated rats. *Horm Metab Res* 1980;12:591–595.

77. Chen Y-DI, Howard J, Huang V, et al: Disassociation between plasma triglyceride concentration and tissue lipoprotein lipase deficiency in insulin-deficient rats. *Diabetes* 1980;29:643–647.

78. Ishikawa A, Murase T, Yamada N, et al: Lipoprotein lipase activity in adipose tissue of streptozotocin-induced diabetic rats. *Endocrinol Jpn* 1982;29:379–381.

79. Tan MH, Bonen A, Garner JB, et al: Physical training in diabetic rats: Effect on glucose tolerance and serum lipids. *J Appl Physiol* 1982;52:1514–1518.

80. Dall'Aglio E, Chang F, Chang H, et al: Effect of exercise and diet on triglyceride metabolism in rats with moderate insulin deficiency. *Diabetes* 1983;32:46–50.

81. Hansen FM, Nilsson P, Hustvedt BE, et al: Significance of hyperinsulinemia in ventromedial hypothalamus-lesioned rats. *Am J Physiol* 1983;244:E203–E208.

82. Gavin LA, McMahon F, Moeller M: Modulation of adipose lipoprotein lipase by thyroid hormone in diabetes. The significance of the low T3 state. *Diabetes* 1985;34:1266–1271.

83. Gavin LA, Cavalieri RR, Moeller M, et al: Brain lipoprotein lipase is responsive to nutritional and hormonal modulation. *Metabolism* 1987;36:919–924.

84. Behr SR, Kraemer FB: Insulin deficiency decreases lipoprotein lipase secretion by murine macrophages. *Diabetes* 1988;37:1076–1081.

85. Feingold KR, Soued M, Staprans I, et al: Effect of tumor necrosis factor (TNF) on lipid metabolism in the diabetic rat. Evidence that inhibition of adipose tissue lipoprotein lipase activity is not required for TNF-induced hyperlipidemia. *J Clin Invest* 1989;83:1116–1121.

86. Deshaies Y, Geloen A, Paulin A, et al: Restoration of lipoprotein lipase activity in insulin-deficient rats by insulin infusion is tissue-specific. *Can J Physiol Pharmacol* 1991;69:746–751.

87. Ramirez I, Severson DL: Effect of diabetes on acid and neutral triacylglycerol lipase and on lipoprotein lipase activities in isolated myocardial cells from rat heart. *Biochem J* 1986;238:233–238.

88. Rodrigues B, Braun JEA, Spooner M, et al: Regulation of lipoprotein lipase activity in control and diabetic rat hearts by plasma lipids. *Am J Physiol* 1992;262:E216–E223.

89. Porte D Jr, Bierman EL: The effect of heparin infusion on plasma triglyceride *in vivo* and *in vitro* with a method for calculating triglyceride turnover. *J Lab Clin Med* 1969; 73:631–648.

90. Bagdade JD, Porte D Jr, Bierman EL: Acute insulin withdrawal and the regulation of plasma triglyceride removal in diabetic subjects. *Diabetes* 1968;17:127–132.

91. Brunzell JD, Porte D Jr, Bierman EL: Abnormal lipoprotein-lipase-mediated plasma triglyceride removal in untreated diabetes mellitus associated with hypertriglyceridemia. *Metabolism* 1979;28:901–907.

92. Haffner SM, Foster DM, Kushwaha RS, et al: Retarded chylomicron apolipoprotein-B catabolism in type II (non-insulin-dependent) diabetic subjects with lipaemia. *Diabetologia* 1984;26:349–354.

93. Vessby B, Selinus I, Lithell H: Serum lipoproteins and lipoprotein lipase in overweight, type II diabetics during and after supplemented fasting. *Arteriosclerosis* 1985; 5:93–100.

94. Georgopoulos A, Phair RD: Abnormal clearance of postprandial Sf100-400 plasma lipoproteins in insulin-dependent diabetes mellitus. *J Lipid Res* 1991;32:1133–1142.

95. Wilson DE, Schreibman PH, Arky RA: Post-heparin lipolytic activity in diabetic patients with a history of mixed hyperlipemia. Relative rates against artificial substrates and human chylomicrons. *Diabetes* 1969;18:563–566.

96. Nikkila EA, Huttunen JK, Ehnholm C: Postheparin plasma lipoprotein lipase and hepatic lipase in diabetes mellitus. Relationship to plasma triglyceride metabolism. *Diabetes* 1977;26:11–21.

97. Nikkila EA, Hormila P: Serum lipids and lipoproteins in insulin-treated diabetes. Demonstration of increased high density lipoprotein concentrations. *Diabetes* 1978; 27:1078–1086.

98. Rubba P, Capaldo B, Falanga A, et al: Plasma lipoproteins and lipoprotein lipase in young diabetics with and without ketonuria. *J Endocrinol Invest* 1985;8:433–436.

99. Eckel RH, Goldberg IJ, Steiner L, et al: Plasma lipolytic activity. Relationship to postheparin lipolytic activity and evidence for metabolic regulation. *Diabetes* 1988; 37:610–615.

100. Dunn FL, Thompson MJ, Eckel RH, et al: Intraperitoneal insulin therapy in IDDM normalizes very low density lipoprotein composition independent of improved glycemic control [abstract]. *Diabetes* 1992;41:26A.

101. Bagdade J, Ritter M, Eckel M, et al: Insulin therapy pathologically alters cholesteryl ester transfer (CET) in insulin-dependent diabetes mellitus (IDDM) [abstract]. *Clin Res* 1992;40:208A.

102. Taskinen M-R, Nikkila EA: Lipoprotein lipase activity of adipose tissue and skeletal muscle in insulin-deficient human diabetes. Relation to high-density and very-low-density lipoproteins in response to treatment. *Diabetologia* 1979;17:351–356.

103. Taskinen M-R, Nikkila EA, Nousianen R, et al: Lipoprotein lipase activity in adipose tissue and skeletal muscle of human diabetics during insulin deprivation and restoration. *Scand J Clin Lab Invest* 1981;41:263–268.

104. Taskinen M-R, Nikkila EA, Ollus O: Serum lipids and lipoproteins in insulin-dependent diabetic subjects during high-carbohydrate, high-fiber diet. *Diabetes Care* 1983; 6:224–230.

105. Lithell H, Jacobs I, Vessby B, et al: Decrease of lipoprotein lipase activity in skeletal muscle in man during a short-term carbohydrate-rich dietary regime: With special reference to HDL cholesterol, apolipoprotein and insulin concentrations. *Metabolism* 1982;31:994–998.

106. Costill DL, Cleary P, Fink WJ, et al: Training adaptations in skeletal muscle of juvenile diabetics. *Diabetes* 1979;28:818–822.

107. Bagdade JD, Porte D Jr, Bierman EL: Diabetic lipaemia. A form of acquired fat-induced lipaemia. *N Engl J Med* 1967;276:427–433.

108. Persson B: Lipoprotein lipase activity of human adipose tissue in health and in some diseases with hyperlipidemia as a common feature. *Acta Med Scand* 1973;193:457–462.

109. Guy-Grand B, Bigorie B: Effect of fat cell size, restrictive diet and diabetes on lipoprotein lipase released by human adipose tissue. *Horm Metab Res* 1975;7:471–475.

110. Brunzell JD, Porte D Jr, Bierman EL: Reversible abnormalities in postheparin lipolytic activity during the late phase of release in diabetes mellitus (postheparin lipolytic activity in diabetes). *Metabolism* 1975;24:1123–1137.

111. Pykalisto OJ, Smith PH, Brunzell JD: Determinants of human adipose tissue lipoprotein lipase. The effect of diabetes and obesity on basal- and diet-induced activity. *J Clin Invest* 1975;56:1108–1117.

112. Taylor KG, Galton DJ, Holdsworth G: Insulin-independent diabetes: A defect in the activity of lipoprotein lipase in adipose tissue. *Diabetologia* 1979;16:313–317.

113. Taskinen M-R, Nikkila EA, Kuusi T, et al: Lipoprotein lipase activity and serum lipoproteins in untreated type II (insulin-independent) diabetes associated with obesity. *Diabetologia* 1982;22:46–50.

114. Agardh C-D, Nilsson-Ehle P, Schersten B: Improvement of the plasma lipoprotein pattern after institution of insulin treatment in diabetes mellitus. *Diabetes Care* 1982; 5:322–325.

115. Agardh C-D, Sartor G, Nilsson-Ehle P: Plasma high density lipoproteins and lipolytic enzyme activities in diabetic patients. *Acta Med Scand* 1983;213:123–128.

116. Arner P, Bolinder J, Engfeldt P, et al: The relationship between the basal lipolytic and lipoprotein lipase activities in human adipose tissue. *Int J Obesity* 1983;7:167–172.

117. Pfeifer MA, Brunzell JD, Best JD, et al: The response of plasma triglyceride, cholesterol, and lipoprotein lipase to treatment in non-insulin-dependent diabetic subjects without familial hypertriglyceridemia. *Diabetes* 1983;32:525–531.

118. Kasim SE, Tseng K, Jen K-LC, et al: Significance of hepatic triglyceride lipase activity in the regulation of serum high density lipoproteins in type II diabetes mellitus. *J Clin Endocrinol Metab* 1987;65:183–187.

119. Pollare T, Vessby B, Lithell H: Lipoprotein lipase activity in skeletal muscle is related to insulin sensitivity. *Arterioscler Thromb* 1991;11:1192–1203.

120. Simsolo RB, Ong JM, Saffari B, et al: Effect of improved diabetes control on the expression of lipoprotein lipase in human adipose tissue. *J Lipid Res* 1992;33:89–96.

121. Lewis GF, O'Meara NM, Soltys PA, et al: Fasting hypertriglyceridemia in non-insulin-dependent diabetes mellitus is an important predictor of postprandial lipid and lipoprotein abnormalities. *J Clin Endocrinol Metab* 1991;72:934–944.

122. Eckel RH, Yost TJ: Weight reduction increases adipose tissue lipoprotein lipase responsiveness in obese women. *J Clin Invest* 1987;80:992–997.

Chapter 6

Reverse Cholesterol Transport, Lecithin:Cholesterol Acyltransferase, and Cholesteryl Ester Transfer in Insulin-Dependent and Non-Insulin-Dependent Diabetes Mellitus

Christopher J. Fielding, PhD

Reverse cholesterol transport is the pathway by which cholesterol in peripheral tissues is returned through the plasma to the liver for catabolism or recycling. Because of the potential of this pathway to limit or reverse an accumulation of cholesterol in the vascular bed, its regulation has been studied not only in healthy individuals, but also in those with a genetic or acquired increased risk of atherosclerotic vascular disease.

Those with diabetes mellitus make up the most numerous group at high risk for macrovascular disease.[1-3] Both insulin-dependent (IDDM; type I) and non-insulin-dependent (NIDDM; type II) diabetics show an increased incidence of coronary and other macrovascular disease compared to the population at large. In type I diabetes the increased risk of coronary artery disease (CAD) is to a significant extent (although not totally) the consequence of impaired renal function. Indeed, in one study insulin-dependent diabetics with renal failure had an estimated 15-fold greater risk of CAD than a comparable IDDM group with normal renal function.[3] Nondiabetic patients with end-stage renal disease are also at high risk of CAD.

The pattern of plasma lipoproteins found in type II diabetics, and type I diabetics after the development of renal failure, is strikingly similar to that found in nondiabetics (including those with renal failure unrelated to diabetes)[4-6] who share an increased risk of atherosclerotic vascular disease (Figure 6.1). It features a decreased ratio of cholesterol mass in high-density lipoprotein (HDL) compared to that in low-density lipoprotein (LDL). The link between insulin deficiency, these lipoprotein abnormalities, and atherosclerosis continues to

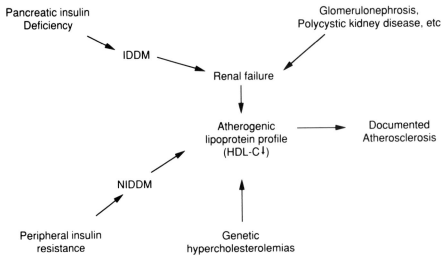

Figure 6.1 Hierarchy of consequences associated with the development of atherosclerosis in NIDDM and IDDM.

arouse interest, although the literature on plasma cholesterol metabolism in diabetes is scattered. It is the purpose of the present chapter to bring together recent research in this area, and to attempt a broad synthesis that may link metabolic defects in individual steps of the reverse cholesterol transport pathway to the accumulation of cholesterol in the vessel wall that is found in many diabetics.

The vessel wall synthesizes little of its own cholesterol.[7] Its cholesterol content represents mainly a balance between cholesterol delivered and removed by different lipoproteins. Atherosclerotic macrovascular disease is commonly considered to result from an increased delivery of lipids, particularly via LDL, to the vascular bed. In the population at large, the risk of atherosclerosis is indeed correlated to the circulating concentration of LDL.[8,9] However, may diabetics are not hypercholesterolemic and do not have increased levels of LDL, yet still develop coronary atherosclerosis at a rate much greater than that of the population at large.[10] Atherogenesis could also result if the return of cholesterol from the periphery (including the vascular bed) to the liver was reduced. The reverse transport of cholesterol most intimately involves the HDL in plasma.[11] Additionally, low HDL levels appear as a strong independent risk factor for the development of atherosclerosis.[12–14] Could the increase in macrovascular disease associated with diabetes mellitus be a direct result, at least in part, of low HDL levels and decreased effectiveness of the reverse cholesterol transport pathway?

Reverse Cholesterol Transport in Normal Subjects

The transport and metabolism of cholesterol in human plasma can be considered as four sequential metabolic steps[15] (Figure 6.2).

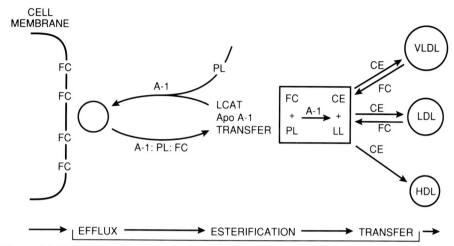

Figure 6.2 The reverse cholesterol transport pathway. CE = cholesteryl ester; FC = free cholesterol; LL = lysolecithin; PL = phospholipid. *(Reprinted, by permission, from Fielding PE, Fielding CJ: in Vance DE, Vance J (eds): Biochemistry of Lipids, Lipoproteins and Membranes. Amsterdam, Elsevier, 1991, pp 427–459.)*

Step 1: Cell-to-Plasma Cholesterol Transport

Animal and human studies in vivo demonstrate the continuous transport of peripheral cell cholesterol to the plasma.[16–18] In human subjects, net cholesterol transport into plasma has been measured in the presence of vascular cells or fibroblasts.[19–21]

Several independent studies have confirmed that the main factor promoting the net transport of free cholesterol from cell membranes to plasma is the HDL fraction of plasma.[22] The HDL fraction is highly heterogeneous, and all HDL species are not alike in their ability to promote cholesterol transport. HDLs containing apolipoprotein A-I but not apolipoprotein A-II are more effective than those containing both apolipoproteins.[19,23,24] Further subfractionation of apo A-I–only HDL by density gradient electrophoresis indicates a special role for a minor fraction of HDL of low molecular weight that has anomalous pre-β electrophoretic migration during electrophoresis (in contrast to the α migration rate of most of HDL).[25,26]

Two mechanisms have been suggested for the special activity of small pre-β HDL in reverse cholesterol transport. The first would involve specific binding of this HDL to the cell surface. A candidate HDL receptor protein with a molecular mass of about 100 kDa has been characterized,[27,28] although its structure has not yet been reported. The second mechanism would depend on the physical properties of the small HDL itself—for example, a greater diffusibility, or an increased ability to bind free cholesterol.[29] Further research is still needed to distinguish the contributions made by these two processes.

Step 2: Esterification of Cholesterol by Lecithin:Cholesterol Acyltransferase

Lecithin:cholesterol acyltransferase (LCAT) catalyzes the transesterification of lecithin and free cholesterol of HDL, resulting in the synthesis of cholesteryl ester and lysolecithin.[15] Cholesteryl ester is insoluble, unlike free cholesterol, which is readily diffusible. Because of this change, the continuing action of LCAT can drive a concentration gradient of free cholesterol between the cell membrane and HDL in the extracellular space or plasma, because the cholesteryl ester formed in the plasma becomes sequestered in the core of the acceptor lipoproteins.

All of the free cholesterol that contributes to the substrate pool of LCAT is not from peripheral cell membranes. Some is secreted as part of the triglyceride-rich very-low-density lipoproteins (VLDLs) and their product, LDL, and is then transferred to HDL for esterification by LCAT (Figure 6.2). Studies of cholesterol balance in whole plasma indicate that LDL contributes most of the lipoprotein free cholesterol esterified by LCAT.[30,31] The relative contributions of cell membranes and LDL under physiologic conditions depend mainly on the proportions of cholesterol in each pool locally, which will be a function of vessel diameter, among other factors. Estimates based on the cholesterol content of endothelial cells and plasma lipoproteins in small vessels suggest that about half of free cholesterol for LCAT activity may normally originate in each under these conditions.[20]

Only the cholesterol that originates from peripheral cells contributes to reverse cholesterol transport. The part of plasma total cholesterol that is secreted from the liver in lipoprotein form, retained in the plasma for esterification, and then returned to the liver for catabolism or recycling does not add to the magnitude of the reverse cholesterol transport pathway.

Step 3: Cholesteryl Ester Transfer Protein Activity

Cholesteryl ester transfer protein (CETP) catalyzes the exchange of cholesteryl esters, triglycerides, or other neutral lipids between all plasma lipoprotein classes.[15] Between two lipoproteins with similar composition of neutral lipids (eg, two HDLs of the same subclass), CETP will promote nonproductive exchange. Between lipoproteins with significantly different compositions, CETP will catalyze a net transfer of cholesteryl ester and triglyceride, with each lipid moving down its own concentration gradient. In normal plasma, net transfer of cholesteryl esters is from HDL to VLDL and LDL. When LCAT and CETP activities have been compared in the same plasma, CETP activity is considerably less than that of LCAT, in both fasting and postprandial plasma.[32,33] Thus cholesteryl ester transfer is not an obligatory step in reverse cholesterol transport, and the majority of cholesteryl ester synthesized by LCAT often remains in HDL.

Two considerations determine the extent to which CETP in plasma promotes net transfer—that is, the exchange of cholesteryl ester for triglyceride. First, the relative proportions of different lipoproteins present in plasma will determine to what extent CETP acts to catalyze the exchange of lipids within the same class of particles (eg, between one HDL and another). Second, the ratio of cholesteryl ester and triglycerides in an individual lipoprotein particle will determine what proportion of total exchange represents a net transfer.[34] For example, if VLDL is secreted already enriched in cholesteryl ester, the net transfer of cholesteryl ester from HDL to VLDL will decrease because a higher proportion of CETP will be involved in the nonproductive exchange of cholesteryl ester for cholesteryl ester between VLDL and other lipoproteins, and a lesser proportion in the exchange of cholesteryl ester for triglyceride—even if the mass of CETP in plasma remains unchanged or is even increased. Under some conditions the transfer promoted by CETP can even become reversed.[35] In this case CETP catalyzes net transfer of cholesteryl ester from VLDL to HDL, rather than the reverse. In human plasma the major part of CETP activity involves the non-productive exchange of lipids of like kind between different lipoprotein particles, and a smaller proportion results in "net" transfer. This proportion cannot be predicted from the circulating mass of CETP, because it depends only on the properties of the donor and acceptor particles.

Step 4: Clearance of Lipoprotein Cholesterol by the Liver

Steps 1 through 3 lead to the accumulation of LCAT-derived cholesteryl ester in HDL and LDL. The proportion of LCAT-derived cholesteryl ester transferred to LDL or retained in HDL varies considerably and depends on the source of the free cholesterol involved.[36] Transfer of cholesteryl ester derived from cellular free cholesterol to LDL appears to be lower (about 10% of that synthesized) than when the free cholesterol originates in VLDL and LDL. This probably indicates that the former is localized in an HDL species that is a relatively poor substrate for CETP. When lipoprotein cholesterol is the source of the free cholesterol esterified by LCAT, 25% to 60% of the cholesteryl esters formed can be recovered in VLDL and LDL.

The mechanism of removal of cholesteryl ester from plasma depends on the type of lipoprotein in which it is contained. LDL is removed mainly via hepatic LDL (apo B, apo E) receptors. In hypercholesterolemia, receptor-independent pathways assume major importance. Some cholesteryl ester may be removed independently of the endocytosis of the intact lipoprotein. In the case of HDL, most of the removal of cholesteryl ester appears to take place without the uptake of the intact lipoprotein.[37] The mechanism of this selective uptake has not been fully elucidated, but appears to involve a direct interaction with the hepatocyte membrane. Some HDL may be removed via the LDL receptor mechanism, if it contains bound apo E. However, apo E–containing HDLs make up a negligible proportion of total HDL in human plasma,[15] and there is little evidence for a unique role for these particles in reverse cholesterol transport.

Reverse Cholesterol Transport in Diabetes Mellitus

Cell-to-Plasma Cholesterol Transport in Diabetes

Cholesterol net transport from standard monolayers of peripheral cells to plasma was found to be severely reduced in the plasma of untreated non-insulin-dependent diabetics, compared to that in plasma from normoglycemic controls (Figure 6.3). In the same study, plasma from insulin-dependent diabetics maintained by conventional insulin therapy, who had hyperglycemia and plasma lipid levels comparable to those in the NIDDM group, had a rate of cholesterol transport that was not significantly reduced from that measured in the plasma.[38]

In the type II (NIDDM) patients, this study also found an increase in cholesterol-rich VLDL containing apo E. When these particles were removed from plasma by anti–apo E immunoaffinity chromatography, cell-to-plasma cholesterol transport was normalized (Figure 6.4). The same procedure in normoglycemic plasma was without effect on transport rates.[38] These data suggest that

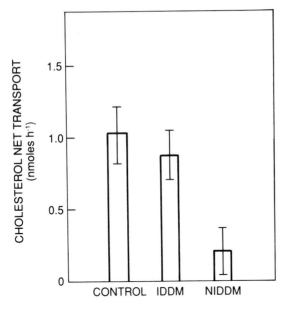

Figure 6.3 Rates of transport of free cholesterol from a cultured fibroblast monolayer to plasma. The plasma was diluted to 1.2% vol/vol before analysis to equalize the free cholesterol present in cell membranes and plasma. *(Reprinted, by permission, from Fielding CJ, Castro GR, Donner C, et al: Distribution of apolipoprotein E in the plasma of insulin-dependent and non-insulin dependent diabetes and its relation to cholesterol transport. J Lipid Res 1986;27:1052–1061.)*

the reduced net transport of cholesterol in the NIDDM subjects was mainly the result of an increased influx of free cholesterol from VLDL into the cells. NIDDM plasma is also characterized by an increase in the level of the apo A-I–only or pre-β HDLs, which promote cholesterol efflux in normal plasma.[39] It is unclear whether this increase is a secondary response to increased influx, or the pre-β HDL is itself poorly functional and a contributor to the reduced reverse cholesterol transport observed.

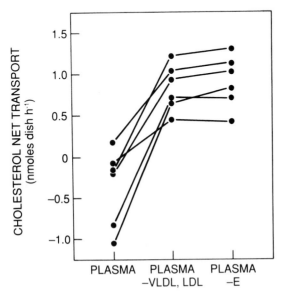

Figure 6.4 The effect of removing VLDL and LDL by heparin–agarose affinity chromatography, or of removing apolipoprotein E by immunoaffinity chromatography, on cholesterol net transport from a cultured fibroblast monolayer to diabetic or control plasma. Assay conditions were as described in the legend to Figure 6.3. *(Reprinted, by permission, from Fielding CJ, Castro GR, Donner C, et al: Distribution of apolipoprotein E in the plasma of insulin-dependent and non-insulin dependent diabetes and its relation to cholesterol transport. J Lipid Res 1986;27:1052–1061.)*

Table 6.1 Plasma LCAT Activity in NIDDM, IDDM, and Normoglycemic Plasma

| | | LCAT Rate (nmol/mL/h) | | |
	Treatment	Diabetic	Control	Ref.
NIDDM	Sulfonylurea	96 ± 7	88 ± 6	40
NIDDM	None	62 ± 9	81 ± 17	43
NIDDM	None	66 ± 23	61 ± 18	38
NIDDM	None	69 ± 12	88 ± 9	42
IDDM	Insulin[a]	67 ± 16	61 ± 18	38
IDDM	Insulin[b]	83 ± 7	82 ± 7	40

[a] Intensive insulin therapy.
[b] Conventional insulin therapy.

LCAT Activity in Diabetes Mellitus

Most studies have found rates of esterification of free cholesterol by LCAT in normoglycemic and diabetic plasma to be similar (Table 6.1). Type I diabetics with normal renal function had plasma LCAT activities within the normal range.[38] There appear to be no published data for type I patients with end-stage renal disease or nephrotic syndrome, although nondiabetic patients with either syndrome were found to have significantly decreased LCAT rates.[41,42] At least in the case of end-stage renal disease, this decrease in activity reflects a decreased circulating level of LCAT protein.[41] Untreated type II diabetics had plasma rates of cholesterol esterification that were normal or slightly (but not significantly) decreased.[38,43,44] Not surprisingly, these rates were unaffected by intensive insulin therapy.[44]

Because the total rate of utilization of plasma free cholesterol by LCAT was similar in NIDDM and normal plasma, but the utilization of cellular cholesterol (ie, reverse cholesterol transport) was decreased, the utilization of lipoprotein free cholesterol for esterification was increased in untreated NIDDM. This was normalized by intensive insulin therapy.

Cholesteryl Ester Transfer in Diabetes Mellitus

Abnormalities of cholesteryl ester net transfer have been reported in both IDDM and NIDDM. In IDDM patients with normal renal function and without clinical symptoms of vascular disease, cholesteryl ester transfer activity was normal in one study and increased in another[45] (Table 6.2). In studies of unidirectional isotopic transfer by CETP, presumably reflecting plasma CETP mass, activity in IDDM plasma was modestly (20%) increased.[46] The increase in isotopic transfer in this assay was greater in IDDM subjects who smoked.[47] In untreated NIDDM patients, cholesteryl ester net transfer rates were significantly reduced.[44,48] Intensive insulin therapy caused some increase in net transfer rates, although normalization was not achieved over 6 weeks.[44]

An increased proportion of free cholesterol in plasma lipoproteins, particularly LDL, is now a recognized characteristic of plasma in those subjects at increased risk of atherosclerotic vascular disease, including those with familial

Table 6.2 Cholesteryl Ester Net Transfer Rates in NIDDM, IDDM, and Normoglycemic Plasma

		Net Transfer (nmol/mL/h)		
	Treatment	Diabetic	Control	Ref.
NIDDM	None	1 ± 4	52 ± 15	44
NIDDM	None	8 ± 6	40 ± 12	48
IDDM	Insulin[a]	34 ± 6	40 ± 12	48
IDDM	Insulin[a]	30–90[b]	10–40[b]	45

[a] Conventional insulin therapy.

[b] Nonlinear kinetics. The range given is for the range of assay periods reported.

hypercholesterolemia,[49] end-stage renal disease,[41] and NIDDM.[48] In NIDDM, the free cholesterol content of both VLDL and LDL (expressed relative to phospholipid) is proportionately increased (Figure 6.5). The free cholesterol–phospholipid ratio of LDL was inversely correlated with the rate of cholesteryl ester transfer in IDDM, NIDDM, and normoglycemic subjects (Figure 6.6).

Although transfer rates did to some extent reflect the proportions of triglyceride and cholesteryl ester in LDL, this is only one of the factors determining net cholesteryl ester transfer rates in native plasma, as discussed above. Not surprisingly, the correlation between transfer rates and LDL triglyceride–cholesteryl ester mass ratio was much weaker than that between transfer rates and the ratio of free cholesterol and phospholipid (Figure 6.7).

The major part of LDL free cholesterol, as of other lipoproteins, is present in the surface monolayer.[50] In phospholipid films, the incorporation of free cho-

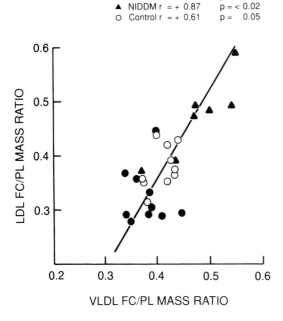

Figure 6.5 The free cholesterol–phospholipid (FC/PL) mass ratio in VLDL and LDL in IDDM, NIDDM, and normoglycemic control subjects. Lipoproteins were fractionated by heparin–agarose affinity chromatography, as described by Fielding et al.[44]

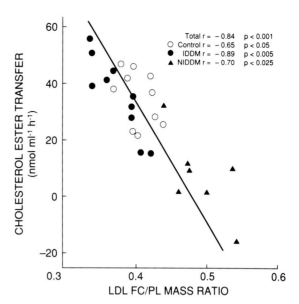

Figure 6.6 The relationship between cholesteryl ester transfer rates and LDL free cholesterol–phospholipid (FC/PL) mass ratio in the plasma of IDDM, NIDDM, and normoglycemic control subjects. *(Adapted from Fielding CJ, Reaven CM, Liu G, et al: Increased free cholesterol in plasma low and very low density lipoproteins in noninsulin-dependent diabetes mellitus: Its role in the inhibition of cholesteryl ester transfer. Proc Natl Acad Sci USA 1984;81:2512–2516.)*

lesterol increases rigidity and decreases permeability and exchange.[51,52] When the composition of VLDL and LDL from diabetic and normoglycemic subjects was plotted according to triangular coordinates, the surface monolayer of NIDDM LDL had a predicted composition that was almost fully saturated with free cholesterol,[48] unlike the situation found for LDL in the IDDM and normoglycemic groups (Figure 6.8). Studies in which NIDDM VLDL and LDL were mixed with HDL from normal plasma, and vice versa, confirmed the conclusion that VLDL

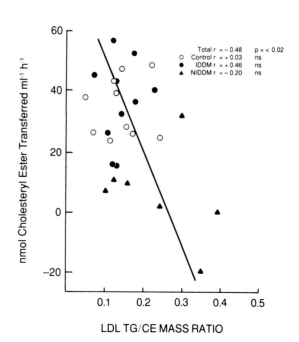

Figure 6.7 The relationship between cholesteryl ester transfer rates and LDL triglyceride–cholesteryl ester (TG/CE) mass ratio in the plasma of IDDM, NIDDM, and normoglycemic control subjects.

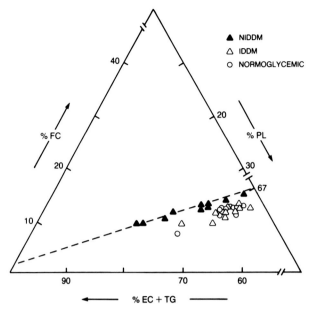

Figure 6.8 The lipid composition of NIDDM, IDDM, and normal LDL calculated on triangular coordinates as described by Miller and Small.[50] The dashed line represents the composition at which the surface monolayer is saturated with free cholesterol.

and LDL of NIDDM plasma were relatively poor acceptors of HDL-derived cholesteryl esters (Figure 6.9).

The suggestion that the free cholesterol content of LDL might be related to reduced cholesteryl ester transfer from HDL in NIDDM[48] has been challenged on the basis of studies in which centrifugally isolated HDL and LDL were modified in lipid composition by incubation with emulsions containing different proportions of lecithin and cholesterol.[53] An increased level of free cholesterol in HDL was found to increase cholesteryl ester transfer to LDL, and it was concluded that free cholesterol was a potent physiologic stimulant of transfer. However, the free cholesterol–phospholipid ratio of NIDDM HDL is decreased, not increased, relative to normal (0.07 versus 0.14).[54] This no doubt contributes to the spontaneous transfer of free cholesterol from LDL to HDL observed in diabetic plasma, even in the absence of LCAT activity.[48] Additionally, the lipid composition of the emulsion-modified LDL was quite different from that of native normal or NIDDM LDL.[47,54]

Effects of Treatment on Reverse Cholesterol Transport in Diabetes

Comparison of cholesterol metabolic data in different studies of human diabetes is difficult. This is not only because of the inherent heterogeneity of the diabetic population. There were also major differences in the means used to achieve diabetic control in individual studies, which could have contributed to the changes in lipid metabolic parameters found independently of their effects on plasma glucose levels. Diabetic control has been reported using insulin or several different oral agents. Therapy with insulin was traditional, intensive, or continuous. The period of effective control varied from a few weeks to many

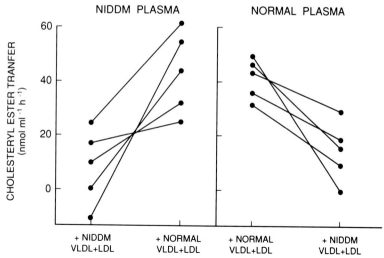

Figure 6.9 Effects of VLDL and LDL from normoglycemic plasma on cholesteryl ester transfer in NIDDM (*left*) and of VLDL and LDL from diabetic plasma on cholesteryl ester transfer in normal subjects (*right*). NIDDM and normal plasma were fractionated by heparin–agarose affinity chromatography to separate the combined VLDL + LDL fraction from the remaining plasma proteins, including HDL. Diabetic VLDL and LDL were then incubated with the remaining fraction of normal or diabetic plasma. For NIDDM plasma, as shown in the left panel, transfer was higher in the presence of normal VLDL and LDL. In the reciprocal experiment, normal VLDL and LDL were incubated with the remaining fraction of NIDDM plasma. As shown in the right panel, for normal plasma transfer was decreased in the presence of diabetic VLDL and LDL. *(Adapted from Fielding CJ, Reaven GM, Liu G, et al: Increased free cholesterol in plasma low and very low density lipoproteins in noninsulin-dependent diabetes mellitus: Its role in the inhibition of cholesteryl ester transfer. Proc Natl Acad Sci USA 1984;81:2512–2516.)*

months in different studies. Finally, factors such as obesity and smoking status no doubt contributed in some studies to the results obtained. Nevertheless, some generalizations can be made:

1. The abnormalities of plasma cholesterol metabolism in NIDDM that have been described in this chapter are clearly not the consequence of hyperglycemia or hypertriglyceridemia per se, because NIDDM and IDDM subjects with comparable plasma glucose and triglyceride levels had different patterns of cholesterol transport.

2. Oral agents alone were ineffective in normalizing abnormal reverse cholesterol transport in NIDDM.

3. Insulin therapy (particularly when intensive) normalized or improved cell-to-plasma cholesterol net transport, cholesteryl ester transfer, HDL cholesterol concentration, and LDL free cholesterol content. Not surprisingly, insulin therapy had little or no effect on plasma LCAT levels, which were usually normal to begin with.

All IDDM patients were under insulin therapy to control ketosis but, if renal function was normal, HDL cholesterol levels, cholesterol transport, LCAT, cholesteryl ester transfer, and LDL free cholesterol were all within normal limits or optimized beyond control levels. Following the development of end-stage renal disease or nephrosis, HDL cholesterol decreased as the risk of CAD increased. It is quite likely that at this point a pattern of abnormal plasma cholesterol metabolism similar to that found in NIDDM emerges, because this pattern is found in nondiabetic renal patients.[41] However, there appear to be no studies directed specifically to plasma cholesterol metabolism in the IDDM patient with renal failure. Studies along these lines could add importantly to our knowledge of the relationship between diabetes and atherosclerosis.

Underlying Mechanisms for the Development of Macrovascular Disease in Diabetes

The pattern of plasma lipoprotein abnormalities in diabetes is also seen in other patient groups with quite different primary metabolic abnormalities, who share an increased risk of atherosclerotic vascular disease that is quantitatively similar. This pattern includes most notably an increased effective level of free cholesterol in VLDL and LDL and reduced cell-to-plasma cholesterol transport. The utilization of free cholesterol by the LCAT reaction appears to be an important branch point in cholesterol transport in normal plasma (Figure 6.2). VLDL and LDL enriched in free cholesterol not only provide substrate for LCAT in competition with cell membrane cholesterol, but they can also mediate the transfer of free cholesterol directly to cell membranes, in opposition to reverse cholesterol transport.

Several studies of cholesterol balance in untreated NIDDM indicate that whole-body cholesterol synthesis is significantly increased.[55–57] Diabetes was associated with an increased fecal loss of steroids. One study found no effect on overall cholesterol balance, but found the same fecal steroid effect.[58] In IDDM without renal disease, whole-body cholesterol synthesis was normal. Effective diabetes control with insulin in NIDDM also normalized whole-body cholesterol synthesis.[56]

The liver is the major site of whole-body cholesterol synthesis. The data

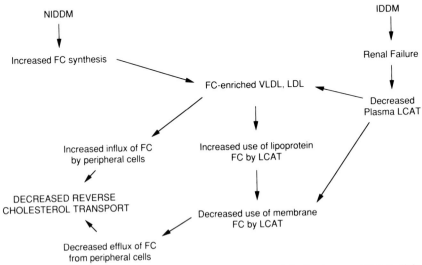

Figure 6.10 Hypothesis on the interrelationship between metabolic abnormalities in diabetic plasma and the development of atherosclerotic vascular disease. FC = free cholesterol.

summarized above suggest that the primary effect of diabetes on reverse cholesterol transport may be mediated in many diabetics, at least in part, via an effect on cholesterol synthesis. VLDL and its product, LDL, are of hepatic origin. Thus an oversynthesis of hepatic cholesterol could lead directly to the secretion of the cholesterol-rich lipoproteins characteristic of uncontrolled NIDDM. As discussed earlier in this section, VLDL and LDL free cholesterol has two potential effects on cholesterol balance in peripheral cells: it can increase cholesterol influx into peripheral cells, and it may decrease cholesterol efflux from these cells by reducing the utilization of cellular free cholesterol for the LCAT reaction. The lower cholesterol content of HDL in untreated NIDDM may itself reflect the reduced transport of cholesterol from cell membranes into this fraction. This hierarchy of effects is shown in Figure 6.10.

Conclusion

As is clear throughout this chapter, our knowledge of plasma cholesterol metabolism in diabetes is still based on relatively few studies. Nevertheless, it seems likely that the abnormalities reported may be closely linked to the increase in large vessel disease that, along with other characteristics, is often found in diabetes. With new developments in our understanding of normal lipoprotein metabolism, we may shortly achieve a much better understanding of these processes at the molecular level.

Acknowledgment

The original research of this laboratory that contributes to this review was supported by the National Institutes of Health through Arteriosclerosis SCOR HL 14237.

References

1. Fein FS, Scheuer J: Heart disease in diabetes, in Rifkin H, Porte D (eds): *Diabetes Mellitus, Theory and Practice*. New York, Elsevier, 1990, pp 812–823.
2. Laakso M, Ronnemaa T, Pyorala K, et al: Atherosclerotic vascular disease and its risk factors in non-insulin-dependent diabetic and nondiabetic subjects in Finland. *Diabetes Care* 1988;11:449–463.
3. Krolewski AS, Kosinski EJ, Warram JH, et al: Magnitude and determinants of coronary artery disease in juvenile-onset, insulin-dependent diabetes mellitus. *Am J Cardiol* 1987;59:750–755.
4. Nikkila EA: High density lipoproteins in diabetes. *Diabetes* 1981;30(suppl 2):82–87.
5. Ruderman NB, Haudenschild C: Diabetes as an atherogenic factor. *Progr Cardiovasc Dis* 1984;26:373–412.
6. Bagdade JD, Albers JJ: Plasma high density lipoprotein concentrations in chronic-hemodialysis and renal-transplant patients. *N Engl J Med* 1977;296:1436–1439.
7. Hashimoto H, Tillemans H, Sarma JSM, et al: Lipid metabolism in perfused human nonatherosclerotic coronary arteries and saphenous veins. *Atherosclerosis* 1974;19: 35–45.
8. Kannel WB, Castelli WP, Gordon T, et al: Serum cholesterol, lipoproteins, and the risk of coronary heart disease. *Ann Intern Med* 1971;74:1–12.

9. Lipid Research Clinics Program: The Lipid Research Clinics Coronary Primary Prevention Trial results. The relationship of reduction in incidence of coronary heart disease to cholesterol lowering. *JAMA* 1984;251:365–374.

10. Shurtleff D: *Some Characteristics Related to the Incidence of C-V Disease and Death: Framingham Study, 18 Year Follow Up.* Washington, DC, U.S. Government Printing Office, 1974, p 30.

11. Miller GJ, Miller NE: Plasma high density lipoprotein concentration and development of ischaemic heart disease. *Lancet* 1975;1:16–19.

12. Miller NE, Thelle DS, Forde OH, et al: The Tromso Heart Study. High density lipoprotein and coronary artery disease: A prospective case-control study. *Lancet* 1977; 1:965–967.

13. Gordon DJ, Probstfield JL, Garrison RJ, et al: High density lipoprotein cholesterol and cardiovascular disease. Four prospective American studies. *Circulation* 1989;79: 8–15.

14. Sweetnam P, Elwood P, Yarnell J, et al: HDL cholesterol and its subfractions in the Caerphilly and Speedwell heart disease studies, in Miller NE (ed): *High Density Lipoproteins and Atherosclerosis.* Amsterdam, Exerpta Medica, 1989, pp 43–50.

15. Fielding PE, Fielding CJ: Dynamics of lipoprotein transport in the circulatory system, in Vance DE, Vance J (eds): *Biochemistry of Lipids, Lipoproteins and Membranes.* Amsterdam, Elsevier, 1991, pp 427–459.

16. Davis RA, Helgerud P, Dueland S, et al: Evidence that reverse cholesterol transport occurs in vivo and requires lecithin-cholesterol acyltransferase. *Biochim Biophys Acta* 1982;689:410–414.

17. Schwartz CC, Zech LA, Vandenbroeck JM et al: Reverse cholesterol transport measure in vivo in man: The central roles of HDL, in Miller NE (ed): *High Density Lipoproteins and Atherosclerosis.* Amsterdam, Exerpta Medica, 1989, pp 321–329.

18. Miller NE, La Ville A, Crook D: Direct evidence that reverse cholesterol transport is mediated by high density lipoprotein in rabbit. *Nature* 1985;314:109–111.

19. Fielding CJ, Fielding PE: Evidence for a lipoprotein carrier in human plasma catalysing sterol efflux from cultured fibroblasts and its relationship to lecithin:cholesterol acyltransferase. *Proc Natl Acad Sci USA* 1981;78:3911–3914.

20. Fielding PE, Davison PM, Karasek MA, et al: Regulation of sterol transport in human microvascular endothelial cells. *J Cell Biol* 1982;94:350–354.

21. Fielding PE, Fielding CJ, Kane JP, et al: Cholesterol net transport, esterification and transfer in human hyperlipidemic plasma. *J Clin Invest* 1983;71:449–460.

22. Johnson WL, Mahlberg FH, Rothblat GH, et al: Cholesterol transport between cells and high density lipoproteins. *Biochim Biophys Acta* 1991;1085:273–298.

23. Barbaras R, Puchois P, Fruchart JC, et al: Cholesterol efflux from cultured adipose cells is mediated by LpAI particles but not by LpAI:AII particles. *Biochem Biophys Res Commun* 1987;142:63–69.

24. Hara H, Yokoyama S: Interaction of free apolipoproteins with macrophages. Formation of high density lipoprotein-like lipoproteins and reduction of cellular cholesterol. *J Biol Chem* 1991;266:3080–3086.

25. Castro GR, Fielding CJ: Early incorporation of cell-derived cholesterol into prebeta-migrating high density lipoprotein. *Biochemistry* 1988;27:25–29.

26. Francone OL, Gurakar A, Fielding CJ: Distribution and functions of lecithin:cholesterol acyltransferase and cholesteryl ester transfer protein in plasma lipoproteins. *J Biol Chem* 1989;264:7066–7072.

27. Graham DL, Oram JF: Identification and characterization of a high density lipoprotein-binding protein in cell membranes by ligand blotting. *J Biol Chem* 1987;262:7439–7442.

28. Tozuka M, Fidge N: Purification and characterization of two high-density-lipoprotein-binding proteins from rat and human liver. *Biochem J* 1989;261:239–244.

29. Phillips MC, Johnson WJ, Rothblat GH: Mechanisms and consequences of cellular cholesterol exchange and transfer. *Biochim Biophys Acta* 1987;906:223–276.

30. Fielding CJ, Fielding PE: Regulation of human plasma lecithin:cholesterol acyltransferase activity by lipoprotein acceptor cholesteryl ester content. *J Biol Chem* 1981; 256:2102–2104.

31. Park MSC, Kudchodkar BJ, Frolich J, et al: Study of the components of reverse cholesterol transport in lecithin:cholesterol acyltransferse deficiency. *Arch Biochem Biophys* 1987;258:545–554.

32. De Parscau L, Fielding CJ: Abnormal plasma cholesterol metabolism in cigarette smokers. *Metabolism* 1986;35:1070–1073.

33. Castro GR, Fielding CJ: Effects of postprandial lipema on plasma cholesterol metabolism. *J Clin Invest* 1985;75:874–882.

34. Morton RE, Zilversmit DB: Interrelationship of lipids transferred by the lipid transfer protein isolated from human lipoprotein-deficient plasma. *J Biol Chem* 1983;258: 11751–11757.

35. Fielding PE, Jackson EM, Fielding CJ: Chronic dietary fat and cholesterol inhibit the normal postprandial stimulation of plasma cholesterol metabolism. *J Lipid Res* 1989; 30:1211–1218.

36. Fielding PE, Miida T, Fielding CJ: Metabolism of low density lipoprotein free cholesterol by human plasma lecithin:cholesterol acyltransferase. *Biochemistry* 1991;30: 8551–8557.

37. Goldberg DI, Beltz WF, Pittman RC: Evaluation of pathways for the cellular uptake of high density lipoprotein cholesterol esters in rabbits. *J Biol Chem* 1991;87:331–346.

38. Fielding CJ, Castro GR, Donner C, et al: Distribution of apolipoprotein E in the plasma of insulin-dependent and noninsulin-dependent diabetes and its relation to cholesterol transport. *J Lipid Res* 1986;27:1052–1061.

39. Ishida BY, Frohlich J, Fielding CJ: Prebeta-migrating high density lipoprotein: Quantitation in normal and hyperlipidemic plasma by solid phase immunoassay following electrophoretic transfer. *J Lipid Res* 1987;28:778–786.

40. Schernthane G, Kostner GM, Dieplinger H, et al: Apolipoproteins (A-I, A-II, B), L_p (a) lipoproteins and lecithin:cholesterol acyltransferase activity in diabetes mellitus. *Atherosclerosis* 1983;49:277–293.

41. Dieplinger H, Schoenfeld PV, Fielding CJ: Plasma cholesterol metabolism in endstage renal diseaase. *J Clin Invest* 1986;77:1071–1083.

42. Nayale SS, Bhaskaranana N, Kamath KS, et al: Serum apolipoproteins A and B, lecithin: cholesterol acyltransferase activities and urinary cholesterol levels in nephrotic syndrome patients before and during steroid treatment. *Nephron* 1990;54:234–239.

43. Yao JK, Palumbo PJ, Dyck PJ: Lecithin:cholesterol acyltransferase and serum fatty acids. *Artery* 1981;9:262–274.

44. Fielding CJ, Reaven GM, Fielding PE: Human noninsulin-dependent diabetes: Identification of a defect in plasma cholesterol transport normalized *in vivo* by insulin and *in vitro* by selective immunoadsorption of apolipoprotein E. *Proc Natl Acad Sci USA* 1982;79:6365–6369.

45. Bagdade JD, Ritter MC, Subbaiah PV: Accelerated cholesteryl ester transfer in patients with insulin-dependent diabetes mellitus. *Eur J Clin Invest* 1991;21:161–167.

46. Dullaart RPF, Groener JEM, Dikkeschei LD, et al: Increased cholesteryl ester transfer activity in complicated type I (insulin-dependent) diabetes mellitus—its relationship with serum lipids. *Diabetologia* 1989;32:14–19.

47. Dullaart, RPF, Groener JEM, Dikkeschei BD, et al: Elevated cholesteryl ester transfer protein activity in IDDM men who smoke. *Diabetes Care* 1991;14:338–341.

48. Fielding CJ, Reaven GM, Liu G, et al: Increased free cholesterol in plasma low and very low density lipoproteins in noninsulin-dependent diabetes mellitus: Its role in the inhibition of cholesteryl ester transfer. *Proc Natl Acad Sci USA* 1984;81:2512–2516.

49. Fielding CJ: The origin and properties of free cholesterol potential gradients in plasma and their relation to atherogenesis. *J Lipid Res* 1984;25:1624–1628.

50. Miller KW, Small DM: Surface-to-core and interparticle equilibrium distributions of triglyceride-rich lipoprotein lipids. *J Biol Chem* 1983;258:13772–13784.

51. Stockton GW, Smith ICP: A deuterium nuclear magnetic resonance study of the condensing effect of cholesterol on egg phosphatidycholine bilayer membranes. *Chem Phys Lipids* 1976;17:251–263.

52. Papahadjopoulos D, Nir S, Ohki S: Permeability properties of phospholipid mixtures: Effect of cholesterol and temperature. *Biochim Biophys Acta* 1971;266:561–583.

53. Morton RE: Free cholesterol is a potent regulator of lipid transfer protein function. *J Biol Chem* 1988;263:12235–12241.

54. Bagdade JD, Buchanan WE, Kuusi T, et al: Persistent abnormalities in lipoprotein composition in noninsulin-dependent diabetes after intensive insulin therapy. *Arteriosclerosis* 1990;10:232–239.

55. Bennion LJ, Grundy SM: Effects of diabetes mellitus on cholesterol metabolism in man. *N Engl J Med* 1977;296:1365–1371.

56. Anderson E, Hellstrom P, Hellstrom K: Cholesterol and bile acid metabolism in middle-aged diabetics. *Diabete et Metab* 1986;12:261–267.

57. Andersen E, Hellstrom P, Hellstrom K: Cholesterol biosynthesis in nonketotic diabetics before and during insulin therapy. *Diabetes Res Clin Pract* 1987;3:207–214.

58. Saudek CD, Brach EL: Cholesterol metabolism in diabetes. The effect of diabetic control on sterol balance. *Diabetes* 1978;27:1059–1064.

Chapter 7

Clinical Picture and Therapy of Dyslipidemia in Diabetes Mellitus

Abhimanyu Garg, MBBS, MD, and
Scott M. Grundy, MD, PhD

Several factors, such as dyslipidemia, hyperglycemia, obesity, hypertension, and abnormalities in hemostasis and platelet functions, may predispose patients with diabetes mellitus to atherosclerosis or its complications. The term "dyslipidemia" includes not only abnormal concentrations of lipids and lipoproteins but also abnormalities in composition and metabolism of lipoproteins. Because prevalence, mechanisms, clinical picture, and therapeutic options for dyslipidemias may differ considerably between insulin-dependent and non-insulin-dependent diabetes mellitus (IDDM and NIDDM), the two types are considered separately in the following discussion on clinical picture and treatment of dyslipidemias.

Clinical Picture of Dyslipidemia

Dyslipidemia in IDDM Patients

Prevalence

Information on the prevalence of dyslipidemia in IDDM patients is incomplete. Recent data suggest that the prevalence of high-risk serum cholesterol levels (greater than 247.5 mg/dL [6.4 mmol/L]) in an unselected group of IDDM patients is similar to that in the nondiabetic population.[1] Comparative studies on a small number of IDDM patients, however, reveal that levels of plasma lipids and lipoproteins are usually "normal" in most patients after good glycemic control with either conventional or intensive insulin therapy.[2,3]

Lipoprotein Abnormalities

Usually patients in poor glycemic control or in ketoacidosis have increased triglyceride levels in very-low-density lipoproteins (VLDLs) and even chylomicrons.[4] Those having chylomicronemia may exhibit eruptive xanthomas, lipemia retinalis, and sometimes acute pancreatitis. The principal causes of diabetic hypertriglyceridemia are low activity of lipoprotein lipase (LPL) and excessive VLDL production, both resulting from insulin deficiency. Poor glycemic control also can raise concentrations of low-density lipoprotein (LDL) cholesterol and decrease levels of high-density lipoprotein (HDL) cholesterol.

Most lipoprotein abnormalities in IDDM mitigate during improved metabolic control with appropriate insulin therapy.[5] Treatment with insulin lowers production rates for VLDL triglyceride and LDL apolipoprotein (apo) B, and treatment with intensive insulin therapy can lead to extremely low levels of total cholesterol and LDL cholesterol.[6,7] Well-controlled IDDM patients typically have normal or low-normal concentrations of plasma triglycerides and relatively high levels of HDL cholesterol. Whether higher HDL cholesterol levels in IDDM patients are due to an increase in HDL_2 cholesterol or HDL_3 cholesterol remains to be determined. Some studies, however, suggest that levels of HDL_2 cholesterol are normal or lower than normal, whereas concentrations of HDL_3 cholesterol are relatively increased.[8,9] Consequently, the ratio of HDL_2 cholesterol to HDL_3 cholesterol may be reduced, and thus, in spite of high HDL cholesterol levels, IDDM patients may not be protected against coronary heart disease (CHD). Still, some investigators[10,11] have observed an increased ratio of HDL_2 to HDL_3 cholesterol in IDDM patients, which could be protective. Further research on HDL metabolism in IDDM obviously is needed.

Abnormalities in composition of apo B-100–containing lipoproteins (VLDL, intermediate-density lipoprotein [IDL], and LDL) further may enhance atherogenesis in IDDM patients despite a "normal" lipoprotein profile. Pietri et al[6] noted an abnormally high ratio of cholesterol to triglycerides in VLDL particles of IDDM patients on conventional therapy, and this abnormality persisted despite intensive insulin therapy. Georgopoulos and Rosengard[12] confirmed the finding of cholesterol-enriched VLDL particles in IDDM patients. More recently, Klein et al[13] and James and Pometta[14] noted increased concentrations of unesterified cholesterol in VLDL particles from IDDM patients. In the study by James and Pometta,[14] LDL subfractions were relatively depleted in esterified cholesterol but were enriched in triglycerides.

Factors Affecting Lipoprotein Levels in IDDM

The factors affecting lipoprotein levels in IDDM are summarized in Table 7.1 and are given in order of relative importance. The need for glycemic control with insulin therapy already has been discussed. Besides the degree of glycemic control, presence or absence of diabetic nephropathy also affects lipoprotein levels in IDDM patients. As compared to IDDM patients with normal excretion rates for urinary albumin, patients with microalbuminuria have higher levels of

Table 7.1 Factors Affecting Lipoprotein Levels in IDDM Patients

1. Level of metabolic control
2. Diabetic nephropathy
3. Obesity
4. Diet composition
5. Route of insulin administration (subcutaneous or intravenous versus intraperitoneal)
6. Genetic forms of dyslipidemia
7. Drug therapy for associated medical conditions
8. Cigarette smoking
9. Alcohol intake

plasma triglycerides, VLDL cholesterol, LDL cholesterol, and apo B and lower levels of HDL cholesterol, in particular HDL$_2$ cholesterol.[15,16] Presence of overt diabetic nephropathy (chronic renal failure and/or nephrotic syndrome) can worsen the lipoprotein profile, and the specific changes depend on whether chronic renal failure or nephrotic syndrome is the predominant manifestation of diabetic nephropathy.

Although obesity generally affects lipoprotein levels more in NIDDM than IDDM, obese IDDM patients often have low levels of HDL subfractions (HDL$_2$ cholesterol in men and HDL$_3$ cholesterol in women) and high levels of VLDL triglycerides.[17] Consumption of diets rich in saturated fats and cholesterol further raises LDL cholesterol levels in IDDM patients. Other factors such as level of physical activity, genetic forms of hyperlipoproteinemia, drugs such as β-adrenergic blockers and diuretics, cigarette smoking, and alcohol intake probably contribute to lipoprotein abnormalities in some IDDM patients as well.

Relationship of Dyslipidemia in IDDM With CHD Risk

Risk of CHD in IDDM is almost equivalent to that of heterozygous familial hypercholesterolemia, being several fold higher than in the nondiabetic subjects. Epidemiologic studies on relatively small numbers of IDDM patients suggest that hypertension and proteinuria are important contributors to CHD in advanced IDDM.[18,19] The role of plasma lipids and lipoproteins was not assessed in the study by Krolewski et al,[18] whereas Jensen et al[19] reported higher levels of both blood pressure and serum cholesterol in IDDM patients who developed CHD than in those who did not; hence high cholesterol levels as well as hypertension probably contribute to CHD in IDDM. Other cross-sectional studies have noted a higher prevalence of dyslipidemia in IDDM patients having CHD as compared to those without.[20,21] Thus, abnormalities in lipoprotein metabolism, particularly higher cholesterol levels, should be added to the list of risk factors responsible for atherosclerotic vascular disease in IDDM patients.

Dyslipidemia in NIDDM Patients

Prevalence

The prevalence of dyslipidemia in NIDDM varies among different populations of diabetic patients. Regardless of the geographic or racial origin, NIDDM patients consistently have a two- to threefold excess of dyslipidemia compared to the corresponding nondiabetic population.[22–25] High frequencies of both hypercholesterolemia and hypertriglyceridemia were reported by the World Health Organization multinational study of vascular disease in diabetic subjects.[26,27] The Framingham Heart Study[23] noted that the excess prevalence of dyslipidemia in adult patients with diabetes mellitus occurred mainly as hypertriglyceridemia, increased VLDL cholesterol levels, and reduced HDL cholesterol levels. A similar picture was reported by Stern et al[25] in both Hispanic and caucasian patients with NIDDM from San Antonio, Texas. In fact lipoprotein abnormalities in patients predisposed to NIDDM may precede onset of overt hyperglycemia by several years and thus may enhance atherogenesis before the diagnosis of NIDDM is ever made.[28] Whether this dyslipidemia of prediabetes is due to an inherited form of insulin resistance or simply to obesity is uncertain. Nonetheless, the testing of first-degree relatives of NIDDM patients to rule out dyslipidemias is prudent.

Lipoprotein Abnormalities

NIDDM patients frequently present with high levels of total triglycerides and VLDL cholesterol.[22-25] HDL cholesterol or apo A-I concentrations also are often reduced in patients with NIDDM. Typically levels of LDL cholesterol are not elevated as a result of NIDDM per se. Hypertriglyceridemia appears to be secondary to both excess production rates of VLDL triglycerides and reduced lipolytic rates for triglyceride-rich lipoproteins; the latter may be related in part to decreased availability of LPL. If metabolic control is severely deranged, some patients even develop severe hypertriglyceridemia and chylomicronemia, which can precipitate acute pancreatitis. Low levels of HDL cholesterol, particularly HDL_2 and apo A-I, probably result from the concomitant defect in triglyceride metabolism.

NIDDM patients, moreover, have several abnormalities in composition of lipoproteins. VLDL and IDL are abnormally rich in triglycerides and unesterified cholesterol. LDL particles are also triglyceride rich. Some patients may have an elevated LDL cholesterol–apo B ratio, indicating enrichment of LDL particles with cholesteryl esters, but markedly hypertriglyceridemic patients have a low LDL cholesterol–apo B ratio, signifying cholesterol-depleted LDL. Fielding et al described an abnormal lipoprotein in the LDL density range, which was rich in unesterified cholesterol and apo E[29]; concentrations of this abnormal lipoprotein fell with improvement in glycemic control. Other investigators using analytic ultracentrifugation have observed an increased frequency of polydisperse LDL in NIDDM, in contrast to a monodisperse pattern in normal subjects.[30] Other studies also suggest a high prevalence of small, dense LDL particles in NIDDM patients,[31] which may be more atherogenic than normal LDL.

Factors Affecting Lipoprotein Levels in NIDDM

The primary determinants of dyslipidemia in NIDDM appear to be the degree of metabolic control, severity of obesity and pattern of distribution of fat, presence or absence of nephropathy, and physical activity and exercise capacity (Table 7.2). Hyperlipoproteinemia of genetic origin also is accentuated by NIDDM. Lipoprotein abnormalities in NIDDM patients, unlike those in IDDM patients, usually do not completely normalize with good glycemic control, whether obtained by

Table 7.2 Factors Affecting Lipoprotein Levels in NIDDM Patients

1. Level of metabolic control
2. Degree of obesity and pattern of body fat distribution
3. Physical activity and exercise capacity
4. Diabetic nephropathy
5. Diet composition
6. Genetic forms of hyperlipoproteinemias
7. Diuretics and β-adrenergic blocker therapy
8. Cigarette smoking
9. Alcohol intake

oral hypoglycemic drugs or insulin therapy. Since NIDDM predisposes to hypertriglyceridemia, even mild to moderate alcohol consumption can accentuate hypertriglyceridemia in diabetic patients. High-carbohydrate intakes likewise raise plasma triglyceride levels and lower HDL cholesterol levels. Heavy smoking also can worsen hypertriglyceridemia. In several patients, drugs such as β-adrenergic blockers, diuretics, corticosteroids, estrogens, and anabolic steroids will accentuate dyslipidemia. Infections sometimes induce severe hypertriglyceridemia in NIDDM patients and put them at risk for acute pancreatitis.

Relationship of Dyslipidemia in NIDDM to CHD Risk

The risk for CHD in NIDDM patients is two to three times that in a comparable nondiabetic population.[23] Although the role of hypertriglyceridemia in causation of CHD is debated, hypertriglyceridemia is a stronger predictor of CHD mortality in NIDDM patients.[27,32,33] These patients may be unusually susceptible to abnormalities in lipoproteins occurring with hypertriglyceridemia that predispose to CHD; these include increased concentrations of chylomicron remnants, VLDL remnants, IDL, and small, dense LDL as well as low levels of HDL. Even mild elevations of LDL may be unusually atherogenic in hypertriglyceridemic patients because of abnormalities in composition and metabolism of LDL particles. Furthermore, the importance of LDL cholesterol as a risk factor in NIDDM patients must not be overlooked. The prevalence of CHD among NIDDM patients from certain populations, such as Pima Indians of Arizona, Japanese, and Chinese, is quite low[26]; all of these populations have low concentrations of total cholesterol and LDL cholesterol as compared to NIDDM patients from Western societies. These low LDL levels may well account for the low rates of CHD in these populations, and this relationship underscores the need to maintain low levels of LDL cholesterol in NIDDM patients to achieve a major reduction in risk of CHD.

Targets for Lipid-Lowering in Patients With Diabetes Mellitus

IDDM Patients

IDDM patients can belong to either pediatric or adult age groups. Because of the high risk of CHD in IDDM, patients belonging to both age groups need evaluation for dyslipidemia. Recently the National Cholesterol Education Program (NCEP) developed guidelines for classification, detection, and treatment of high cholesterol levels in adults[34] and young people.[35] The NCEP panels focused on LDL as the primary lipid risk factor and established targets for LDL lowering. Classifications for adults and for children and adolescents based on total cholesterol or LDL cholesterol levels are shown in Tables 7.3 and 7.4, respectively. Treatment decisions are modified according to the risk status of patients; more aggressive therapy is indicated when patients have CHD or two CHD risk factors. Diabetes mellitus is counted as a risk factor, as is male sex. If these recommendations are followed, active intervention with either diet or drugs should be instituted in diabetic men but not in diabetic women having borderline levels of LDL cholesterol. In contrast, because diabetes mellitus seemingly wipes out any protection against CHD afforded by female sex,[23] we recently proposed that

Table 7.3 Classification of Total and LDL Cholesterol Levels in Adults: National Cholesterol Education Program[a]

	Total Cholesterol		LDL Cholesterol	
	mg/dL	mmol/L	mg/dL	mmol/L
Desirable	<200	<5.2	<130	<3.4
Borderline-high	200–239	5.2–6.2	130–159	3.4–4.0
High	≥240	≥6.2	≥160	≥4.1

[a] Treatment decisions with either diet or drugs therapy are based on the risk status of the patients, whether they already have definite CHD, or if they have any two of the following risk factors: male sex, family history of premature CHD, cigarette smoking, hypertension, low HDL cholesterol level, diabetes mellitus, definite cerebrovascular or peripheral vascular disease, or severe obesity.

diabetic women with borderline LDL cholesterol levels should be treated similarly to men.[36] In other words, the presence of diabetes essentially counted as two risk factors, and sex was disregarded.

Since increased concentrations of VLDL and its remnants may be as atherogenic as LDL particles in patients with diabetes mellitus,[13] we further proposed that both VLDL and LDL be included in risk assessment and therapeutic goals.[36] The combined fraction, called non-HDL cholesterol, may be considered as the target of therapy in patients with diabetes mellitus.

Thus, in line with the recommendations of the NCEP panels, we have proposed therapeutic goals for adults and children with diabetes mellitus (Tables 7.5 and 7.6, respectively). The minimum goal of therapy in adults with IDDM may be a non-HDL cholesterol level of less than 4.1 mmol/L (160 mg/dL), with the ideal goal being 3.4 mmol/L (130 mg/dL). In children and adolescents with IDDM, the minimum goal of therapy may be a non-HDL cholesterol level less

Table 7.4 Classification of Total and LDL Cholesterol Levels in Children and Adolescents From Families with Hypercholesterolemia or Premature Cardiovascular Disease: National Cholesterol Education Program

	Total Cholesterol		LDL Cholesterol	
	mg/dL	mmol/L	mg/dL	mmol/L
Acceptable	<170	<4.4	<110	<2.8
Borderline	170–199	4.4–5.1	110–129	2.8–3.3
High	≥200	≥5.2	≥130	≥3.4

Table 7.5 Proposed Therapeutic Goals for Adults With Diabetes Mellitus[a]

	Minimum		Ideal	
	mg/dL	mmol/L	mg/dL	mmol/L
Total cholesterol	<200	<5.2	~170	~4.4
LDL cholesterol	<130	<3.4	~100	~2.6
Non-HDL cholesterol	<160	<4.1	~130	~3.4

[a] Recommendations are for both men and women.

Table 7.6 Proposed Minimum Therapeutic
Goals for Children and Adolescents With
Diabetes Mellitus[a]

	mg/dL	mmol/L
Total cholesterol	<170	<4.4
LDL cholesterol	<110	<2.8
Non-HDL cholesterol	<125	<3.2

[a] Recommendations are the same for both sexes.

than 3.2 mmol/L (125 mg/dL) and the ideal goal may be 2.3 mmol/L (90 mg/dL).

NIDDM Patients

The proposed therapeutic goals for adults with diabetes mellitus should be used for patients with NIDDM because almost all of them are adults (Table 7.5). Since hypertriglyceridemia is the most prevalent lipid abnormality and may be a predictor of CHD in NIDDM patients, it seems reasonable to recommend a reduction of triglyceride levels to the normal range (less than 2.8 mmol/L or 250 mg/dL).

Dietary Therapy for Diabetic Dyslipidemia

IDDM Patients

For patients with IDDM, the American Diabetes Association[37] recommends a high-carbohydrate diet that is low in total fat, saturated fatty acids, and cholesterol. The major purpose of this diet is to reduce LDL cholesterol levels. Certainly replacing saturated fatty acids with carbohydrates in diet will reduce plasma cholesterol levels in IDDM patients.[38,39] One of these studies,[38] however, reported that a high-carbohydrate diet raised plasma triglyceride levels and markedly lowered HDL cholesterol levels, which may not be desirable.

Recently, we proposed an alternative approach to diet therapy in NIDDM patients, that of using diets rich in monounsaturated fatty acids instead of carbohydrates.[40] This dietary approach may also be extended to IDDM patients. In fact, in a short-term study in IDDM patients, Perotti et al[41] observed improvement in plasma glucose profile on the high-monounsaturated-fat diet as compared to the usual high-carbohydrate diet. The plasma lipids and lipoproteins remained the same on the two diets. Thus, a diet rich in monounsaturated fatty acids may be a suitable alternative to a high-carbohydrate diet for IDDM patients.

Besides the composition of the diet and the total amount of energy consumed by the patients, an important aspect of dietary therapy in IDDM patients is to match the timing and the content of various meals to the time of administration of insulin and the dose of insulin. A consistent pattern of dietary habits is helpful for keeping good metabolic control. Care should be taken to provide extra energy for underweight patients, growing children, and pregnant patients with IDDM. Some patients who may be obese need to carefully reduce energy intake and possibly insulin dose.

NIDDM Patients

The best diet for patients with NIDDM would be one that minimizes hypergly-cemia, optimizes plasma levels of lipids and lipoproteins, and reduces obesity. The diets currently recommended for NIDDM patients by the American Diabetes Association[37] and the NCEP[34,35] to achieve these aims are similar; they consist of high-carbohydrate diets with reduced amounts of saturated fatty acids (less than 10% of the total energy intake) and cholesterol (less than 300 mg/d).

In spite of broad acceptance of these recommendations, there is not a uni-versal agreement that high-carbohydrate diets are most appropriate for NIDDM patients.[42] At a recent Consensus Development Conference on Diet and Exercise in NIDDM, sponsored by the National Institutes of Health,[42] it was pointed out that high-carbohydrate diets increase plasma triglyceride and VLDL cholesterol concentrations and reduce HDL cholesterol levels; consequently they may not be appropriate for all NIDDM patients. For this reason, we recently compared two types of diets in NIDDM patients, a high-carbohydrate diet and a low-car-bohydrate diet rich in monounsaturated fatty acids.[36] Both diets had similarly low contents of saturated fatty acids and cholesterol. The diet high in mon-ounsaturated fatty acids improved glycemic control, reduced plasma triglyceride and VLDL cholesterol levels, and raised levels of HDL cholesterol compared to the high-carbohydrate diet (Figure 7.1) This finding again throws into question whether high-carbohydrate diets are necessarily best for NIDDM patients. Pre-liminary results of a recent multicenter study in NIDDM patients revealed per-sistence of beneficial effects of high-monounsaturated-fat diets on plasma tri-glyceride and VLDL cholesterol levels for more than 3 months, when compared to high-carbohydrate diets.[43]

One other reason for advocating high-carbohydrate diets is the claim that they improve glucose tolerance in nondiabetic individuals[44] and possibly in patients with mild NIDDM or impaired glucose tolerance.[45] Nonetheless, recent studies by our group[40] as well as others[46] indicate that high-carbohydrate intakes often worsen hyperglycemia in moderately severe NIDDM. Indeed, even in pa-tients with mild NIDDM, we did not find an improvement in insulin sensitivity or glycemic control when a high-carbohydrate diet was compared to a low-carbohydrate diet.[47]

Therefore, replacement of saturated fatty acids with monounsaturated fatty acids, instead of carbohydrates, may be preferable for many patients with NIDDM. NIDDM patients who may benefit from diets higher in monounsaturates are those with hypertriglyceridemia, those with low HDL cholesterol levels, el-derly patients with poor compliance to the high-carbohydrate diets, and preg-nant women, who have increased energy requirements. The major potential disadvantage of a diet higher in total fats is that it may interfere with weight reduction, which is needed for obese NIDDM patients. However, fat apparently promotes satiety more than carbohydrate, and for this reason, higher fat diets should be just as efficacious as high-carbohydrate diets provided that strict attention is given to total caloric intake.

Another nutrient class that has evoked a great deal of interest recently includes the ω-3 polyunsaturated fatty acids (eicosapentaenoic and docosah-exaenoic acids) from fish oils.[48] The ω-3 polyunsaturated fatty acids, when given in a dose of 3 to 10 g/d, will lower plasma triglyceride levels in markedly hy-pertriglyceridemic patients.[49,50] In addition, these fatty acids affect platelet me-

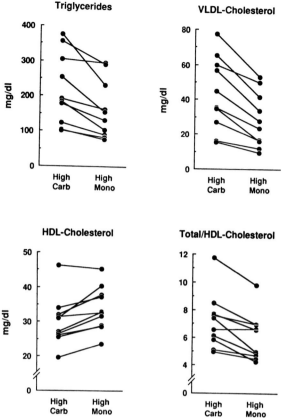

Figure 7.1 Mean levels of plasma triglycerides, VLDL cholesterol, and HDL cholesterol, and total cholesterol–HDL cholesterol ratio in ten NIDDM patients during the high-carbohydrate (High Carb) and the high-monounsaturated-fat (High Mono) diet periods. *(Reprinted, by permission, from Garg A: Role of monounsaturated fatty acids in nutrition for patients with non-insulin-dependent diabetes mellitus, in Proceedings of the 14th International Diabetes Federation Congress, Amsterdam Elsevier Science Publishers BV, to be published.)*

tabolism and have antithrombotic properties. The appropriate intake of ω-3 polyunsaturates for diabetic patients, however, has not been determined. In high intakes, these fatty acids may exacerbate insulin resistance and thus can have deleterious effects on glycemic control.[51,52] This finding seemingly offsets the potential benefit of the triglyceride-lowering effect of ω-3 polyunsaturates in patients with NIDDM.

Beyond the composition of diet, patients with NIDDM should restrict energy intake to reduce adiposity. Most NIDDM patients are obese, and even those who are considered as nonobese often have maldistribution of adiposity (ie, more central and intra-abdominal fat than peripheral or gluteofemoral fat). Daily exercise combined with low-calorie diets will help to reduce central adiposity. Weight reduction in NIDDM patients improves glycemic control and causes a marked lowering of plasma triglycerides and VLDL cholesterol levels, but unfortunately only a modest increase in HDL cholesterol levels.[53–55] Diet and exercise in conjunction with hypoglycemic agents should be tried for a period of 3 to 6 months before initiating lipid-lowering drugs. Patients with severe dyslipidemia resulting from genetic disorders in lipoprotein metabolism are an exception, and lipid-lowering drugs can be started simultaneously with other measures such as diet and exercise.

Glycemic Control for Diabetic Dyslipidemia

IDDM Patients

In most patients with IDDM, management of hyperglycemia with insulin therapy should help to correct dyslipidemia as well. Several studies have shown that glycemic control using intensive insulin therapy, either with multiple subcutaneous injections or with continuous subcutaneous insulin infusion by insulin pumps, generally is effective for achieving normal or below-normal levels of plasma lipids in IDDM patients.[5,6] There are, however, limitations to intensive insulin therapy, as observed in the ongoing Diabetes Control and Complications Trial[56]; the most important side effect, of course, is severe hypoglycemia. Thus practical considerations often preclude use of intensive insulin therapy, and consequently patients remain mildly hyperlipidemic because of their IDDM per se.

NIDDM Patients

In NIDDM patients, good glycemic control likewise will improve dyslipidemia. This may be achieved by either insulin or oral hypoglycemic agents. In the United States, only sulfonylureas are available as oral agents, whereas in other countries biguanide derivatives, such as metformin, also can be used. In most patients with mild to moderate hyperglycemia, sulfonylureas are used, whereas for severe hyperglycemia, or for primary or secondary failure of sulfonylurea therapy, insulin therapy is indicated. In some patients with NIDDM, proper glycemic control with diet, weight reduction, and appropriate use of hypoglycemic agents may normalize levels of lipids and lipoproteins. Unfortunately, residual dyslipidemia persists in many patients in spite of these measures.[57] Persistent dyslipidemia can be the result of either concomitant genetic hyperlipoproteinemias or insufficient correction of hyperglycemia. Still, achieving the best glycemic control practical is essential before turning to lipid-lowering drugs. Whether insulin therapy offers for patients with mild to moderate hyperglycemia any advantage over sulfonylureas for normalizing levels of lipids and lipoproteins is not clear from experimental evidence, although it should be possible to achieve better glycemic control with insulin therapy, and hence better dyslipidemia control. Practicality, however, will favor the use of oral agents for the majority of patients with NIDDM.

Lipid-Lowering Drugs for Diabetic Dyslipidemia

IDDM Patients

A general approach for use of lipid-lowering drugs in IDDM patients is presented. Unfortunately, this approach is not based on a large body of experimental evidence but must be inferred from general principles derived from nondiabetic subjects and patients with NIDDM. The advantages and disadvantages of each category of drugs in patients with diabetes mellitus are discussed in detail in the following section dealing with NIDDM patients.

Since patients with IDDM generally are young, if a decision is made to use lipid-lowering drugs, one must take into account that therapy will be required for many years. Furthermore, there are limited data to indicate which drugs are most effective and safe in IDDM patients. According to the NCEP,[35] the only drugs recommended for lowering serum cholesterol in children and adolescents are the bile acid sequestrants and niacin. Other drugs, such as hydroxyme-thylglutaryl coenzyme A (HMG CoA) reductase inhibitors, probucol, gemfibrozil, and clofibrate, generally are not recommended for routine use in children and adolescents. Nicotinic acid can be used in patients who do not achieve desirable cholesterol levels with bile acid sequestrant therapy, but only under careful expert guidance. Recommendations for children and adolescents with IDDM can be assumed to be the same.

When adult IDDM patients have elevated LDL cholesterol levels (the most common lipoprotein abnormality), the most appropriate therapy probably is use of bile acid sequestrants or HMG CoA reductase inhibitors. Unfortunately, experience with these two drugs in IDDM is limited. Cholestyramine can be tried first. Whether cholestyramine therapy will also normalize abnormalities in composition of LDL particles in IDDM remains to be studied. HMG CoA reductase inhibitors in general are highly effective in lowering cholesterol levels, but they have not been studied in IDDM patients. Nicotinic acid deteriorates glycemic control in NIDDM patients,[58] and it may worsen hyperglycemia and increase insulin requirements in IDDM as well; to date, however, there are no reports of its use in IDDM. Fibric acid derivatives (bezafibrate and clofibrate) have been tried in patients with IDDM[59,60] and found to be effective in reducing both VLDL and LDL levels. However, the LDL-lowering effects of these drugs are relatively small. Still, for IDDM patients with marked hypertriglyceridemia who do not respond to diet and insulin therapy, fibric acid derivatives may be considered. Nicotinic acid probably should be avoided in IDDM patients until further studies are carried out to demonstrate efficacy and safety.

NIDDM Patients

The NCEP[34] recommends bile acid binding resins and nicotinic acid as first-line drugs in the treatment of hypercholesterolemia in nondiabetic patients. Patients with NIDDM, however, have unique metabolic derangements, and therefore the choice of lipid-lowering drugs in diabetic patients may not be the same as that for nondiabetic subjects. In a series of clinical studies, we have evaluated various categories of drugs for therapy of dyslipidemia in NIDDM patients. The risks and benefits of each category of lipid-lowering drugs for NIDDM patients are discussed in the following sections. Since the approach to management of NIDDM patients with hyperchylomicronemia syndrome or those with diabetic nephropathy could be different than that for other NIDDM patients, these topics are discussed separately.

HMG CoA Reductase Inhibitors

Lovastatin, pravastatin, simvastatin, and fluvastatin belong to this new class of lipid-lowering drugs. The first three drugs are currently available in the United States. These drugs inhibit hepatic HMG CoA reductase, the rate-limiting enzyme

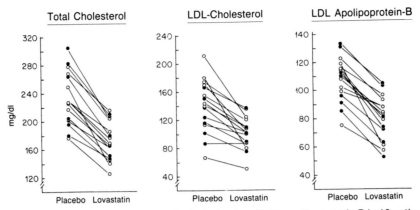

Figure 7.2 Plasma levels of total and LDL cholesterol and LDL apolipoprotein B in 16 patients with NIDDM during the placebo and lovastatin periods. Each symbol represents the mean of five daily determinations. Solid circles represent mean values in patients on insulin therapy, and open circles represent mean values in patients on glyburide therapy. *(Reprinted, by permission, from Garg A, Grundy SM: Lovastatin for lowering cholesterol levels in non-insulin-dependent diabetes mellitus. N Engl J Med 1988;318:81–86.)*

in cholesterol synthesis, which secondarily increases LDL receptor activity.[61] This increase in hepatic LDL receptors enhances clearance of both LDL and VLDL remnants and lowers their plasma levels. In general, these drugs do not change the composition of VLDL or LDL particles. Effects on HDL cholesterol concentrations are variable, but overall a slight increase is observed.

We have evaluated the efficacy of lovastatin (20 mg twice daily) for treatment of dyslipidemia in NIDDM patients and found it to be highly effective in lowering lipid levels.[62] Lovastatin therapy reduced plasma total cholesterol levels by 26%, LDL cholesterol levels by 28%, and LDL apo B levels by 26% (Figure 7.2). Lovastatin therapy also lowered plasma triglyceride and VLDL cholesterol levels, particularly in patients with borderline hypertriglyceridemia (Figure 7.3). This drug, however, did not raise levels of HDL cholesterol (Figure 7.3). Most patients were able to achieve the proposed therapeutic goal for non-HDL cholesterol levels (Table 7.5). Glycemic control was not affected by lovastatin therapy.

Yoshino et al[63] have evaluated pravastatin therapy for NIDDM patients with dyslipidemia and have found it to be moderately effective, although a low dose of pravastatin (5 mg twice daily) was used, which may not have shown the drug's true potential. Recently, in another study of pravastatin therapy (10 to 20 mg/ d) in NIDDM patients, they further confirmed our observation that HMG CoA reductase inhibitors do not adversely affect glycemic control.[64] Since HMG CoA reductase inhibitors reduce lithogenicity of bile,[65] they could be especially beneficial in NIDDM patients, who are known to be at high risk of developing cholesterol gallstones.[66] Lovastatin produces cataracts in dogs when given in very high doses. Although extensive clinical investigation in nondiabetic patients has revealed no increase in lens opacities during protracted lovastatin therapy,[67] the fact that NIDDM patients are at increased risk of cataracts means there is the outside possibility that these drugs may increase cataractogenesis in diabetic patients. Long-term studies therefore are needed to rule out any adverse effect of these drugs on cataract formation in NIDDM patients. This remote possibility, however, does not preclude their use in NIDDM patients at the present time.

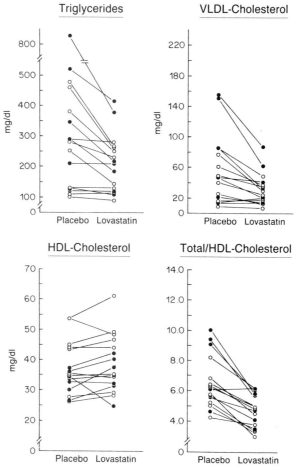

Figure 7.3 Plasma levels of triglycerides, VLDL cholesterol, and HDL cholesterol, and the ratio of total cholesterol to HDL cholesterol in 16 patients with NIDDM during the placebo and lovastatin periods. Each symbol represents the mean of five daily determinations. Solid circles represent mean values in patients on insulin therapy, and open circles represent mean values in patients on glyburide therapy. *(Reprinted, with permission, from Garg A, Grundy SM: Lovastatin for lowering cholesterol levels in non-insulin-dependent diabetes mellitus. N Engl J Med 1988;318:81–86.)*

Other side effects of HMG CoA reductase inhibitors include minor gastrointestinal upsets and reversible increases in alanine aminotransferase and aspartate aminotransferase levels. These agents also can cause myopathy, which can manifest as muscle weakness, soreness, elevated creatine kinase levels, and rarely rhabdomyolysis, myoglobinuria, and acute renal failure.[68] Although the precise mechanisms for myopathy are not known, it probably occurs only when serum levels of the drug become elevated. Therefore, use of these agents should be avoided in patients with moderately severe renal insufficiency resulting from diabetic nephropathy or in patients with hepatic disease; both of these conditions may interfere with disposal of these drugs and thus raise their serum levels. Also, concomitant use of HMG CoA reductase inhibitors with other drugs such as cyclosporin, gemfibrozil, erythromycin, and nicotinic acid also increases the risk of myopathy, and in general these combinations should be avoided. Other minor side effects of reductase inhibitors are headache, skin rash, and possibly sleep disturbances.

Overall, HMG CoA reductase inhibitors appear to be safe and effective drugs for treatment of dyslipidemia in NIDDM patients. In fact, they may be the drug of choice for NIDDM patients with high LDL cholesterol levels and normal or moderately elevated serum triglycerides. HMG CoA reductase inhibitors, however, should not be used in patients with marked hypertriglyceridemia because they are largely ineffective.

Fibric Acid Derivatives

This category of drugs includes several agents: gemfibrozil, clofibrate, fenofibrate, bezafibrate, clinofibrate, and ciprofibrate. Only gemfibrozil and clofibrate are currently available in the United States. Fibric acids lower plasma triglyceride concentrations, mainly by increasing activity of LPL and possibly by reducing hepatic VLDL synthesis.[69] When triglyceride levels fall, HDL cholesterol concentrations are increased modestly. In patients with normal triglyceride levels, the fibric acids lower LDL cholesterol by 5% to 15%. In hypertriglyceridemic patients, however, the fall in triglyceride levels usually is accompanied by an increase in LDL cholesterol levels.[70] This increase, interestingly, can reflect a normalization of LDL composition (ie, an increase in LDL cholesterol–apo B ratios to the normal range).[70] With this change comes a reduction in heterogeneity of LDL particles and elimination of the small, dense LDL particles characteristic of hypertriglyceridemic patients.[71] It is worth noting that in the Helsinki Heart Study,[72] gemfibrozil therapy, when compared with placebo therapy, reduced rates of CHD primarily in patients with hypertriglyceridemia, despite the fact that many had an increase in LDL cholesterol levels. Therefore, in spite of causing small increases in LDL cholesterol levels in NIDDM patients with hypertriglyceridemia, these agents could still reduce risk of CHD.

In our study,[73] gemfibrozil was highly effective for lowering triglycerides in NIDDM patients with marked hypertriglyceridemia and thus reduced the risk of acute pancreatitis (Figure 7.4). A simultaneous increase in HDL cholesterol levels also was noted. As stated earlier, LDL cholesterol levels rose on gemfibrozil therapy, although levels of LDL apo B did not increase. Gemfibrozil therapy did not adversely affect glycemic control. We further evaluated the effectiveness of a combination of gemfibrozil with lovastatin for treatment of marked hypertriglyceridemia in NIDDM patients.[73] Although this combination was highly effective in lipid lowering, recent information indicates that it may be accompanied by increased risk for myopathy.[68] The combination of gemfibrozil and lovastatin therefore cannot be used routinely in NIDDM patients, and only carefully selected patients should be considered for such therapy. Close monitoring is required to prevent development of severe myopathy with accompanying myoglobinuria and acute tubular necrosis, which could be catastrophic for a patient with NIDDM.

Interestingly, one fibric acid, clofibrate, has been reported to improve glucose tolerance.[74] Even so, use of clofibrate has declined in recent years because of the report of long-term side effects in the World Health Organization study.[75] Paradoxically, more patients in the clofibrate group developed diabetes mellitus

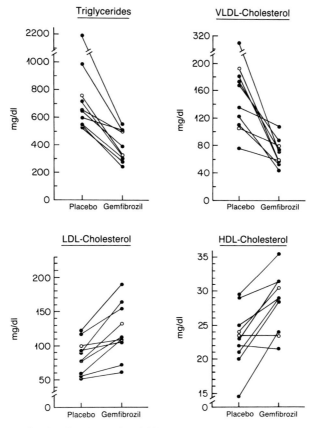

Figure 7.4 Plasma levels of triglycerides, VLDL cholesterol, LDL cholesterol, and HDL cholesterol during placebo and gemfibrozil therapy in ten NIDDM patients with marked hypertriglyceridemia. Symbols represent means of two determinations. Solid circles represent mean values in patients on insulin therapy, and open circles represent mean values in patients on glyburide therapy. *(Reprinted, by permission, from Garg A, Grundy SM: Gemfibrozil alone and in combination with lovastatin for treatment of hypertriglyceridemia in NIDDM. Diabetes 1989;38:364–372. Copyright 1989, American Diabetes Association, Inc.)*

than in the placebo group in this study, but whether this association is causal remains to be determined.

Fibric acid therapy increases risk for cholesterol gallstones,[75,76] and in NIDDM patients, a group that already is predisposed to cholelithiasis, this may be a disadvantage. Since renal excretion is an important major route of elimination of fibric acids, these drugs should be used with caution, if at all, in patients with diabetic nephropathy and chronic renal failure because of increased risk of drug retention and development of myopathy. Other side effects of fibric acids include various gastrointestinal symptoms, occasional changes in hematologic parameters, and abnormal liver function tests. A slight increase in incidence of malignancies of the biliary tract and small intestine was reported with clofibrate therapy in the World Health Organization study.[75] Whether the association was causal is uncertain, however, since a recent reanalysis of the trial data has thrown this association into question. In the Helsinki Heart Study,[77] gemfibrozil therapy was not associated with increased rate of malignancy. The fibric acids potentiate the action of oral anticoagulants, and patients receiving the latter should be carefully monitored.

Fibric acid derivatives are the first choice of therapy for NIDDM patients with marked hypertriglyceridemia and chylomicronemia. Also, in diabetic patients with concomitant type III hyperlipoproteinemia, these agents probably are the drug of choice.

Nicotinic Acid and Analogues

Because nicotinic acid effectively lowers plasma triglyceride and VLDL levels and raises HDL cholesterol concentrations, at first glance it might be considered an ideal drug for treatment of diabetic dyslipidemia. This possibility necessitates a closer look at nicotinic acid. Although precise mechanisms for its lipid-lowering properties are not known, nicotinic acid has been reported to inhibit lipolysis from adipose tissue and thereby reduce flux of free fatty acids to the liver. Reduced availability of free fatty acids, which are substrates for triglyceride synthesis in the liver, causes reduction in VLDL triglyceride synthesis.[78] Besides lowering VLDL triglycerides, nicotinic acid therapy changes the composition of VLDL particles by reducing their cholesteryl ester content.[79] The increase in HDL cholesterol levels occurring with nicotinic acid is due primarily to an increase in HDL_2 cholesterol concentrations.[80] In patients without hypertriglyceridemia, nicotinic acid therapy is moderately effective for lowering LDL cholesterol levels.

We recently showed that nicotinic acid (4.5 g/d in divided doses) is indeed efficacious for lowering triglyceride and raising HDL levels in NIDDM patients (Figure 7.5).[58] In these patients, however, a deterioration of glycemic control occurred (Figure 7.6). Nicotinic acid therapy also raised plasma uric acid levels, increasing the risk of gout in patients already predisposed to it (Figure 7.6). Induction of hyperuricemia potentially may induce renal dysfunction, particularly in patients with diabetic nephropathy. It is our view, therefore, that nicotinic acid therapy generally should be avoided in NIDDM patients.

Nicotinic acid analogues—acipimox (5-methylpyrazine carboxylic acid) and niceritrol (pentaerythritol tetranicotinate)—are available outside the United States. Acipimox is not as effective for lowering plasma lipids as nicotinic acid[81,82] but, on the positive side, preliminary studies suggest no deterioration of glycemic control in NIDDM subjects given 250 mg of acipimox three times daily.[83] However, worsening of glucose tolerance was reported in glucose-intolerant subjects receiving higher doses of acipimox.[82] Niceritrol therapy also can worsen glycemic control and insulin resistance.[84] Therefore, more investigation is required before acipimox or niceritrol can be safely recommended for treatment of the dyslipidemia of NIDDM.

Nicotinic acid therapy is accompanied by several other side effects. Flushing of skin occurs immediately after initiating drug therapy, but the severity of flushing episodes declines after several weeks of therapy. Aspirin may lessen the severity of flushing. Nicotinic acid and its analogues further can exacerbate peptic ulcer and cause abnormalities in liver function tests. The slow-release preparations of nicotinic acid seemingly are more hepatotoxic than the regular crystalline form of the drug.[85] Other less common side effects of nicotinic acid therapy include postural hypotension, toxic amblyopia, pruritus, acanthosis nigricans, and skin pigmentation.

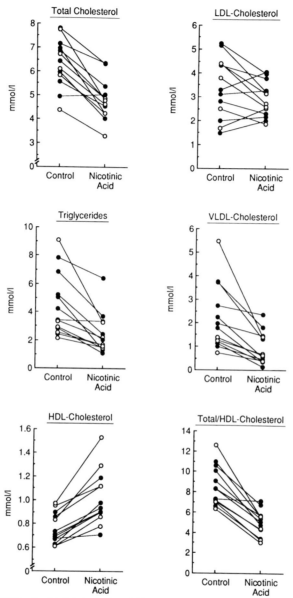

Figure 7.5 Plasma levels of total cholesterol, LDL cholesterol, triglycerides, VLDL cholesterol, and HDL cholesterol and the ratio of total cholesterol to HDL cholesterol during the control and the nicotinic acid periods in 13 NIDDM patients with dyslipidemia. Each circle represents the mean of five daily determinations. Solid circles indicate mean values in patients receiving insulin therapy; open circles, values in patients receiving glyburide therapy or diet alone. *(Reprinted, by permission, from Garg A, Grundy SM: Nicotinic acid as therapy for dyslipidemia in non-insulin-dependent diabetes mellitus. JAMA 1990;264:723–726. Copyright 1990, American Medical Association.)*

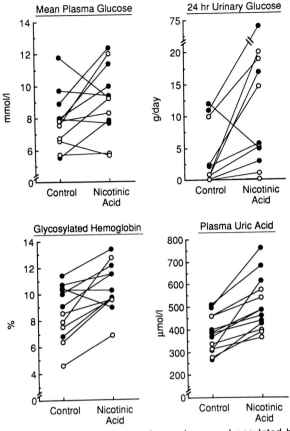

Figure 7.6 Mean plasma glucose, 24-hour urinary glucose, glycosylated hemoglobin, and plasma uric acid levels during the control and the nicotinic acid periods in 13 NIDDM patients with dyslipidemia. Solid circles indicate mean values in patients receiving insulin therapy; open circles, values in patients receiving glyburide therapy or diet alone. *(Reprinted, by permission, from Garg A, Grundy SM: Nicotinic acid as therapy for dyslipidemia in non-insulin-dependent diabetes mellitus. JAMA 1990;264:723–726. Copyright 1990, American Medical Association.)*

Bile Acid Binding Resins

The bile acid binding resins, cholestyramine or colestipol, interrupt enterohepatic circulation of bile acids and cause an increase in hepatic LDL receptor activity. Consequently, their major action is to lower LDL cholesterol levels. The resins, however, have not been evaluated systematically in NIDDM patients.[86,87] Because they tend to raise serum triglyceride levels, this may be a disadvantage in that NIDDM patients already are prone to hypertriglyceridemia.[88] Preliminary results of an ongoing trial of cholestyramine therapy in hypercholesterolemic NIDDM patients in our laboratory suggest that cholestyramine therapy effectively reduces LDL cholesterol levels without appreciably raising triglyceride levels.[89] Interestingly, in our patients, cholestyramine therapy caused slight improvement in glycemic control; this improvement occurred without any changes in body weight or doses of hypoglycemic drugs. Bile acid binding resins therefore may be useful for NIDDM patients with normal triglyceride levels. Serum triglyceride levels, however, should be monitored closely in patients receiving these drugs.

Since constipation is the major side effect of resin therapy, it may be best to avoid these drugs in patients with diabetic autonomic neuropathy. In contrast, rare patients who have diarrhea as a manifestation of autonomic neuropathy could have a symptomatic benefit from resin therapy. Other gastrointestinal side effects of these drugs are abdominal discomfort, flatulence, heartburn, and indigestion. A mild steatorrhea and deficiency of fat-soluble vitamins and folic acid also may occur with long-term use. In children and adolescents, height and weight should be closely monitored, and appropriate analyses should be performed to ensure that specific vitamin deficiencies are prevented. Some investigators recommend routine use of folate supplements in children receiving bile acid sequestrants. Sequestrants also are known to interfere with intestinal absorption of various drugs and should be used cautiously in patients taking multiple medications.

Probucol

Probucol lowers LDL cholesterol levels through increased clearance of LDL, most likely by nonreceptor pathways.[90] Probucol does not reduce serum triglyceride concentrations; it does, however, lower levels of HDL cholesterol. Even though probucol reduces HDL levels, it has been reported to cause regression of xanthomas in hypercholesterolemic patients.[91] Besides lowering serum cholesterol, probucol is an effective antioxidant.[92] The drug is carried in LDL particles and prevents oxidative modification of LDL. According to some investigators, oxidation and other modifications of lipoproteins are essential for atherogenesis. If so, probucol might prevent atherosclerosis by virtue of its antioxidant properties. Indeed, in hypercholesterolemic animals, probucol therapy inhibits development of atherosclerosis.[93,94] The antioxidant property of probucol could be beneficial in patients with diabetes mellitus because their lipoproteins and other matrix proteins are more prone to glycosylation as well as oxidation. However, for lack of sufficient in vivo evidence in support of this theory of atherosclerosis, probucol therapy cannot be justified solely for its antioxidant properties at the present time. Thus, for NIDDM patients, the use of probucol is problematic. If future clinical trials in humans demonstrate retarded atherogenesis with probucol, the drug might be especially useful for NIDDM patients.

One side effect of probucol is a widening of the Q-T interval on the electrocardiogram; such a widening may be of particular concern for diabetic patients with autonomic neuropathy, who already may have a prolonged Q-T interval. Other side effects include gastrointestinal symptoms (particularly diarrhea), headache, and rash.

Hyperchylomicronemia Syndrome (Type V Hyperlipoproteinemia)

Hyperchylomicronemia syndrome is characterized by high levels of both VLDL and chylomicrons, and triglyceride concentrations usually exceed 11.3 mmol/L (1,000 mg/dL). It can occur in either NIDDM or IDDM patients. Risk of acute pancreatitis is high, and the primary therapeutic consideration is to avoid pancreatitis or, if it has already occurred, to prevent future attacks.[95] Although poor glycemic control is primarily responsible for hyperchylomicronemia in most diabetic patients, other factors, such as moderate to heavy alcohol consumption, increased caloric intake, severe obesity, β-adrenergic blocker therapy, and estrogen-containing oral contraceptives may have an important contribution. Often diabetic patients with severe hypertriglyceridemia have concomitant genetic forms of hyperlipoproteinemias that are exacerbated by poor glycemic control.

The first goal of therapy in such patients is to reduce plasma triglyceride levels to below 5.6 mmol/L (500 mg/dL) so as to prevent acute pancreatitis. Patients presenting with acute pancreatitis should discontinue oral intake and should be managed by parental nutrition without lipid emulsions. When oral intake is restarted, very-low-fat diets are required to minimize chylomicron formation, the key factor responsible for development of pancreatitis. Insulin therapy should be instituted promptly to achieve euglycemia. In most patients, severe chylomicronemia can be eliminated by good glycemic control. If hypertriglyceridemia persists, other exacerbating factors should be removed. Fibric acids are useful for lowering triglyceride levels in chylomicronemic patients.[73] However, they should be instituted only after achieving good glycemic control because they may not be very effective in hyperglycemic patients. The ω-3 polyunsaturated fatty acids may be tried in patients not tolerating fibric acids, but long-term experience with these agents in patients with diabetes mellitus is not available. Furthermore, ω-3 polyunsaturated fatty acids may enhance insulin resistance and worsen glycemic control in some patients.

Dyslipidemia in Diabetic Nephropathy

Diabetic nephropathy accentuates lipoprotein disorders in both IDDM and NIDDM patients. The pattern of dyslipidemia depends on the presentation of diabetic nephropathy (ie, microalbuminuria, nephrotic syndrome, or chronic renal insufficiency). With chronic renal failure, the major pattern is hypertriglyceridemia and low HDL cholesterol, which seemingly are due to reduced activity of LPL.[96] With the nephrotic syndrome, elevations of LDL cholesterol are the predominant abnormality, but many patients also have hypertriglyceridemia. Hepatic overproduction of lipoproteins apparently is a contributing factor to hyperlipidemia in the nephrotic syndrome, but other abnormalities also occur. The catabolism of VLDL is impaired in many patients,[97] and hepatic uptake of LDL also may be sluggish. Nephrotic hyperlipidemia thus appears to be multifactorial in origin. In several patients with diabetic nephropathy, a combined picture of nephrotic syndrome and chronic renal failure exists and a spectrum of lipoprotein abnormalities may be present.

Restriction of protein intake usually is advised for patients with diabetic nephropathy. In dyslipidemic patients, restriction of saturated fatty acids and cholesterol should be undertaken. Patients with nephrotic syndrome, however, often are poorly responsive to these usual dietary modifications. If dyslipidemia persists despite good glycemic control and dietary modification, consideration can be given to lipid-lowering drugs.

In patients with chronic renal insufficiency, the safety and efficacy of lipid-lowering drugs has not been well studied. In those with the nephrotic syndrome, bile acid binding resins and probucol appear to be safe, but desirable levels of LDL cholesterol often are not achieved with these agents alone.[98,99] HMG CoA reductase inhibitors are effective in nondiabetic patients with nephrotic syndrome and can be considered for treating diabetic patients with nephrotic syndrome and mild renal insufficiency.[97,98,100] The safety of HMG CoA reductase inhibitors in patients with moderately severe renal insufficiency has not been evaluated, and these drugs should be used with caution in such patients because of the danger of severe myopathy.

For lowering serum triglyceride levels in patients with chronic renal insufficiency, low-dose fibric acid derivatives have been recommended.[101] Because these drugs are excreted mainly by the kidneys, even low doses can precipitate myopathy.[102] Therefore, a careful monitoring of patients is required if fibric acid derivatives are used in patients with chronic renal insufficiency. The ω-3 polyunsaturated fatty acids are another option for lowering triglycerides in patients with chronic renal failure; their efficacy in diabetic patients with nephropathy, however, has not been studied systematically.

Conclusion

To summarize, although the clinical picture and prevalence of dyslipidemia in IDDM patients are different than those in NIDDM patients, the lipoprotein abnormalities seemingly play an important role in causation of CHD and other atherosclerotic vascular manifestations in both types of diabetes mellitus. Therefore, equal emphasis should be given to normalization of dyslipidemia and control of hyperglycemia. Therapeutic goals for serum cholesterol reduction should be lower in diabetic patients that in nondiabetic patients, and the goals for children with diabetes mellitus may be different than those for adults with diabetes mellitus. Because of peculiar metabolic derangements in patients with diabetes mellitus, the therapeutic interventions may not be same as those for nondiabetic patients.

Dietary therapy along with weight reduction, an exercise program, and good metabolic control with oral hypoglycemic agents or insulin therapy should be employed before turning to lipid-lowering medications. For children with IDDM, bile acid binding resins are the drug of choice; other drugs should be tried under the guidance of a lipid specialist. In adults with diabetes mellitus, HMG CoA reductase inhibitors may be the drug of choice for patients with elevated LDL cholesterol who have normal or borderline-high levels of plasma triglycerides. Fibric acid derivatives appear preferable in patients with marked hypertriglyceridemia. Bile acid binding resins may be tried in normotriglyceridemic patients with isolated increase in LDL cholesterol. Nicotinic acid should be avoided in patients with diabetes mellitus. The role of probucol for dyslipidemia in patients with diabetes mellitus is not clear.

References

1. Haaber AB, Kofoed-Enevoldsen A, Jensen T: The prevalence of hyperlipidemia and its relationship with albuminuria in insulin dependent diabetic patients: An epidemiologic study. *Diabetic Med* 1992;9:557–561.
2. Sosenko JM, Breslow JL, Miettinen OS, et al: Hyperglycemia and plasma lipid levels.

A prospective study of young insulin-dependent diabetic patients. *N Engl J Med* 1980;302:650–654.

3. Strobl W, Widhalm K, Schober E, et al: Apolipoproteins and lipoproteins in children with type I diabetes: Relation to glycosylated serum protein and HbA1. *Acta Paediatr Scand* 1985;74:966–971.

4. Bagdade JD, Porte D, Bierman EL: Diabetic lipemia. *N Engl J Med* 1967;276:427–433.

5. Rosenstock J, Strowig S, Cercone S, et al: Reduction in cardiovascular risk factors with intensive diabetes treatment in insulin-dependent diabetes mellitus. *Diabetes Care* 1987;10:729–734.

6. Pietri AO, Dunn FL, Grundy SM, et al: The effect of continuous subcutaneous insulin infusion on very-low-density lipoprotein triglyceride metabolism in type I diabetes mellitus. *Diabetes* 1983;32:75–81.

7. Rosenstock J, Vega GL, Raskin P: Effect of intensive diabetes treatment on low-density lipoprotein apolipoprotein B kinetics in type I diabetes. *Diabetes* 1988;37:393–397.

8. Durrington PN: Serum high density lipoprotein cholesterol subfractions in type I (insulin-dependent) diabetes mellitus. *Clin Chim Acta* 1982;120:21–28.

9. Bagdade JD, Subbaiah PV: Whole-plasma and high-density lipoprotein subtraction surface lipid concentration in IDDM men. *Diabetes* 1989;38:1226–1230.

10. Helve E: High density lipoprotein subfractions during continuous insulin infusion therapy. *Atherosclerosis* 1987;64:173–180.

11. Mattock MB, Sakter AM, Fuller JH et al: High density lipoprotein subfractions in insulin-dependent diabetic and normal subjects. *Atherosclerosis* 1982;45:67–79.

12. Georgopoulos A, Rosengard AM: Abnormalities in the metabolism of postprandial and fasting triglyceride-rich lipoprotein subfractions in normal and insulin-dependent diabetic subjects: Effects of sex. *Metabolism* 1989;38:781–789.

13. Klein RL, Lyons TJ, Lopes-Virella MF: Interaction of very-low-density lipoprotein isolated from type I (insulin-dependent) diabetic subjects with human monocyte-derived macrophages. *Metabolism* 1989;38:1108–1114.

14. James RW, Pometta D: Differences in lipoprotein subfraction composition and distribution between type I diabetic men and control subjects. *Diabetes* 1990;39:1158–1164.

15. Vannini P, Ciavarella A, Flammini A, et al: Lipid abnormalities in insulin-dependent diabetic patients with albuminuria. *Diabetes Care* 1984;7:151–154.

16. Winocour PH, Durrington PN, Ishola M, et al: Influence of proteinuria on vascular disease, blood pressure, and lipoproteins in insulin-dependent diabetes mellitus. *BMJ* 1987;294:1648–1651.

17. Laakso M, Pyorala K: Adverse effects of obesity on lipid and lipoprotein levels in insulin-dependent and non-insulin-dependent diabetes. *Metabolism* 1990;39:117–122.

18. Krolewski AS, Kosinski EJ, Warram JH, et al: Magnitude and determinants of coronary artery disease in juvenile-onset, insulin-dependent diabetes mellitus. *Am J Cardiol* 1987;59:750–755.

19. Jensen T, Borch-Johnsen K, Kofoed M, et al: Coronary heart disease in young type I (insulin-dependent) diabetic patients with and without diabetic nephropathy: Incidence and risk factors. *Diabetologia* 1987;30:144–148.

20. Laakso M, Pyorala K, Sarlund H, et al: Lipid and lipoprotein abnormalities associated with coronary heart disease in patients with insulin-dependent diabetes mellitus. *Arteriosclerosis* 1986;6:679–684.

21. Taskinen MR, Syvanne TK, Syvanne M: Lipid changes in macrovascular disease in diabetes, in Andreani D, Gueriguian J, Striker G (eds): *Diabetic Complications. Epidemiology and Pathogenetic Mechanisms*. New York, Raven Press, 1991, pp 313–326.

22. Hanefeld M, Schulze J, Fischer S, et al: The diabetes intervention study (DIS): A

cooperative multi-intervention trial with newly manifested type II diabetics: Preliminary results. *Monogr Atheroscler* 1985;13:98–103.

23. Wilson PWF, Kannel WB, Anderson KM: Lipids, glucose intolerance and vascular disease: The Framingham Study. *Monogr Atheroscler* 1985;13:1–11.

24. Assman G, Schulte H: The Prospective Cardiovascular Munster (PROCAM) study: Prevalence of hyperlipidemia in persons with hypertension and/or diabetes mellitus and the relationship to coronary heart disease. *Am Heart J* 1988;116:1713–1724.

25. Stern MP, Patterson JK, Haffner SM, et al: Lack of awareness and treatment of hyperlipidemia in type II diabetes in a community survey. *JAMA* 1989;262:360–364.

26. Diabetes Drafting Group: Prevalence of small vessel and large vessel disease in diabetic patients from 14 centres: The World Health Organisation multinational study of vascular disease in diabetics. *Diabetologia* 1985;28(suppl 1):615–640.

27. West KM, Ahuja MMS, Bennett PH, et al: The role of circulating glucose and triglyceride concentrations and their interactions with other "risk factors" as determinants of arterial disease in nine diabetic population samples from the WHO multinational study. *Diabetes Care* 1983;6:361–369.

28. Haffner SM, Stern MP, Hazuda HP, et al: Cardiovascular risk factors in confirmed prediabetic individuals. Does the clock for coronary heart disease start ticking before the onset of clinical diabetes? *JAMA* 1990;263:2893–2898.

29. Fielding CJ, Castro GR, Donner C, et al: Distribution of apolipoprotein E in the plasma of insulin-dependent and noninsulin-dependent diabetics and its relation to cholesterol net transport. *J Lipid Res* 1986;27:1052–1062.

30. Fisher WR: Heterogeneity of plasma low density lipoproteins: Manifestations of the physiologic phenomenon in man. *Metabolism* 1983;32:283–291.

31. Kissebah AH: Low density lipoprotein metabolism in non-insulin-dependent diabetes mellitus. *Diabetes Metab Rev* 1987;3:619–651.

32. Fontbonne A, Eschwege E, Cambien F, et al: Hypertriglyceridemia as a risk factor of coronary heart disease mortality in subjects with impaired glucose tolerance or diabetes: Results from the 11-year follow-up of the Paris prospective study. *Diabetologia* 1989;32:300–304.

33. Ronnemaa T, Laakso M, Pyorala K, et al: High fasting plasma insulin is an indicator of coronary heart disease in non-insulin-dependent diabetic patients and nondiabetic subjects. *Arterioscler Thromb* 1991;11:80–90.

34. National Cholesterol Education Program Expert Panel, National Heart, Lung, and Blood Institute: Report of the National Cholesterol Education Program Expert Panel on detection, evaluation, and treatment of high blood cholesterol in adults. *Arch Intern Med* 1988;148:36–69.

35. National Cholesterol Education Program: *Report of the Expert Panel on Blood Cholesterol Levels in Children and Adolescents*, NIH publ No 91-2732. Washington, DC, U.S. Department of Health and Human Services, 1991.

36. Garg A, Grundy SM: Management of dyslipidemia in NIDDM. *Diabetes Care* 1990;13:153–169.

37. American Diabetes Association: Nutritional recommendations and principles for individuals with diabetes mellitus. *Diabetes Care* 1986;10:126–132.

38. Hollenbeck CB, Connor WE, Riddle MC, et al: The effects of a high-carbohydrate low-fat cholesterol-restricted diet on plasma lipid, lipoprotein, and apoprotein concentrations in insulin-depenent (type 1) diabetes mellitus. *Metabolism* 1985;6:559–566.

39. Simpson RW, Mann JI, Eaton J, et al: High-carbohydrate diets and insulin-dependent diabetics. *BMJ* 1979;2:523–525.

40. Garg A, Bonanome A, Grundy SM, et al: Comparison of a high-carbohydrate diet with a high-monounsaturated-fat diet in patients with non-insulin-dependent diabetes mellitus. *N Engl J Med* 1988;391:829–834.

41. Perrotti N, Santoro D, Genovese S, et al: Effect of digestible carbohydrates on glucose control in insulin-dependent diabetic patients. *Diabetes Care* 1984;7:354–359.

42. National Institutes of Health: Consensus development conference on diet and exercise in non-insulin-dependent diabetes mellitus. *Diabetes Care* 1987;10:639–644.

43. Garg A, Reaven GM, Bantle JP, et al: Long-term effects of high-carbohydrate versus high-monounsaturated fat diets in NIDDM [abstract]. *Diabetes* 1992;41(suppl 1):72A.

44. Himsworth HP: The dietetic factor determining the glucose tolerance and sensitivity to insulin of healthy men. *Clin Sci* 1935;2:67–94.

45. Brunzell JD, Lerner RL, Hazzard WR, et al: Improved glucose tolerance with high carbohydrate feeding in mild diabetes. *N Engl J Med* 1971;284:521–524.

46. Coulston AM, Hollenbeck CB, Swislocki ALM, et al: Deleterious metabolic effects of high-carbohydrate, sucrose-containing diets in patients with non-insulin-dependent diabetes mellitus. *Am J Med* 1987;82:213–220.

47. Garg A, Grundy SM, Unger RH: Comparison of effects of high and low carbohydrate diets on plasma lipoproteins and insulin sensitivity in patients with mild NIDDM. *Diabetes* 1992;41:1278–1285.

48. Grundy SM, Garg A: Cardiovascular actions of fish oils and omega-3 fatty acids. *Prog Cardiol* 1991;4:21–37.

49. Phillipson BE, Rothrock DW, Connor WE, et al: Reduction of plasma lipids, lipoproteins, and apoproteins by dietary fish oils in patients with hypertriglyceridemia. *N Engl J Med* 1985;312:1210–1216.

50. Nozaki S, Garg A, Vega GL, et al: Post-heparin lipolytic activity and plasma lipoprotein response to ω-3 polyunsaturated fatty acids in patients with primary hypertriglyceridemia. *Am J Clin Nutr* 1991;53:638–642.

51. Glauber H, Wallace P, Griver K, et al: Adverse metabolic effect of omega-3 fatty acids in non-insulin-dependent diabetes mellitus. *Ann Intern Med* 1988;108:663–668.

52. Friday KE, Childs MT, Tsunehara CH, et al: Elevated plasma glucose and lowered triglyceride levels from omega-3 fatty acid supplementation in type II diabetes. *Diabetes Care* 1989;12:276–281.

53. Kennedy L, Washe K, Hadden DR, et al: The effect of intensive dietary therapy on serum high density lipoprotein-cholesterol in patients with type 2 non-insulin-dependent diabetes mellitus: A prospective study. *Diabetologia* 1982;23:24–27.

54. Wolf R, Grundy SM: Influence of weight reduction on plasma lipoproteins in obese patients. *Arteriosclerosis* 1983;3;160–169.

55. Hughes TA, Gwynne JT, Switzer BR, et al: Effects of caloric restriction and weight loss on glycemic control, insulin release and resistance, and atherosclerotic risk in obese patients with type II diabetes mellitus. *Am J Med* 1984;77:7–17.

56. The Diabetes Control and Complications Trial (DCCT) Research Group: Epidemiology of severe hypoglycemia in the Diabetes Control and Complications Trial. *Am J Med* 1991;90:450–459.

57. Hollenbeck CB, Chen Y-DI, Greenfield MS, et al: Reduced plasma high density lipoprotein-cholesterol concentrations need not increase when hyperglycemia is controlled with insulin in non-insulin-dependent diabetes mellitus. *J Clin Endocrinol Metab* 1985;62:605–608.

58. Garg A, Grundy SM: Nicotinic acid as therapy for dyslipidemia in non-insulin-dependent diabetes mellitus. *JAMA* 1990;264:723–726.

59. Narduzzi JV, Danowski TS, Weir TF, et al: Laboratory indices in clofibrate therapy of juvenile-onset diabetes. *Clin Pharmacol Ther* 1967;8:817–823.

60. Winocour PH, Durrington PN, Bhatnagar D, et al: Double-blind placebo-controlled study of the effects of bezafibrate on blood lipids, lipoproteins, and fibrinogen in hyperlipidaemic type 1 diabetes mellitus. *Diabetic Med* 1990;7:736–743.

61. Grundy SM: HMG-CoA reductase inhibitors for treatment of hypercholesterolemia. *N Engl J Med* 1988;319:24–33.

62. Garg A, Grundy SM: Lovastatin for lowering cholesterol levels in non-insulin-dependent diabetes mellitus. *N Engl J Med* 1988;318:81–86.

63. Yoshino G, Kazumi T, Kasama T, et al: Effects of CS-514, an inhibitor of 3-hydroxy-

3-methylglutaryl coenzyme A reductase, on lipoprotein and apolipoprotein in plasma of hypercholesterolemic diabetics. *Diabetes Res Clin Pract* 1986;2:179–181.

64. Yoshino G, Kazumi T, Iwai M, et al: Long-term treatment of hypercholesterolemic non-insulin-dependent-diabetes mellitus (NIDDM) with pravastatin (CS-514). *Atherosclerosis* 1989;75:67–72.

65. Duane WC, Hunninghake DB, Freeman ML, et al: Simvastatin: A competitive inhibitor of HMG CoA-reductase, lowers cholesterol saturation index of gallbladder bile. *Hepatology* 1988;8:1147–1150.

66. Bennion LJ, Grundy SM: Effects of diabetes mellitus on cholesterol metabolism in man. *N Engl J Med* 1977;296:1365–1371.

67. Hunninghake DB, Miller VT, Goldberg I, et al: Lovastatin: Follow-up ophthalmologic data. *JAMA* 1988;259:354–355.

68. Pierce LR, Wysowski DK, Gross TP: Myopathy and rhabdomyolysis associated with lovastatin-gemfibrozil combination therapy. *JAMA* 1990;264:71–75.

69. Saku K, Gartside PS, Hynd BA, et al: Mechanism of action of gemfibrozil on lipoprotein metabolism. *J Clin Invest* 1985;75:1702–1712.

70. Vega GL, Grundy SM: Gemfibrozil therapy in primary hypertriglyceridemia associated with coronary heart disease. Effects on metabolism of low-density lipoproteins. *JAMA* 1985;253:2398–2403.

71. Eisenberg S, Gavish D, Oschry Y, et al: Abnormalities in very low, and high density lipoproteins in hypertriglyceridemia. Reversal toward normal with bezafibrate treatment. *J Clin Invest* 1984;74:470–482.

72. Manninen V, Elo MO, Frick MH, et al: Lipid alterations and decline in the incidence of coronary heart disease in the Helsinki Heart Study. *JAMA* 1988;260:641–651.

73. Garg A, Grundy SM: Gemfibrozil alone and in combination with lovastatin for treatment of hypertriglyceridemia in NIDDM. *Diabetes* 1989;38:364–372.

74. Kobayashi M, Shigeta Y, Hirata Y, et al: Improvement of glucose tolerance in NIDDM by clofibrate: A randomized double-blind study. *Diabetes Care* 1988;11:495–499.

75. Committee of Principal Investigators: WHO Cooperative trial on primary prevention of ischaemic heart disease with clofibrate to lower serum cholesterol: Final mortality follow-up. *Lancet* 1984;2:600–604.

76. Leiss O, von Bergman K, Gnasso A, et al: Effect of gemfibrozil on biliary lipid metabolism in normolipidemic subjects. *Metabolism* 1985;34:74–82.

77. Frick MH, Elo MO, Haapa K, et al: Helsinki Heart Study: Primary prevention trial with gemfibrozil in middle-aged men with dyslipidemia. *N Engl J Med* 1987;317:1237–1245.

78. Grundy SM, Mok HYI, Zech L, et al: Influence of nicotinic acid on metabolism of cholesterol and triglycerides in man. *J Lipid Res* 1981;22:24–36.

79. Tornvall P, Hamsten A, Johansson J, et al: Normalisation of the composition of very low density lipoprotein in hypertriglyceridemia by nicotinic acid. *Atherosclerosis* 1990;84:219–227.

80. Shepherd J, Packard CJ, Patsch JR, et al: Effects of nicotinic acid on plasma high-density lipoprotein subfraction distribution and composition and on apolipoprotein A metabolism. *J Clin Invest* 1979;63:858–867.

81. Crepaldi G, Avogaro P, Descovich GC, et al: Plasma lipid lowering activity of acipimox in patients with type II and type IV hyperlipoproteinemia. Results of a multicenter trial. *Atherosclerosis* 1988;70:115–121.

82. Taskinen M-R, Nikkila EA: Effects of acipimox on serum lipids, lipoproteins and lipolytic enzymes in hypertriglyceridemia. *Atherosclerosis* 1988;69:249–255.

83. Lavezzari M, Milanesi G, Oggioni E, et al: Results of a phase IV study carried out with acipimox in type II diabetic patients with concomitant hyperlipoproteinaemia. *J Int Med Res* 1989;17:373–380.

84. Lithell H, Vessby B, Hellsing K: Changes in glucose tolerance and plasma insulin during lipid-lowering treatment with diet, clofibrate and niceritrol. *Atherosclerosis* 1982;43:177–184.

85. Rader JI, Calvert RJ, Hathcock JN: Hepatic toxicity of unmodified and time-release preparations of niacin. *Am J Med* 1992;92:77–81.
86. Bandisode MS, Boshell BR: Hypocholesterolemic activity of colestipol in diabetes. *Curr Ther Res* 1975;18:276–284.
87. Duntsch VG: Langzeittherapie der hypercholesterinamie beim diabetiker mit colestipol. *Fortschr Med* 1981;99:73–75.
88. Crouse JR: Hypertriglyceridemia: A contraindication to the use of bile acid binding resins. *Am J Med* 1987;83:243–248.
89. Garg A, Grundy SM: Cholestyramine therapy for dyslipidemia in NIDDM. *Clin Res* 1992;40:239A.
90. Kesaniemi YA, Grundy SM: Influence of probucol on cholesterol and lipoprotein metabolism in man. *J Lipid Res* 1984;25:780–790.
91. Yamamoto A, Matsuzawa Y, Yokoyama S, et al: Effects of probucol on xanthomata regression in familial hypercholesterolemia. *Am J Cardiol* 1986;57:29H–35H.
92. Parthasarathy S, Young S, Witztum JL, et al: Probucol inhibits oxidative modification of low density lipoprotein. *J Clin Invest* 1986;77:641–644.
93. Kita T, Nagano Y, Yokode M, et al: Probucol prevents the progression of atherosclerosis in Watanabe heritable hyperlipidemic rabbit, an animal model for familial hypercholesterolemia. *Proc Natl Acad Sci USA* 1987;84:5928–5931.
94. Carew TE, Schwenke DC, Steinberg D: Antiatherogenic effect of probucol unrelated to its hypocholesterolemic effect: Evidence that antioxidants in vivo can selectively inhibit low density lipoprotein degradation in macrophage-rich fatty streaks and slow the progression of atherosclerosis. *Proc Natl Acad Sci USA* 1987;84:7725–7729.
95. Miller A, Lees RS, McCluskey MA, et al: The natural history and surgical significance of hyperlipemic abdominal crisis. *Ann Surg* 1979;190:401–408.
96. Bagdade JD, Porte D, Bierman EL: Hypertriglyceridemia: A metabolic consequence of chronic renal failure. *N Engl J Med* 1968;279:181–185.
97. Vega GL, Grundy SM: Lovastatin therapy in nephrotic hyperlipidemia: Effects on lipoprotein metabolism. *Kidney Int* 1988;33:1160–1168.
98. Rabelink AJ, Erkelens DW, Hene RJ, et al: Effects of simvastatin and cholestyramine on lipoprotein profile in hyperlipidemia of nephrotic syndrome. *Lancet* 1988;2:1335–1338.
99. Iida H, Izumino K, Asaka M, et al: Effect of probucol on hyperlipidemia in patients with nephrotic syndrome. *Nephron* 1987;47:280–283.
100. Golper TA, Illingworth DR, Morris CD, et al: Lovastatin in the treatment of multifactorial hyperlipidemia associated with proteinuria. *Am J Kidney Dis* 1989;13:312–320.
101. Goldberg AP, Sherrard DJ, Haas LB, et al: Control of clofibrate toxicity in uremic hypertriglyceridemia. *Clin Pharmacol Ther* 1977;21:317–325.
102. di Giulio S, Boulu R, Nicolai A, et al: Clofibrate treatment of hyperlipidemia in chronic renal failure. *Clin Nephrol* 1977;8:504–509.

Part **2**

Diabetes and Atherosclerosis

Chapter 8

Reaction of the Muscular and Fibroelastic Artery Wall in Diabetes

Thomas Ledet, MD, PhD, and Robert W. Wissler, MD, PhD

For many years large vessel disease in diabetic patients has been a neglected research field, with only sporadic and infrequent publications that give insight into the recognizably specific pathogenesis of large and medium-sized arterial reactions in these individuals. Twenty years ago the term "diabetic macroangiopathy" was introduced.[1] This phrase indicates the presence of more or less characteristic and non-atherosclerotic reactions in the larger arteries in diabetic patients. As a part of diabetic angiopathy, diabetic macroangiopathy implies much more than accelerated or more severe atherosclerosis. It represents a variety of reactions some of which are present in the entire blood vascular system. Therefore, diabetic macroangiopathy is not a complication of diabetes mellitus but rather a part of this systemic disease. Clinically, it is often manifest late in the disease course.

The present chapter focuses on large (elastic) and medium-sized (muscular) artery disease in diabetic patients, mostly in the context of current views about diabetic macroangiopathy and its relationship to atherosclerosis in diabetes mellitus. In the opinion of most research workers, atherosclerosis is in one way or another related to lipoprotein alterations and/or abnormal passage of lipoprotein into the artery wall, with predilections for certain sites in the arterial systems.

Structural and Biochemical Changes in Diabetic Macroangiopathy

The composition of the arterial wall has been subjected to much histologic, histochemical, and biochemical analysis, particularly in recent years. These studies follow and build on the results of a multinational study of large arteries in which it was demonstrated that more extensive and more advanced lesions occur more frequently in arteries from diabetic than nondiabetic subjects.[2]

Quantitative histochemical approaches have indicated that there is an ac-

147

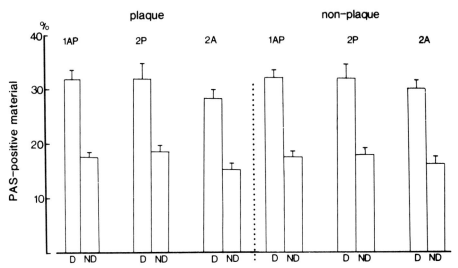

Figure 8.1 The area fraction of a PAS-positive glycoprotein in the coronary arteries from a group of diabetic (D) and nondiabetic (ND) subjects. 1AP = the first 2 to 3 cm of the anterior descending left and posterior decending right coronary arteries. 2A and 2P = the middle part of the anterior and posterior coronary artery, respectively. Bar = SEM (standard error of the mean).

cumulation of periodic acid–Schiff (PAS)-positive glycoprotein (Figure 8.1), but this is accompanied by a decrease in glycosaminoglycan-poor (Alcian blue–negative) material (Figure 8.2) in the tunica media of the extramural coronary arteries from type II diabetic individuals. There is little doubt that this reaction is a manifestation of diabetes, but there are other equally pathognomonic reactions that will be presented. This manifestation is accompanied by an increased amount of connective tissue.[3] It is noteworthy that this lesion is *also seen in areas without atherosclerosis*. More recently, quantitative immunohistochemical data indicate that at least part of the PAS-positive material seen in diabetic arteries in segments without atherosclerosis is identical to fibronectin.[4] Moreover, analyses of tunica media using the same quantitative techniques indicate that the basement membrane components, type IV collagen and laminin, occupy larger areas of the vessel wall in the arteries of diabetic individuals as compared to similar arteries of nondiabetic individuals (L.M. Rasmussen, L. Heickendorff, and T. Ledet, unpublished data). These alterations in this arterial tunica media were also found to be diffuse and unrelated to intimal lesions. Recent biochemical data have shown that the amount of type IV collagen is increased in the aortas from diabetic subjects (L.M. Rasmussen and T. Ledet, unpublished data).

It appears from these biochemical analyses of the structure of the arterial wall that a number of changes can be demonstrated in areas that do not display classic atherosclerosis. Some of these alterations in the larger arteries appear to be a part of a general vascular reaction because they are not directly related to the atherosclerotic lesions and because the accumulation of PAS-positive substances with reduced content of glycosaminoglycans in the small vessels and capillaries is known as the classic indicator of diabetic microangiopathy. Thus, for the first time, there is developing evidence of pathologic common denominators in the vascular manifestation of the disease.

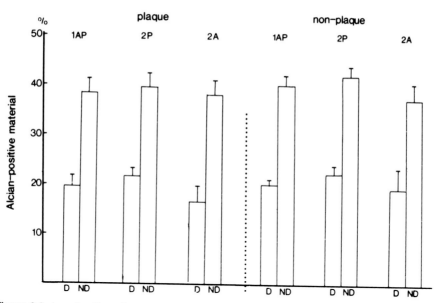

Figure 8.2 Area fraction obtained of glycosaminoglycan-poor (alcian blue–positive) material in the coronary arteries from a group of diabetic (D) and nondiabetic (ND) subjects. 1AP = the first 2 to 3 cm of the anterior descending left and posterior descending right coronary arteries. 2A and 2P = the middle part of the anterior and posterior coronary artery, respectively. Bar = SEM (standard error of the mean).

Macroangiopathy in Experimental Diabetes

Many observations concerning the pathogenesis of diabetic large vessel disease have been reported from studies in animals with experimental or spontaneous diabetes mellitus. The influence of diabetes and increased serum cholesterol was analyzed in alloxan-diabetic squirrel monkeys. The incidence of gross lesions in large vessels was higher than among the control animals.[5] Later it was shown that *Macaca nigra* monkeys at the Oregon Regional Primate Center developed genetically related diabetes mellitus similar to type I diabetes in humans.[6] They also showed larger sudanophilic aortic lesions when fed a normal stock diet as compared to controls that had not developed diabetes. Another noteworthy observation in the same study was the correlation between the incidence and severity of lesions and the degree of abnormality in the intravenous glucose tolerance test. These results suggest that factor(s) in the diabetic metabolism may be of importance in the development of the internal lesions.

These diabetic *M. nigra* monkeys were sustained on a well-balanced low-fat, cholesterol-free ration in an almost ideal natural habitat. The detailed histopathologic observations, which were published in 1984, indicated that many of these spontaneously diabetic primates developed severe atherosclerotic lesions and that, in general, these plaques were rich in proliferated intimal and medial smooth muscle cells, as well as the collagen and elastin these cells synthesize.[7] As might be expected, there was much less deposited lipid as compared to that usually found in rhesus monkeys (*Macaca mulata*) fed a high-fat, high-cholesterol atherogenic ration.[8]

It has also been reported that the number of cells in the walls of the coronary arteries was increased in a group of rats with long-term and poorly controlled diabetes as compared to nondiabetic and well-controlled diabetic rats.[9] More studies are needed in order to clarify the influence of experimental diabetes on the vessel wall.

In the late 1960s the increased serum insulin induced by treatment was put forward as a cause for the development of vessel damage in diabetic subjects.[10] The concept received support from studies in nondiabetic rats and chickens treated with large doses of insulin.[11,12] It was demonstrated that insulin enhanced the synthesis of cholesterol in the aorta. The cholesterol synthesis effects have not been confirmed using KK – mice, which usually have increased levels of serum insulin, or in diabetic rats treated with insulin.[13] It has not been possible to demonstrate an effect of insulin on the transfer of cholesterol from plasma to the arterial wall in aorta from nondiabetic rabbits.[14] In another study also using pieces of aorta from nondiabetic rabbits, only a modest and slow effect has been demonstrated. The transport of amino acids and carbohydrate into the vessel wall was only slightly affected.[15]

Cell Proliferation Studies In Vitro

The modern tissue culture technique was introduced in the 1950s and was used early on to study arterial wall cells in vitro.[16–21] In the early 1970s this approach was used to study interactions of arterial cells with hyperlipidemic serum and lipoproteins in an attempt to elucidate various aspects of the development of atherosclerotic lesions.[22–25] It was demonstrated at that time that insulin causes increased growth of the arterial smooth muscle cells in culture. However, many of the data were obtained after starvation of the cells by serum deprivation before an insulin effect could be seen. Moreover, the insulin concentration was rather high (200 to 2,500 μU/mL).[26–28]

The results of other investigations utilizing diabetic rats and combining in vitro and in vivo techniques indicated that insulin did not appear to affect the lipid metabolism in the arterial wall.[29] In the laboratory of one of us (T.L.) in Denmark, it has not been possible to demonstrate a growth effect of insulin, and other groups have arrived at the same conclusion.[30,31] It is important to note that serum from patients with juvenile diabetes of recent onset and a serum insulin concentration of 0 to 6 μU/mL still increased the growth of arterial smooth muscle cells significantly more than serum from nondiabetic individuals.[30] Insulin treatment has also been observed to be associated with a reduction of cell numbers in the intima of coronary arteries from rats with long-term diabetes that was well controlled.[9] A number of studies have demonstrated the lack of effect of insulin on the growth of arterial smooth muscle cells.

In contrast, it has now been shown in many laboratories that serum from patients with diabetes and from animals with experimental diabetes contains a factor or factors that stimulate(s) the arterial smooth muscle cells in culture to increased growth.[31–34] It has also been demonstrated that it is not the increased glucose that enhances the growth rate of the smooth muscle cell, nor is it the level of insulin in the cell culture media that affects the growth of the arterial smooth muscle cell explants under these conditions.[25,32] In a study in which serum from type I diabetics was ultrafiltrated, a growth factor(s) with a molecular weight between 3,000 and 30,000 was present.[31] In another analysis of serum

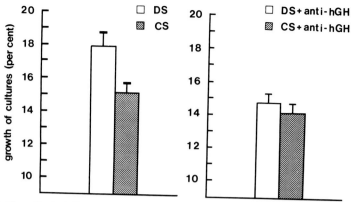

Figure 8.3 The effect of diabetic and nondiabetic serum with and without antiserum to human growth hormone (hGH). DS = diabetic serum (n = 10). CS = nondiabetic serum (n = 8). Bar = SEM (standard error of the mean).

from type II diabetics, the data showed the presence of a growth factor with a molecular weight less than 3,500, which was active after heating and not affected by a lipid dissolving agent.[33,34]

One factor long considered as active in the development of diabetic angiopathy has been the presence of increased levels of growth hormone.[35] The effect of growth hormone on the growth of arterial smooth muscle cells was analyzed in vitro. The data demonstrated stimulation of increased growth at 1 ng/mL. When antigrowth hormone serum was added to the culture media, the increased growth effect of diabetic serum was abolished[36,37] (Figure 8.3). It is noteworthy that Bettmann et al[38] have demonstrated that reduced proliferation of cells occurs in tunica intima after hypophysectomy in rats with vessel wall alterations.

Studies of Arterial Wall Metabolism in Diabetes

Serum from diabetic subjects seems to contain factor(s) that promote(s) the secretion of type I collagen and fibronectin but not type III collagen when arterial smooth muscle cells are grown in culture.[39] The fibronectin production could also be enhanced by human growth hormone (5 ng/mL), whereas collagen secretion was unchanged. High concentrations of glucose or ketones did not affect

Table 8.1 The Effect of Ketones (0.2 mM) and Human Growth Hormone (hGH; 1 ng/mL) on Arterial Procollagens Type I and Type III, and Fibronectin (Expressed as cpm/µg Cell Protein, Mean ± SEM)

	Control	+Ketones	N^a	p^b	Control	+hGH	N^a	p^b
Type I	20.08 ± 1.14	20.24 ± 1.01	22	—	26.24 ± 1.29	32.65 ± 2.13	20	<.02
Type III	27.25 ± 1.41	27.77 ± 1.73	21	—	25.57 ± 1.90	26.68 ± 2.92	19	—
Fibronectin	38.15 ± 2.16	36.99 ± 2.06	21	—	24.73 ± 1.36	31.23 ± 1.62	19	<.01

$^a N$ = number of paired cultures.
$^b p$ = Paired comparison.

Table 8.2 The Effect of Glucose (150 mg/dL) and Insulin (100 U/mL) on Arterial Procollagens Type I and Type II and Fibronectin (Expressed as cpm/μg Cell Protein, Mean ± SEM)

	Control	+ Glucose	N^a	p^b	Control	+ Insulin	N^a	p^b
Type I	23.98 ± 2.42	18.36 ± 1.53	16	<.05	25.11 ± 1.97	21.51 ± 1.71	22	<.05
Type III	28.34 ± 3.04	24.81 ± 2.79	14	>.05	33.44 ± 2.91	27.89 ± 2.62	23	<.05
Fibronectin	25.07 ± 1.94	23.67 ± 2.08	14	>.05	55.04 ± 3.48	45.92 ± 3.20	23	<.02

[a] N = number of paired cultures.
[b] p = Paired comparison.

the secretion, whereas insulin (100 μU/mL) reduced the elaboration of collagen and fibronectin (Tables 8.1 and 8.2).

Fibronectin is a component of the basement membrane surrounding the arterial smooth muscle cells.[40,41] Using serum from type I and type II diabetic subjects, the basement membrane production from cultures of arterial smooth muscle cells was increased compared to the effect of nondiabetic serum.[42] The results could not be ascribed to the levels of glucose in the incubation medium. However, human growth hormone (1 ng/mL) was able to enhance the accumulation of basement membrane–like material,[43] whereas insulin, ketones, or glucagon had no effect.[44] The results of further studies on the effects of diabetic serum or growth hormone employing radioactive tracers (^{35}S) demonstrated that the production of glycosaminoglycans was reduced. Recently, it was shown that the amount of heparan sulfate proteoglycan secreted from the arterial smooth muscle cells was relatively reduced after growth hormone addition (V. Thoegersen, L. Heickendorff, and T. Ledet, unpublished data).

Altered Low-Density Lipoprotein and Diabetic Macroangiopathy

Previous studies have shown that low-density lipoprotein (LDL) can be glycosylated in vitro with a reduced binding to the receptors of cultured human fibroblasts.[45] However, LDL isolated from type I and type II diabetics with average glucose value of 12.6 mmol/L revealed no difference in binding and degradation compared to LDL from ten nondiabetic subjects.[46] A small but significant increase in the synthesis of cholesteryl ester and cholesterol accumulation could be demonstrated in human monocyte-derived macrophages after incubation with glycosylated LDL from type I diabetic individuals.[47]

Recently there have been numerous reports of investigations that reopened the long-standing interest[48,49] in immunologic reactions that alter the pathogenesis of atherosclerosis. These studies emphasize the effects of sustained circulating immune complexes on the acceleration of the progression of atherosclerosis and the altered microarchitecture of the lesions so that concentric, intramural, inflammatory atheroarteritis results,[50] as well as the role of T lymphocytes and the cytokines in the altered atherogenesis.[51,52] In diabetes there is reason to believe that both increased oxidation of LDL and glycosylation of LDL may be occurring.[53,54] In some cases these may be present to the extent that they can trigger changes in cellular lipid metabolism[47] or initiate autoimmune mechanisms that may, in turn, play a role in accelerating atherogenesis.[55]

The Unclear Role of Insulinlike Growth Factor 1

In recent years, growth factor 1 (IGF-1), or somatomedin C, has been considered in relation to diabetic angiopathy.[56] Although the serum concentration of IGF-1 is normal or reduced in diabetes,[57] the level around the various cells is unknown. Several years ago we were not able to demonstrate a growth effect of somatomedins A and B.[37] Infusion of IGF-1 to rats that had lesions in the aorta after intimal injury with a balloon catheter revealed increased proliferation in the smooth muscle cells.[56] It is still unclear if IGF-1 takes part in the pathogenesis of diabetic angiopathy. Studies utilizing a limited number of nondiabetic rabbits with antibodies against glycosylated LDL demonstrated that the clearance rate of glycosylated LDL was greatly accelerated. Furthermore, it also was shown that the uptake into the aorta was considerably lower as compared to that with native LDL.[58]

Hypertriglyceridemia

Hypertriglyceridemia is one of the most consistent disturbances of lipid metabolism in diabetes that can be reflected in the diabetic artery wall and influence the development of accelerated atherosclerosis. It is associated with elevation of triglyceride-rich very-low-density lipoproteins (VLDLs). Many consider this to be a hallmark of diabetes. Recent evidence indicates that part of the trigger that may account for this hyperlipidemia is related to insulin resistance and the effect of the diabetic state on hepatic VLDL and triglyceride synthesis,[59] but the more precise molecular mechanisms involved are not yet clear.

Summary

This brief review of relatively recent work emphasizes a few of the common denominators that may be active in both the macro- and microarterial involvement in diabetes. These rather remarkable findings certainly do not explain all of the factors that may be active in accelerating and augmenting the severity of atherosclerosis in human diabetes. The findings that have been presented in this chapter include:

The factors that are involved in the excess proliferation of arterial smooth muscle cells, the results of which are observed in both small and large artery disease, and the accumulating factors, are closely related to or identical with growth hormone. There may be a second separate growth-stimulating factor for cell proliferation that is dialyzable and separate from glucose, insulin, and platelet-derived growth factor.

Both the media and the intima are involved not only in the proliferative reaction of the smooth muscle cells but also in their excess synthesis of extraordinary amounts of collagen, elastin, and proteoglycans.

There is clear-cut evidence of excessive basement membrane synthesis around capillaries as well as around individual smooth muscle cells in large and medium-sized arteries.

Rapidly emerging evidence indicates that immune reactions to glycated or oxidized LDLs may be immunogenic and lead to injury of both endothelium and smooth muscle cells. These interactions may result in augmented and accelerated inflammatory responses in both intima and media,[48,60] and may be a prominent factor in some cases of accelerated atherogenesis in diabetes.

It appears that the modern approaches to the investigation of the artery wall and its reaction are leading to an integrated understanding of the major vascular changes that are associated with diabetes mellitus.

References

1. Lundbaek K: Blood vessel disease. *Acta Diabetol Lat* 1971;8(suppl 1):34.
2. Robertson WB, Strong JP: Atherosclerosis in persons with hypertension and diabetes mellitus. *Lab Invest* 1968;18:78–91.
3. Dybdahl H, Ledet T: Diabetic macroangiopathy. Quantitative histopathological studies of the extramural coronary arteries from type 2 (non-insulin dependent) diabetic patients. *Diabetologia* 1987;30:882–886.
4. Rasmussen LM, Heickendorff L: Accumulation of fibronectin in aortas from diabetic patients. A quantitative immunohisto-chemical and biochemical study. *Lab Invest* 1989;61:440–446.
5. Lehner NDM, Clarkson TB, Lofland HB: The effect of insulin deficiency, hypothyroidism, and hypertension on atherosclerosis in the squirrel monkey. *Exp Mol Pathol* 1971;15:230–244.
6. Howard CF Jr: Aortic atherosclerosis in normal and spontaneously diabetic *Macaca nigra. Atherosclerosis* 1979;33:479–493.
7. Howard CF Jr, Vesselinovitch D, Wissler RW: Correlations of aortic histology with gross aortic atherosclerosis and metabolic measurements in diabetic and non-diabetic *Macaca nigra. Atherosclerosis* 1984;53:85–100.
8. Wissler RW: Recent progress in studies of experimental primate atherosclerosis. *Prog Biochem Pharmacol* 1968;4:378–392.
9. Baandrup U, Ledet T, Rasch R: Experimental diabetic cardiopathy preventable by insulin treatment. *Lab Invest* 1981;45:169–173.
10. Stout RW, Vallance-Owen J: Insulin and atheroma. *Lancet* 1969;1:1078–1080.
11. Stout RW: Insulin stimulation of cholesterol synthesis by arterial tissue. *Lancet* 1969; 2:476–478.
12. Stout RW: The effect of insulin on the incorporation of sodium (1-^{14}C) acetate into the lipids of the rat aorta. *Diabetologia* 1971;7:367–372.
13. Chattopadhyay DF, Martin JM: Effect of insulin on the in vitro synthesis of sterol and fatty acid by aorta and liver from diabetic rats. *J Atheroscler Res* 1969;10:131–134.
14. Christensen S, Jensen J: Uptake of labelled cholesterol from plasma by aortic intima-media in control and insulin injected rabbits. *J Atherscler Res* 1975;5:258–259.
15. Arnqvist HJ: *Metabolism in Vascular and Intestinal Smooth Muscle Action of Insulin,* Medical Dissertation No 16. Linköping University, Sweden, 1973.
16. Pollak OJ, Kokubu T: Normal rabbit aortic and myocardial cells cultured in various media. *Circulation* 1960;22:685.
17. Simms HS, Kirk JE, Pollak OJ: *Tissue Culture.* Monographs on Atherosclerosis, Basel, Karger, 1969, vol 1.

18. Robertson AL: Transport of plasma lipoproteins and ultrastructure of human arterial intimacytes in culture. *Wistar Symp Monogr* 1967;6:115.
19. Robertson AL: Role of circulating lipproteins in the proliferative phase of atherogenesis. *Am J Pathol* 1974;74:94a.
20. Rutstein DD, Ingenito EF, Craig JM, et al: Effects of linolenic and stearic acids on cholesterol-induced lipoid deposition in human aortic cells in tissue culture. *Lancet* 1958;1:545–552.
21. Rutstein DD, Castelli WP, Sullivan JC, et al: Effects of fat and carbohydrate ingestion in human beings on serum lipids and intracellular lipid deposition in tissue culture. *N Engl J Med* 1964;271:1–11.
22. Kao VCY, Wissler RW, Dzoga K: The influence of hyperlipidemic serum on the growth of medial smooth muscle cells of rhesus monkey aorta *in vitro*. *Circulation* 1968; 38(suppl VI):12.
23. Fischer-Dzoga K, Jones K, Vesselinovitch D, et al: Ultrastructural and immunohistochemical studies of primary cultures of aortic medial cells. *Exp Mol Pathol* 1973; 18:162–175.
24. Fischer-Dzoga K, Fraser R, Wissler RW: Stimulation of proliferation in stationary primary cultures of monkey and rabbit aortic smooth muscle cells. Effects of lipoprotein fractions of hyperlipemic serum and lymph. *Exp Mol Pathol* 1976;24:346–359.
25. Ross R: The smooth muscle cell. II Growth of smooth muscle in culture and formation of elastic fibres. *J Cell Biol* 1971;50:172–186.
26. Stout RW, Bierman EL, Ross R: Effect of insulin on the proliferation of cultured primate arterial smooth muscle cell. *Circ Res* 1975;36:319–327.
27. Pheifle B, Ditschuneit HH, Ditschuneit H: Insulin as a cellular growth regulator of rat arterial smooth muscle cells in vitro. *Horm Metab Res* 1980;12:381–385.
28. King GL, Buzney SM, Kahn CR, et al: Differential responsiveness to insulin of endothelial and support cells from micro- and macrovessels. *J Clin Invest* 1983;71:974–979.
29. Capron L, Jarnet J: Effects of injury and insulin on lipid synthesis from glucose by the rat thoracic aorta. *Arterioscler Thromb* 1991;11:91–96.
30. Ledet T: Growth hormone stimulating the growth of arterial medial cells in vitro. Absence of effect of insulin. *Diabetes* 1976;25:1011–1018.
31. Ledet T: Growth of rabbit aortic smooth muscle cells in serum of patients with juvenile diabetes. *Acta Pathol Microbiol Scand* [A] 1976;84:508–516.
32. Ledet T, Fischer-Dzoga K, Wissler RW: Growth of rabbit aortic smooth muscle cell cultured in media containing diabetic and hyperlipemic serum. *Diabetes* 1976;25:207–215.
33. Koschinsky T, Bunting CE, Schwippert B, et al: Increased growth of human fibroblasts and arterial smooth muscle cells from diabetic patients related to diabetic serum factors and cell origin. *Atherosclerosis* 1979;33:245–252.
34. Koschinsky T, Bunting CE, Rutter R, et al: Sera from type 2 (non-insulin dependent) diabetic and healthy subjects contain different amounts of a very low molecular weight growth peptide for vascular cells. *Diabetologia* 1985;28:223–228.
35. Lundbaek K, Christensen NJ, Jensen VA, et al: Diabetes, diabetic angiopathy and growth hormone. *Lancet* 1970;2:131–133.
36. Ledet T: Growth hormone antiserum suppresses the growth effect of diabetic serum. Studies on rabbit aortic medial cell cultures. *Diabetes* 1976;26:798–803.
37. Ledet T: Diabetic macroangiopathy and growth hormone. *Diabetes* 1981;30(suppl): 14–17.
38. Bettmann MA, Stemerman MB, Ransil BJ: The effect of hypophysectomy on experimental endothelial cell regrowth and intimal thickening in the rat. *Circ Res* 1981;48: 907–912.
39. Ledet T, Vuust J: Arterial procollagen type I, type III, and fibronectin. Effects of diabetic serum, glucose, insulin, ketones and growth hormone studied on rabbit aortic myomedial cell cultures. *Diabetes* 1980;29:964–970.

40. Heickendorff L, Ledet T: Arterial basement membrane-like material isolated and characterized from rabbit aortic myomedial cell cultures. *Biochem J* 1983;211:397–404.

41. Heickendorff L, Ledet T: The carbohydrate components of arterial basement membrane-like material. Studies on rabbit aortic myomedial cell in culture. *Biochem J* 1983;211:735–741.

42. Rasmussen LM, Ledet T: Serum from diabetic patients enhances the synthesis of arterial basement membrane-like material studied on rabbit aortic myomedial cell culture. *Acta Pathol Microbiol Scand* 1988;96:77–83.

43. Ledet T, Heickendorff L: Growth hormone effect on accumulation of arterial basement membrane like material studied on rabbit aortic myomedial cell cultures. *Diabetologia* 1985;28:922–927.

44. Ledet T, Heickendorff L: Insulin, ketones, glucose and glucagon: Effects on the arterial basement membrane in vitro. *Acta Endocrinol (Copenh)* 1987;115:139–143.

45. Gonen B, Jacobsen D, Farraf P, et al: In vitro glycosylation of low density and high density lipoproteins. *Diabetes* 1981;30:875–878.

46. Kraemer FB, Chen YDT, Cheung RMC, et al: Are the binding and degradation of low density lipoprotein altered in type 2 (non-sinulin dependent) diabetes mellitus? *Diabetologia* 1982;23:28–33.

47. Lyons TJ, Klein RL, Baynes JW, et al: Stimulation of cholesteryl ester synthesis in human monocyte derived macrophages by low-density lipoproteins from type 1 (insulin dependent) diabetic patients: The influence of non-enzymatic glycosylation of low density lipoproteins. *Diabetologia* 1987;30:916–923.

48. Hollander W, Colombo MA, Kramsch DM, et al: Immunological aspects of atherosclerosis. Comparative pathology of the heart. *Adv Cardiol* 1974;13:192–207.

49. Minick CR: Immunologic arterial injury in atherogenesis. Ann N Y Acad Sci 1976;275:210–227.

50. Wissler RW, Vesselinovith D, Davis HR, et al: A new way to lok at atherosclerotic involvement of the artery wall and the functional effects. *Ann N Y Acad Sci* 1985;454:9–22.

51. Hansson GK, Jonasson L, Seifert PS, et al: Immune mechanisms in atherosclerosis. *Arteriosclerosis* 1989;9:567–578.

52. Libby P, Hansson GK: Involvement of the immune system in human atherogenesis: Current knowledge and unanswered questions. *Lab Invest* 1991;64:5–15.

53. Witztum JL, Steinbrecher UP, Kesaniemi YA, et al: Autoantibodies to glucosylated proteins in the plasma of patients with diabetes mellitus. *Proc Natl Acad Sci USA* 1984;81:3204–3208.

54. Palinski W, Yla-Herttuala S, Rosenfeld ME, et al: Antisera and monoclonal antibodies specific for epitopes generated during oxidative modification of low density lipoprotein. *Arteriosclerosis* 1990;10:325–335.

55. Steinberg D, Parthasarathy S, Carew T, et al: Beyond cholesterol: Modifications of low-density lipoprotein that increase its atherogenicity. *N Engl J Med* 1989;320:915–924.

56. Bornfeldt KE, Arnqvist HJ, Capron L: In vivo proliferation of rat insulin-like growth factor I and insulin. *Diabetologia* 1991;35:104–108.

57. Flyvbjerg A, Frystyk J, Sillesen IF, et al: Growth hormone and insulin-like growth factor I in experimental and human diabetes, in Alberti KGMN, Krall LP (eds): *The Diabetes Annual* ed 6. Amsterdam, Elsevier, 1991, pp 562–590.

58. Wiklund O, Witztum JL, Carew TE, et al: Turnover and tissue sites of degradation of glucosylated low density lipoprotein in normal and immunized rabbits. *J Lipid Res* 1987;28:1098–1109.

59. Reaven GM, Olefsky JLM: The role of insulin resistance in pathogenesis of diabetes mellitus. *Adv Metab Disord* 1978;9:313–331.

60. Gimbrone MA Jr: Vascular endothelium: Nature's blood compatible container. *Ann N Y Acad Sci* 1987;516:5–11.

Chapter 9

Hyperinsulinemia, the Insulin Resistance Syndrome, and the Pathogenesis of Atherosclerosis

Karl E. Sussman, MD

This review considers the possible importance of hyperinsulinemia in the pathogenesis of atherosclerosis. The concept that insulin may play a role in accelerating atherogenesis is not new; in fact, this possible relationship was first suggested in the 1960s.[1] This subject has been well reviewed over the years since the relationship was first described.[2,3] The rationale for relating accelerated atherosclerosis to hyperinsulinemia is largely derived from three lines of evidence:

1. Epidemiologic studies demonstrating that hyperinsulinemia is a risk factor for the development of atherosclerotic cardiovascular disease.
2. The existence of a "syndrome" of diverse cardiovascular risk abnormalities associated with hyperinsulinemia.
3. Animal and isolated tissue studies demonstrating that insulin could promote or accelerate the development of atherosclerosis by impacting on various biochemical pathways thought to enhance atherogenesis.

Epidemiologic Studies of Hyperinsulinemia and Atherosclerosis

Previous investigations have demonstrated increased insulin levels in patients with coronary, cerebral, and peripheral vascular disease.[4-8] This early evidence suggested a relationship between hyperinsulinemia and accelerated atherosclerosis, but the significance of this association was unclear. It is evident that these subjects may have been patients with diabetes mellitus otherwise at risk for the development of atherosclerosis and who also may have been hyperinsulinemic as a consequence of insulin therapy or may have had increased insulin levels as a result of associated obesity. Thus, the association of hyperinsulinemia and accelerated atherosclerosis in these studies did not establish causality. In an extensive cross-sectional study in Israel, the association between cardiovascular disease, glucose intolerance, obesity, and hypertension and hyperinsulinemia was examined recently in a representative sample ($n = 1,263$) of the Jewish population of ages 40 to 70 years.[9] Previously known diabetics were excluded. Cardiovascular disease was identified in 97 men and 39 women. The study found that hyperinsulinemia was associated with excess cardiovascular risk in men but not in women. Furthermore, the excess cardiovascular risk in men was confined to hyperinsulinemic subjects in the presence of glucose intolerance, obesity, or hypertension. Hyperinsulinemia in nonobese, normoglycemic, normotensive men is not a cardiovascular risk factor.[9]

Prospective studies also suggested a relationship between insulin levels and subsequent cardiovascular morbidity and mortality in various population groups. In the Helsinki Policemen Study, 982 men ages 35 to 64 years were followed from 1971 to 1980.[10] Insulin and glucose levels were obtained at the outset of the study. Twenty-six men died from coronary heart disease and 37 men experienced nonfatal myocardial infarction. The incidence of these events showed a positive nonlinear correlation with both plasma insulin and blood glucose values. The 5-year follow-up data showed that fatal and nonfatal myocardial infarctions were most common in those subjects who had the highest initial fasting, 1-hour, 2-hour, and total plasma insulin responses to glucose. Fasting plasma insulin levels alone did not appear to be a good predictor of ischemic heart disease. Multivariate analysis revealed that the 1- and 2-hour plasma insulin levels were good independent predictors of coronary heart disease when body mass index (BMI), blood glucose, plasma triglycerides, cholesterol, and systolic blood pressure were controlled for in the data analysis. Excess coronary heart disease events occurred largely at the top 10% of values for plasma insulin.[10]

In the Paris Prospective Study, Fontbonne and associates examined a large cohort of working men and found that the fasting and 2-hour postload plasma insulin levels were good major independent predictors of coronary heart disease.[11–13] The Paris Prospective Study was initiated in the late 1960s on a cohort of middle-aged men (ages 43 to 54). The baseline cohort consisted of 7,028 men. A 75-g glucose tolerance test was given to 6,903 subjects with no known diabetes and to 99 patients with diabetes. Plasma glucose and insulin levels were measured fasting and 2 hours after the glucose load. The subjects underwent cardiovascular examinations; measurement of blood pressure, BMI, serum cholesterol, and triglyceride; and recording of cigarette consumption. After a mean follow-up of 11 years, 126 coronary heart disease deaths were recorded. Major independent predictors of coronary heart disease deaths were blood pressure, smoking, plasma cholesterol level, and fasting and 2-hour postload plasma insulin levels. In the subset of patients with abnormal glucose tolerance, plasma triglyceride was the strongest independent predictor of deaths resulting from coronary heart disease. In the 15-year follow-up report, fasting insulin was no longer an independent predictor of death by coronary heart disease.[13] The 2-hour postload plasma insulin level, when entered as a categorical variable (below or above 452 pmol/L), was still a good independent predictor of deaths resulting from coronary heart disease. Fontbonne et al believe that hyperinsulinemia reflects insulin resistance, which may contribute to coronary heart disease mortality.[13] They expressed the view that circulating insulin per se is not a direct cause of arterial complications.

In the Busselton, West Australia, study, over 3,300 subjects were studied, with both men and women being equally represented. Blood glucose and serum insulin levels were measured 1 hour after glucose load. The circulating insulin level correlated very well with the 6-year incidence of and the 12-year mortality from coronary heart disease in men 60 to 69 years old. This relationship persisted with the analysis of men at all ages. However, there was no association between serum insulin levels and coronary heart disease incidence or mortality in women at any age.[14]

The prospective epidemiologic studies do indeed yield more definitive information concerning the usefulness of plasma insulin level as a marker indicating increased risk for coronary heart disease morbidity and mortality. However, Fontbonne and Eschwege pointed out the need for caution in using these studies in attempting to establish causality.[12] These investigators noted that any measured and identified risk factor at baseline may be related to other more significant risk factors that, because they either were not identified or were not measured at the start of the study, could not be taken into account for the prediction of outcome. Thus, epidemiologic associations per se can never be taken as causal.

Relationship of Hyperinsulinemia and Atherosclerosis

Given the plethora of studies relative to the possible association of hyperinsulinemia with coronary heart disease, several issues arise concerning this relationship. By what mechanisms is elevated plasma insulin placing patients at increased risk for atherosclerosis and/or coronary heart disease? Is it a special population who are predisposed to the development of atherosclerosis, as evidenced by the presence of hyperinsulinemia?

Assuming that insulin may predispose individuals to develop accelerated atherosclerosis, it still remains unknown how insulin may be exerting its effects in humans. There are least four possibilities:

1. Excess insulin and its role in increasing circulating lipids and promoting lipid deposition.
2. Insulin enhancing smooth muscle cell growth.
3. Insulin altering the level of blood coagulation factors.
4. Hyperinsulinemia conceivably inducing hypertension, a known cardiovascular risk factor.

Results of Animal and Tissue Studies

Insulin may exert direct effects on vascular tissue in promoting atherogenesis.[2] Studies have demonstrated the ability of insulin to augment vascular smooth muscle proliferation in cell cultures.[15-19] Platelet-derived growth factor and insulin seem to exert an additive effect on smooth muscle cell proliferation.[19] Whether these effects of insulin are related to atherosclerosis remains subject to some debate.

Insulin treatment has been shown to stimulate lipid synthesis in aortic cells of the diabetic rat.[20] This latter effect may be due to the action of insulin in increasing hydroxymethylglutaryl coenzyme A reductase activity in arterial smooth muscle cells. Insulin also increases the ability of fibroblasts to bind and degrade low-density lipoprotein (LDL), conceivably by regulating the number of LDL receptors.[21] In chickens fed a low-cholesterol diet following high cholesterol intake, insulin suppressed the regression of atherosclerotic lesions that would have occurred with this dietary change.[22] Insulin also appears to inhibit the protective effect of estrogens in the prevention of diet-induced atherosclerosis.[23] In the diabetic animal, insulin could be shown to lower cholesterol levels but did not necessarily decrease the incidence or the severity of atherosclerotic lesions.[23] In alloxan-diabetic monkeys fed high-cholesterol diets, insulin therapy resulted in hypercholesterolemia and accelerated atherosclerosis.[24] Nevertheless, in the setting in which induced insulin deficiency has been restored by insulin, atherosclerosis is decreased. It seems that, in experimental diabetes, there may be a critical balance between the accelerated atherosclerosis caused by insulin deficiency as opposed to atherogenesis induced by hyperinsulinemia. Insulin, by exerting effects on the process of blood coagulation, could also augment atherosclerosis. Insulin has been shown to increase the level of tissue plasminogen activator inhibitor, perhaps providing another potential link between the presence of insulin resistance and associated hyperinsulinemia and atherothrombotic disease.[25,26]

It is evident that hyperinsulinemia can impact on other cardiovascular risk factors predominately affecting circulating lipid levels and also possibly contributing to the risk for developing hypertension. Insulin and triglyceride levels are closely related in subjects with normal and impaired glucose tolerance, endogenous hypertriglyceridemia, and/or obesity.[27–31] Hypertriglyceridemia and hyperinsulinemia frequently coexist in patients. Recent evidence suggests that hyperinsulinemia is also related to increased very-low-density lipoprotein (VLDL) and LDL cholesterol levels and also decreased high-density lipoprotein (HDL) cholesterol.[30–33] Barakat and associates suggested that the risk of coronary heart disease in patients with impaired glucose tolerance or non-insulin-dependent diabetes mellitus (NIDDM) may be further exacerbated by the prevalence of smaller, denser LDL particles.[34] They also reported that LDL size correlated negatively with plasma insulin levels in these patients, independent of triglyceride levels, age, or BMI.[34]

Elevated blood pressure alone does not induce atherosclerosis in experimental animals.[35] However, hypertension has been shown to augment atherosclerotic plaque formation in the presence of hyperlipidemia.[36,37] Recent experimental studies have demonstrated that the presence of hypertension may sustain atherosclerotic progression despite reduction in hypercholesterolemia.[38] Various studies have emphasized the relationship between hypertension and hyperinsulinemia.[7,39–45] This association of hypertension and hyperinsulinism can be seen in subjects who are not obese, although it is the overweight patients who are more likely to have elevated blood pressures and also increased circulating insulin levels.[46] Ferrannini and associates have demonstrated that patients with essential hypertension are insulin resistant, and that this may account for the presence of hyperinsulinemia in this subset of hypertensive subjects.[47] In contrast, this relationship seemed to be only apparent in subjects who have both hypertension and NIDDM.[48]

In a more recent study, this association between hyperinsulinemia and hypertension was not observed in Pima Indians or blacks.[49] Similarly, Collins and associates did not find any association between insulin levels and hypertension in the Micronesian (Nauru), Polynesian (Western Samoa), and Melanesian (New

Caledonians) Pacific islanders.[50] These authors suggest that hyperinsulinemia is not the pathologic link between obesity, NIDDM, and hypertension.[50] It is evident that ethnic factors may impact on the expression of the relationship between hyperinsulinemia and hypertension. However, in a study of insulin-dependent diabetes mellitus (IDDM) patients, blood pressure levels were similar in the patients who were receiving insulin therapy (and who were presumably constantly relatively hyperinsulinemic) and sibling controls, suggesting again that factors other than insulin per se are contributing to the expression of hypertension in hyperinsulinemic subjects.[51]

Insulin Resistance Syndrome

In recent years, considerable attention has been directed at the coexistence of various metabolic abnormalities of carbohydrate and lipid metabolism and an increased predilection for the development of atherosclerosis.[33,52,53] Figure 9.1 depicts the various elements in this relationship and how they may be interrelated. In numerous reports, the relationship of hyperinsulinemia, hypertension, insulin resistance, increased plasma triglycerides, decreased HDL cholesterol, and increased risk for coronary artery disease has been noted.[52] Particularly striking are the studies of Zavaroni and associates, who studied subjects with normal glucose tolerance and hyperinsulinemia.[54] This group had elevated blood pressure levels, increased fasting triglycerides, and diminished HDL cholesterol.[54] More recently, this coexistence of abnormalities has been referred to as syndrome X.[52] There exists some controversy as to whether obesity is an integral part of this disease complex. It does seem clear that the syndrome can occur in the absence of significant obesity. Other investigators, however, have highlighted the presence of central adiposity in this network of metabolic abnormalities.[55–63]

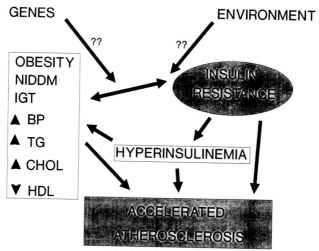

Figure 9.1 Schematic showing components of the insulin resistance syndrome. Depicted are some of the possible interrelationships between the various elements. IGT = impaired glucose tolerance; BP = blood pressure; TG = triglycerides; CHOL = cholesterol; HDL = HDL cholesterol.

Various questions arise when one considers the development and evolution of the abnormalities of the insulin resistance syndrome. Some of the abnormalities seem to present unassociated with the other manifestations of the syndrome, although admittedly various abnormalities could evolve over a period of time. The concomitant expression of the various abnormalities of this syndrome may be causally related (ie, one abnormality leads to the development of another manifestation of the syndrome). The other possibility is that diverse genetic influences lead to the coexpression of various phenotypic manifestations of the syndrome. Presumably, the coexistence of insulin resistance and hyperinsulinemia could lead to hypertriglyceridemia. Conversely, other manifestations of the syndrome may represent independent manifestations of diverse genetic abnormalities.

Jarrett et al have raised questions concerning the putative atherogenic role of insulin.[64] They noted that, although a number of studies have demonstrated a relationship between hyperinsulinemia and atherogenesis, the data are not particularly consistent between the studies. For example, in some reports it seems that the fasting insulin level is the best predictor of coronary heart disease, whereas in others, constituting the majority of the articles, it appears the post–glucose load insulin value correlates best with cardiac events.[3] In still other investigations, no relationship has been discernible between plasma insulin levels and coronary heart disease.[64–66] The study done in Busselton, West Australia, is of note insofar as an association of insulin levels and coronary heart disease is totally lacking in women.[14] Modan and associates also found no association of insulin levels and cardiovascular disease in females.[9]

Several other clinical circumstances suggest that the relationship between insulin levels and coronary heart disease must involve other risk factors as yet undefined. In patients with insulin-secreting tumors, accelerated atherosclerosis does not seem to be a major clinical problem even though they may have been exposed to elevated insulin levels for extended intervals of time. Another reason to cast doubt on this apparent linkage relates to the University Group Diabetes Program study reported a number of years ago.[67] These data certainly did not indicate that insulin-treated diabetic patients were at a special risk for developing coronary heart disease, either in the group of patients who received a fixed dose of insulin or in the subjects who were maintained on a variable insulin dosage regimen.

The evidence does not seem particularly persuasive that exogenous insulin therapy per se imposes an increased risk for atherosclerosis. In the frequently quoted study from the Schwabing Hospital in Munich, macrovascular disease and coronary heart disease were more frequent in those diabetic patients with higher C-peptide levels, expressed either in absolute terms or in relation to body weight.[68] Those subjects with persistent endogenous hyperinsulinemia are likely to be insulin resistant. Of interest, it was these same patients who were also receiving higher insulin doses and who were at increased risk for developing macrovascular disease.[68] Either the higher dose of insulin administered predisposed these patients to atherosclerosis or, more likely, the risk for developing macrovascular disease may have been an expression of insulin resistance (with its associated metabolic abnormalities), as evidenced by the elevated C-peptide levels.

In a similar study in Finland among insulin-treated patients with late-onset diabetes, atherosclerotic vascular disease prevalence was higher in subjects with persistent endogenous insulin secretion (NIDDM) than in those patients with low or no insulin secretion (IDDM).[69] In this study, the C-peptide response to glucagon was measured as an index of insulin secretory capacity. Both groups of subjects were taking approximately the same dose of insulin as therapy. Thus, the patients at greatest risk for accelerated atherosclerosis were those who had NIDDM and were thought to be insulin resistant. In this study, the dose of exogenous insulin was not a critical factor in determining the risk of developing atherosclerotic vascular disease. In this same group of NIDDM patients, other cardiovascular risk factors were present, including low HDL cholesterol and elevated triglyceride levels.[69]

Recapitulation and a Global View

One is led to believe, in reviewing this subject, that the risk for developing atherosclerosis may be an inherent feature of the insulin resistance syndrome, in which hyperinsulinemia is also present. Hyperinsulinemia may be an aggravating factor, although this case remains to be established. In the San Antonio Heart Study, a longitudinal, population-based survey of 2,930 subjects, the authors found underlying insulin resistance (as determined by the presence of hyperinsulinemia) in all subjects manifesting obesity, NIDDM, impaired glucose tolerance, hypertension, hypertriglyceridemia, or hypercholesterolemia.[70] This grouping of abnormalities and their interrelationships are also depicted in Figure 9.1. In the whole group of subjects presenting with one of the aforementioned conditions (1,881 subjects), they found marked fasting or postglucose hyperinsulinemia, high BMI, increased waist–hip ratio, fasting and postglucose glycemia, increased systolic and diastolic blood pressure levels, hypertriglyceridemia, increased total cholesterol, and decreased HDL cholesterol.

Ferrannini and associates referred to this latter network of metabolic abnormalities as the "syndrome of insulin resistance."[70] These authors considered whether insulin resistance is a common result of the six conditions noted above (referred to as the sextet), or is a basic cellular defect contributing to the development of the sextet. Furthermore, these authors raised the issue of whether the insulin resistance syndrome is a predisposing or an aggravating factor in the pathogenesis of the sextet. It is apparent that both genetic and acquired factors may condition or modify the expression of the insulin resistance syndrome and the development of the sextet.

To this concept, one might add that the genetics of the insulin resistance syndrome are undoubtedly complex, probably being multifactorial or polygenic. On the one hand, various components of the insulin resistance syndrome are genetically determined and interrelated. For example, in relating insulin resistance and NIDDM to hypertension, genetic factors are likely to be operative. Normotensive offspring of parents with essential hypertension tend to be more resistant to insulin than those whose parents are normotensive.[71] Normoglycemic, nonobese middle-aged men with a strong family history of NIDDM had significantly higher blood pressure than men without such a family history.[72] On the other hand, it is patently clear that genetic factors, as of this moment unknown, may modify or negate the penetrance of the genes controlling the various components of the insulin resistance syndrome. As an example, the phenotypic expression of hypertension may well be conditioned by genetic factors controlling ion regulation.[73] The presence of hyperinsulinemia may not always be associated with hypertension.

Hyperinsulinemia is a powerful marker of the insulin resistance syndrome and to a minor extent may exert certain actions in enhancing cardiovascular risk. This review has suggested possible sites at which insulin may be exerting action in promoting atherosclerosis. However, the primary abnormality seems to be one of insulin resistance, with its varied expression of diverse metabolic and other abnormalities that place the patient at increased risk for atherosclerosis. Fontbonne also is of the view that hyperinsulinemia is not the culprit in the development of cardiovascular disease.[74] Rather, as already noted, it may simply be a marker indicating the presence of the insulin resistance syndrome.

It has been suggested that insulin administered as therapy may predispose the patient to macrovascular disease. This seems unlikely but cannot be discounted entirely on the basis of available evidence. There is no evidence that switching an insulin-requiring patient to other therapy (eg, sulfonylurea agents) will render that patient less susceptible to the development of atherosclerosis or coronary heart disease, notwithstanding the efforts of some to attempt to establish this case.[2,33]

References

1. Stout RW, Vallance-Owen J: Insulin and atheroma. *Lancet* 1969;1:1078–1080.
2. Stolar MW: Atherosclerosis in diabetes: The role of hyperinsulinemia. *Metabolism* 1988;37(suppl 1):1–9.
3. Stout RW: Insulin and atheroma: 20-year perspective. *Diabetes Care* 1990;13:631–654.
4. Peters N, Hales CN: Plasma-insulin concentrations after myocardial infarction. *Lancet* 1965;1:1144–1145.
5. Tzagournis M, Chiles R, Ryan JM, et al: Interrelationships of hyperinsulism and hypertriglyceridemia in young patients in coronary heart disease. *Circulation* 1968;38:1156–1163.
6. Malherbe C, de Gasparo M, Berthet P, et al: The pattern of plasma insulin rsponses to glucose in patients with a previous myocardial infarction—the respective effects of age and disease. *Eur J Clin Invest* 1970;1:265–270.
7. Welborn TA, Breckenridge A, Rubenstein AH, et al: Serum-insulin in essential hypertension and in peripheral vascular disease. *Lancet* 1966;1:1336–1337.
8. Lichenstein MJ, Yarnell JWG, Elwood PC, et al: Sex hormones, insulin, lipids and prevalent ischemic heart disease. *Am J Epidemiol* 1987;126:647–657.
9. Modan M, Or J, Karasik A, et al: Hyperinsulinemia, sex, and risk of atherosclerotic cardiovascular disease. *Circulation* 1991;84:1165–1175.
10. Pyorala K, Savolainen E, Kaukola S, et al: Plasma insulin as coronary heart disease risk factor: Relationship to other risk factors and predictive value during 9 ½-year followup of the Helsinki Policemen Study population. *Acta Med Scand (Suppl)* 1985;70:38–52.
11. Ducimetiere P, Eschwege E, Papoz L, et al: Relationship of plasma insulin levels to the incidence of myocardial infarction and coronary heart disease mortality in a middle-age population. *Diabetologia* 1980;19:205–210.
12. Fontbonne AM, Eschwege EM: Insulin and cardivoascular disease: Paris Prospective Study. *Diabetes Care* 1991;14:461–469.
13. Fontbonne A, Charles MA, Thibult N, et al: Hyperinsulinaemia as a predictor of coronary heart disease mortality in a healthy population: The Paris Prospective Study, 15-year follow-up. *Diabetologia* 1991;34:356–361.

14. Welborn TA, Wearne K: Coronary heart disease incidence and cardiovascular mortality in Busslton with reference to glucose and insulin concentration. *Diabetes Care* 1979;2:154–160.

15. Stout RW, Bierman EL, Ross R: Effect of insulin on the proliferation of cultured primate arterial smooth muscle cells. *Circ Res* 1975;36:319–327.

16. Pfeifle B, Ditschuneit H: Effect of insulin on growth of cultured human arterial smooth muscle cells. *Diabetologia* 1981;20:155–158.

17. King GL, Goodman AD, Buzney S, et al: Receptors and growth-promoting effects of insulin and insulinlike growth factors on cells from bovine retinal capillaries and aorta. *J Clin Invest* 1985;75:1028–1036.

18. Banskota NK, Taub R, Zellner K, et al: Characterization of induction of protooncogene c-myc and cellular growth in human vascular smooth muscle cells by insulin and IGF-I. *Diabetes* 1989;38:123–129.

19. Banskota NK, Taub R, Zellner K, et al: Insulin, insulin-like growth factor I and platelet-derived growth factor interact additively in the induction of the protooncogene c-myc and cellular proliferation in cultured bovine aortic smooth muscle cells. *Mol Endocrinol* 1989;3:1183–1190.

20. Stout RW: The effect of insulin and glucose on sterol synthesis in cultured rat arterial smooth muscle cells. *Atherosclerosis* 1977;27:271–278.

21. Chait A, Bierman EL, Albers JJ: Regulatory role of insulin in the degradation of low density lipoprotein by cultured human skin fibroblasts. *Biochim Biophys Acta* 1978; 529:292–299.

22. Stamler J, Pick R, Katz LN: Effect of insulin in the induction and regression of atherosclerosis in the chick. *Circ Res* 1960;8:572–576.

23. Wilson RB, Martin JM, Hartroft WS: Failure of insulin therapy to prevent cardiovascular lesions in diabetic rats fed an atherogenic diet. *Diabetes* 1969;18:225–231.

24. Lehner NDM, Clarkson TB, Lofland HB: The effect of insulin defiency, hypothyroidism, and hypertension on atherosclerosis in the squirrel monkey. *Exp Mol Pathol* 1971; 15:230–244.

25. Juhan-Vague I, Alessi MC, Joly P, et al: Plasma plasminogen activator inhibitor-1 in angina pectoris: Influence of plasma insulin and acute phase response. *Arteriosclerosis* 1989;9:362–367.

26. Juhan-Vague I, Alessi MC, Vague P: Increased plasma plasminogen activator inhibitor 1 levels. A possible link between insulin resistance and atherothrombosis. *Diabetologia* 1991;34:457–462.

27. Reaven GM, Lerner RL, Stern MP, et al: Role of insulin in endogenous hypertriglyceridemia. *J Clin Invest* 1967;46:1756–1767.

28. Kyner JL, Levy RI, Soeldner JS, et al: Lipid, glucose and insulin interrelationships in normal, prediabetic, and chemical diabetic subjects. *J Lab Clin Med* 1976;88:345–358.

29. Orchard TJ, Becker DJ, Bates M, et al: Plasma insulin and lipoprotein concentrations: An atherogenic association? *Am J Epidemiol* 1983;118:326–330.

30. Zavaroni I, Dall'Aglio E, Alpi O, et al: Evidence for an independent relationship between plasma insulin and concentration of high density lipoprotein cholesterol and triglycerides. *Atherosclerosis* 1985;55:259–266.

31. Abbott WGH, Lillioja S, Young AA, et al: Relationships between plasma lipoprotein concentrations and insulin action in an obese hyperinsulinemic population. *Diabetes* 1987;36:897–904.

32. Modan M, Halkin H, Lusky A, et al: Hyperinsulinemia is characterized by jointly disturbed plasma VLDL, LDL, and HDL levels: A population-based study. *Arteriosclerosis* 1988;8:227–236.

33. DeFronzo RA, Ferrannini E: Insulin resistance. A multifaceted syndrome responsible for NIDDM, obesity, hypertension, dyslipidemia, and atherosclerotic cardiovascular disease. *Diabetes Care* 1991;14:173–194.

34. Barakat HA, Carpenter JW, McLendon VD, et al: Influence of obesity, impaired glucose tolerance, and NIDDM on LDL structure and composition. Possible link between hyperinsulinemia and atherosclerosis. *Diabetes* 1990;39:1527–1533.
35. Chobanian AV: The influence of hypertension and other hemodynamic factors in atherogenesis. *Prog Cardiovasc Dis* 1983;26:177–196.
37. McGill HC Jr, Carey KD, McMahan CA, et al: Effects of two forms of hypertension on atherosclerosis in the hyperlipidemic baboon. *Arteriosclerosis* 1985;5:481–493.
38. Bretherton KN, Day AJ, Skinner SL: Hypertension-accelerated atherogenesis in cholesterol-fed rabbits. *Atherosclerosis* 1977;27]:79–87.
39. Xu C, Glagov S, Zatina MA, et al: Hypertension sustains plaque progression despite reduction of hypercholesterolemia. *Hypertension* 1991;18:123–129.
40. Reaven GM, Hoffman BB: A role for insulin in the aetiology and course of hypertension. *Lancet* 1987;2:435–436.
41. Schroll M, Hagerup L: Relationship of fasting blood glucose to prevalence of ECG abnormalities and 10 yr risk of mortality from cardiovascular diseases in men born in 1914: From the Glosterup population studies. *J Chronic Dis* 1979;32:699–707.
41. Modan M, Halkin H, Almog S, et al: Hyperinsulinemia. A link between hypertension, obesity and glucose intolerance. *J Clin Invest* 1985;75:809–817.
42. Christlieb AR, Krowlewski AS, Warram JH, et al: Is insulin the link between hypertension and obesity? *Hypertension* 1985;7(suppl 2):54–57.
43. Uusitupa M, Niskanen L, Siitonen O, et al: Hyperinsulinemia and hypertension in patients with newly diagnosed non-insulin-dependent diabetes. *Diabetes Metab* 1987; 13:369–374.
44. Rocchini AP, Katch V, Schork A, et al: Insulin and blood pressure during weight loss in obese adolescents. *Hypertension* 1987;10:267–273.
45. Shen DC, Shieh S-M, Fuh MT, et al: Resistance to insulin-stimulated glucose uptake in patients with hypertension. *J Clin Endocrinol Metab* 1988;66:580–583.
46. Pollare T, Lithell H, Berne C: Insulin resistance is a characteristic feature of primary hypertension independent of obesity. *Metabolism* 1990;39:167–174.
47. Ferrannini E, Buzzigoli G, Bonnadonna R, et al: Insulin resistance in essential hypertension. *N Engl J Med* 1987;317:350–357.
48. Mbanya J-CN, Thomas TH, Wilkinson R, et al: Hypertension and hyperinsulinaemia: A relation in diabetes but not essential hypertension. *Lancet* 1988;1:733–734.
49. Saad MF, Knowler WC, Pettit DJ, et al: Insulin and hypertension: Relationship to obesity and glucose tolerance in Pima Indians. *Diabetes* 1990;39:1430–1435.
50. Collins VR, Dowse GK, Finch CF, et al: An inconsistent relationship between insulin and blood pressure in three Pacific island populations. *J Clin Epidemiol* 1990;43: 1369–1378.
51. Tarn AC Drury PL: Blood pressure in children, adolescents and young adults with type I (insulin-dependent) diabetes. *Diabetologia* 1986;29:275–281.
52. Reaven GM: Role of insulin resistance in human disease. *Diabetes* 1988;37:1595–1607.
53. Kaplan NM: The deadly quartet: Upper body obesity, glucose intolerance, hypertriglyceridemia, and hypertension. *Arch Intern Med* 1989;149:1514–1520.
54. Zavaroni I, Bonora E, Pagliara M, et al: Risk factors for coronary artery disease in healthy people with hyperinsulinemia and normal glucose tolerance. *N Engl J Med* 1989;320:202–206.
55. Kissebah AH, Vyelingum N, Murray R, et al: Relationship of body fat distribution to metabolic complications of obesity. *Clin Endocrinol Metab* 1982;54:254–260.
56. Evans DJ, Hoffman RG, Kalkoff RK, et al: Relationship of body fat topography to insulin sensitivity and metabolic profiles in premenopausal women. *Metabolism* 1984;33:68–75.
57. Peiris AN, Hennes MI, Evans DJ, et al: Relationship of anthropometric measurements of body fat distribution to metabolic profile in premenopausal women. *Acta Med Scand Suppl* 1988;723:179–188.

58. Peiris AN, Sothmann MS, Hoffman RG, et al: Adiposity, fat distribution and cardiovascular risk. *Ann Intern Med* 1989;110:867–872.

59. Krotkiewski M, Bjorntorp P, Sjostrom L, et al: Impact of obesity in metabolism in men and women: Importance of regional adipose tissue distribution. *J Clin Invest* 1983;72:1150–1162.

60. Bjorntorp P: The association between obesity, adipose tissue distribution and disease. *Acta Med Scand Suppl* 1988;723:121–134.

61. Bjorntorp P: Classification of obese patients and complications related to distribution of surplus fat. *Am J Clin Nutr* 1987;45:1120–1125.

62. Bjorntorp P: Abdominal obesity and the development of non-insulin dependent diabetes mellitus. *Diabetes Metab Rev* 1988;4:615–622.

63. Zimmet P, Baba S: Central obesity, glucose intolerance and other cardiovascular disease risk factors: An old syndrome rediscovered. *Diabetes Res Clin Pract* 1990;10: S167–S171.

64. Jarrett RJ, McCartney P, Keen H: The Bedford survey. Ten year mortality rates in newly diagnosed diabetics and normoglycaemic controls and risk indices for coronary heart disease in borderline diabetics. *Diabetologia* 1982;22:79–84.

65. Hockaday TDR: Serum insulin concentrations and anticipatory factors of cardiomyopathy in NIDDM. *Diabete Metab* 1987;13:354–358.

66. Bergstrand R, Wiklund O, Holm G, et al: Glucose tolerance, plasma insulin and lipoproteins in young male myocardial infarction survivors compared with controls matched on serum cholesterol concentration. *Eur J Clin Invest* 1979;9:381–384.

67. Knatterud GL, Klimt CR, Levin ME, et al: Effects of hypoglycemic agents on vascular complications in patients with adult-onset diabetes VII. Mortality and selected nonfatal events with insulin treatment. *JAMA* 1978;240:37–42.

68. Standl E, Janka HU: High serum insulin concentrations in relation to other cardiovascular risk factors in macrovascular disease of type 2 diabetes. *Horm Metab Res Suppl* 1985;15:46–51.

69. Ronnemaa T, Laakso M, Puukka P, et al: Atherosclerotic vascular disease in middle-aged insulin-treated, diabetic patients: Association with endogenous insulin secretory capacity. *Arteriosclerosis* 1988;8:237–244.

70. Ferrannini E, Haffner SM, Mitchell BD, et al: Hyperinsulinemia: The key feature of a cardiovascular and metabolic syndrome. *Diabetologia* 1991;34:416–422.

71. Ferrari P, Weidmann P: Insulin, insulin sensitivity and hypertension. *J Hypertens* 1990; 8:491–500.

72. Berntorp K, Lindgard F: Familial aggregation of type 2 diabetes mellitus as an etiological factor in hypertension. *Diabetes Res Clin Pract* 1985;1:307–313.

73. Aviv A, Gardner J: Racial differences in ion regulation and their possible links to hypertension in blacks. *Hypertension* 1989;14:584–589.

74. Fontbonne A: Insulin: A sex hormone for cardiovascular risk. *Circulation* 1991;84: 1442–1444.

Chapter 10

Glycosylation-Related Mechanisms

Timothy J. Lyons, MD, MRCP, and
Maria F. Lopes-Virella, MD, PhD

Nonenzymatic glycosylation of proteins involves the covalent binding of glucose to reactive amino groups, usually located on lysine side chains and NH_2-terminal amino acid residues. Subsequently, a complex series of reactions takes place, leading to the formation of a wide variety of stable end products. These reactions are collectively termed "the browning reaction" or "the Maillard reaction," and the final products are termed "browning products," "Maillard reaction products," or "advanced glycosylation end products" (AGE).

The chemistry of the initial stage of glycosylation, and the subsequent formation of the known products of the browning reaction, are shown in Figure 10.1. The initial glucose-to-lysine adduct is known as fructose–lysine because of the shift in position of the carbonyl group during the glycosylation reaction. In humans, whether diabetic or not, fructose–lysine is thought *not* to accumulate with age, even in long-lived proteins, but rather to exist in a steady state relationship with ambient glucose concentration.[1] Metabolic alterations directly attributable to fructose–lysine are perhaps most likely to affect short-lived proteins, since these do not exist long enough to accumulate high levels of browning products. In this chapter, we discuss the consequences of fructose–lysine formation in plasma proteins, especially lipoproteins, and their possible role in atherogenesis in diabetes.

The browning process, which is complex and far from being fully understood, has been the subject of several recent review articles.[2–4] It is known that browning products, all of which are derived from fructose–lysine, are numerous, and include species that are colored and fluorescent and that constitute cross-links. However, only two have been identified conclusively (Figure 10.1): N^ϵ-carboxymethyllysine (CML)[5] (and the closely related species N^ϵ-carboxymethylhydroxylysine and 3-(N^ϵ-lysino)-lactic acid[6]), and pentosidine.[7]

CML is formed by oxidative cleavage of fructose–lysine, and was first identified by Ahmed et al in 1986.[5] It is not fluorescent, and is stable and unreactive: it is not involved in cross-link formation *in vivo*. Although it is now known that CML can be formed from species other than glucose (including other

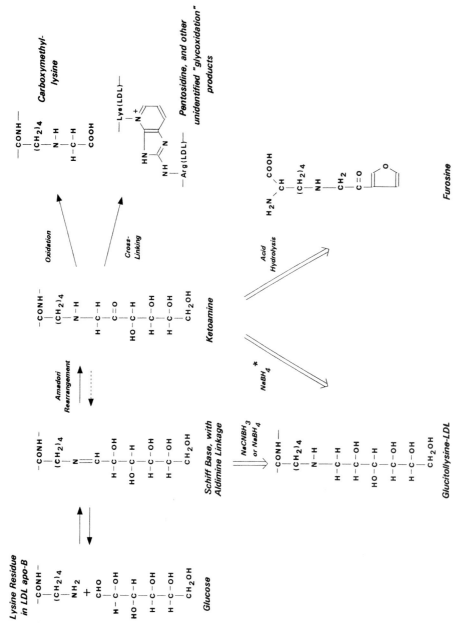

Figure 10.1 Reactions of glycosylation and browning. Solid arrows indicate processes occurring in vivo, and open arrows, processes occurring in vitro. *The reduction of the ketoamine product by sodium borohydride yields a mixture of glucitol–lysine and its stereoisomer, mannitol–lysine. (Reprinted by permission, from Lyons TJ: Lipoprotein glycation and its metabolic consequences. *Diabetes* 1992;41(suppl):67.)

sugars and ascorbate),[8] its formation always involves a free radical oxidation reaction.

Pentosidine is a lysine–arginine cross-link whose structure was first determined by Sell and Monnier in 1989.[7] Originally it was believed that the cross-link was derived mainly from pentoses, but now, like CML, it is known that pentosidine can also be formed during interactions between proteins and other species, including glucose.[9] These studies also demonstrated that the formation of pentosidine, like CML, is dependent on the presence of an oxidative environment. Unlike CML, pentosidine is intensely fluorescent[7,10,11] and it may be considered a "biomarker" for total collagen browning.[11]

It can be appreciated that both of these structurally identified browning products are formed by sequential glycosylation and oxidation reactions, and it is now known that browning and cross-linking of proteins does not occur to any significant extent in an antioxidant environment.[12] To emphasize the close interrelationship of glycosylation and oxidation in the browning process, the final products have been collectively termed "glycoxidation products."[13] Because structural proteins tend to be the longest lived in the body, they are thought to be the most affected by these reactions, which are slow but irreversible. In long-lived proteins, glycoxidation products, unlike fructose–lysine, accumulate with age in a linear fashion, and, like rust on a car, their formation is thought to be irreversible. Two of the current theories to explain the aging process are the "glucose theory of aging"[14–16] and the "free radical (oxidative) theory of aging."[17] It is of interest that both theories are relevant to the formation of glycoxidation products. In this chapter, we concentrate on the consequences of browning in vascular wall structural proteins.

In diabetes, the glycosylation and subsequent browning (or glycoxidation) reactions are enhanced by elevated glucose concentrations. It is unclear whether the diabetic state per se also induces an increase in the generation of free radicals (ie, whether the glycoxidation process is enhanced just by increased glycosylation or whether increased "oxidative stress" is also involved). There is some evidence, however, that glycosylation itself may induce the formation of free radicals.[18] Diabetes is therefore a disease characterized by accelerated biochemical aging of long-lived proteins. In terms of the two theories of aging mentioned above, the accelerated aging is certainly glucose mediated, but perhaps enhanced oxidation-mediated aging may also be involved.

Increased glycosylation, and subsequent glycoxidation, has provided the basis for an attractive hypothesis to explain the development of diabetic complications.[19] It is proposed that these processes, by inducing structural changes, may lead to functional abnormalities of circulating and tissue proteins. Furthermore, such modification of proteins may render them immunogenic[20–22] and result in the formation of immune complexes. As discussed below, glycosylation, oxidation, and glycoxidation may all contribute, in interrelated ways, to the acceleration of atherosclerosis in diabetes. The initial glycosylation reaction product, fructose–lysine, may play its most significant and direct role by causing alterations in the metabolism of short-lived plasma constituents, particularly lipoproteins. This is discussed in some detail below. Free radical–mediated oxidative damage, perhaps enhanced by glycosylation, also affects lipoproteins. However, glycoxidation, or browning, is most significant in the long-lived structural proteins of vessel walls, and is discussed in the second half of this chapter.

Glycosylation and Plasma Proteins

Lipoprotein Glycosylation and Its Effect on Lipoprotein Metabolism

It is well established that lipoproteins are implicated in the development of atherosclerosis, and that diabetes, for reasons that are not yet fully understood, is an independent risk factor for the development of this condition.[23] The possibility that increased glycosylation of lipoproteins may contribute to the problem of macrovascular disease in diabetes has therefore been the subject of extensive research. Many questions arise: Do apolipoproteins indeed undergo increased glycosylation in the diabetic state? Which lipoproteins are affected, and is there differential modification of the various apolipoproteins within the same particle? How do lipoproteins that have undergone modification in vitro (in model systems) and in vivo (in diabetic patients) interact with relevant cell types (ie, cells that are found in the arterial intima and media)? Because lipoproteins are short-lived plasma proteins, is it only the initial stage of glycosylation that is relevant to any altered interactions with cells, or are other factors such as oxidation of constituent lipids, the browning process, or compositional alterations also involved? Finally, since oxidized lipoproteins seem to play a important role in the pathogenesis of atherosclerosis, does glycosylation of the apoprotein predispose the protein and/or lipid portions of the particles to oxidative damage?

The results of studies investigating these questions are summarized below. Not all the answers are available as yet. One major obstacle is the difficulty in measuring apolipoprotein glycosylation. In comparison with other plasma proteins, the procedures are complicated by the presence of the lipid moiety, and by the fact that all lipoproteins, except low-density lipoprotein (LDL), have more than one apoprotein. Since the half-lives and metabolism of the individual apoproteins in very-low-density lipoprotein (VLDL), intermediate-density lipoprotein (IDL), and high-density lipoprotein (HDL) differ, they are likely to have undergone different degrees of glycosylation. It may be important to distinguish these differences in order to investigate possible metabolic consequences. This consideration applies not only to the measurement of apoprotein glycosylation that has occurred in vivo (ie, in lipoproteins isolated from human subjects), but also to the preparation of in vitro–glycosylated particles for studies of cell–lipoprotein interactions in culture. Partly for this reason, most studies have concentrated on LDL, which has only one apoprotein, apo B-100.

Apolipoproteins were first shown to undergo increased glycosylation when exposed to elevated glucose concentrations, either in vitro or in vivo, by Schleicher et al in 1981.[24] Incubating human lipoproteins (LDL and HDL) with [^{14}C]glucose in vitro, they found that the extent of incorporation of glucose into the apolipoprotein components of the particles (apo A-I, A-II, B, C, and E) was directly proportional to the period of incubation and to the ambient concentration of glucose. They also demonstrated a twofold increase in apo B glycosylation in LDL from diabetic compared to nondiabetic human subjects. To measure glycosylation, they used the "furosine method," in which furosine, a product of weak acid hydrolysis of fructose-lysine (Figure 10.1), is assayed. These authors were the first to suggest that increased glycosylation of lipoproteins in vivo might have significant metabolic consequences.

Interactions of Glycosylated LDL with Human Fibroblasts and Murine Macrophages

Studies by Gonen et al,[25] Witztum et al,[26] and Sasaki and Cottam[27] followed, aiming to investigate the abnormal metabolism of glycosylated LDL. These workers examined the interactions of in vitro–glycosylated LDL with cultured human fibroblasts and mouse peritoneal macrophages. LDL was glycosylated in vitro using glucose concentrations varying from 5 to 100 mmol/L for periods of 1 or 2 weeks. In some cases the reducing agent sodium cyanoborohydride was added to increase the degree of glycosylation of LDL. Cyanoborohydride reduces and stabilizes an intermediate product (Schiff base) during the formation of fructose-lysine (Figure 10.1). Since Schiff base formation is readily reversible, its stabilization by chemical reduction accelerates and amplifies the in vitro modification. However, the resulting adduct (glucitol–lysine) does differ slightly from the fructose–lysine formed in vivo. The metabolic studies confirmed that recognition of this "reductively glycosylated" LDL by cells is altered. With normal human fibroblasts, which possess the classic LDL receptor, there was impaired binding and degradation of glycosylated compared to control LDL, the impairment being proportional to the extent of glycosylation. Degradation of LDL by fibroblasts was impaired when only 6% to 8% of lysine residues were modified, and more extensive modification abolished recognition of the lipoprotein particles altogether. In vivo, there was a threefold increase in glycosylation of LDL in diabetic patients, and, in later studies in which LDL was glycosylated in vitro to simulate the extent of glycosylation occurring in vivo in diabetes, Steinbrecher and Witztum[28] found that modification of a few as 2% to 5% of lysine residues, in the absence of cyanoborohydride, decreased LDL catabolism by human fibroblasts by 5% to 25%. Again, the extent of the decrease in catabolism was proportional to the degree of glycosylation. When radiolabeled LDL was injected into guinea pigs and rabbits, the fractional catabolic rate of glycosylated LDL was found to be significantly lower than that of control LDL. In contrast to the findings with fibroblasts, murine peritoneal macrophages failed to distinguish between control and glycosylated LDL. The macrophage is a scavenger cell, but the scavenger receptor of the murine peritoneal macrophage, which recognizes heavily modified acetyl-LDL, did not bind glycosylated LDL.[25,26]

These studies suggested that recognition of in vitro–glycosylated LDL by the classic LDL receptor is impaired. The impairment was detectable when the extent of glycosylation was similar to that occurring in diabetes in vivo, and could therefore contribute to the elevation of plasma LDL cholesterol levels in diabetic patients in poor glycemic control. In contrast, the murine macrophage did not recognize glycosylated LDL as being abnormal.

Interactions of In Vivo–Glycosylated LDL with Human Macrophages

Subsequent studies by our group built on these observations. We demonstrated that the extent of glycosylation of LDL correlates well with other short- and medium-term indicators of glycemic control (mean plasma glucose, plasma protein glycosylation, and hemoglobin [Hb] A_{ic}), and that increased LDL glycosylation is present even in normolipidemic diabetic patients in satisfactory glycemic control.[29] The extent of the increase in apo B glycosylation in diabetic compared to control patients (1.6-fold higher) was of the same order as that for hemoglobin (1.5-fold) and total plasma proteins (2.2-fold).[29] We extended

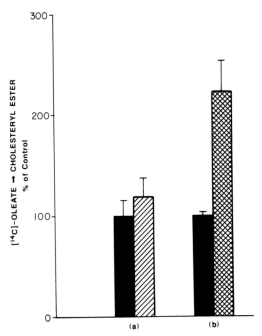

Figure 10.2 Rates of synthesis of [^{14}C]cholesteryl oleate by human monocyte-derived macrophages incubated (A) with LDL (100 μg/mL) isolated from ten type I diabetic patients (▨) and ten control subjects (■), and (B) with in vitro–glycosylated (⊠) and control LDL (■) (100 μg/mL). Rates of synthesis are expressed as percentages of the rates determined with control LDL. The rate of synthesis of [^{14}C]cholesteryl oleate by cells incubated in the absence of LDL averaged 8.6 ± 1.1% of that observed in cells incubated with control LDL.

the studies of cell–lipoprotein interactions using LDL isolated from diabetic and control patients. We showed that recognition of LDL from diabetic patients by human fibroblasts was impaired, although the extent of glycation was not determined.[30] Of direct relevance to the development of atherosclerosis, we also investigated the interactions of LDL isolated from diabetic patients with cultured human plasma monocyte-derived macrophages, the main precursors of foam cells in human atherosclerosis.[31] We found that the human monocyte-derived macrophages behaved quite differently from their murine counterparts. LDL from typical type I diabetic patients (HbA$_{ic}$ range, 6.4% to 10.5%), as shown in Figure 10.2A, was found to stimulate more cholesteryl ester synthesis in human monocyte-derived macrophages than LDL from nondiabetic control subjects. The composition of LDL was similar in the two groups, and the particles appeared to differ only in the extent of apoprotein glycosylation, which was increased 1.4-fold in the diabetic patients. Furthermore, cholesteryl ester synthesis in the macrophages correlated with the extent of LDL glycosylation. In concert with the increased cholesteryl ester synthesis, intracellular cholesteryl ester accumulation was also increased in macrophages exposed to LDL from diabetic patients. In a later study,[32] we investigated human monocyte-derived macrophage interactions with LDL isolated from patients with type II diabetes and matched nondiabetic control subjects. Here, no difference was found in the rate of cholesteryl ester synthesis by macrophages exposed to LDL from the two groups. However, the type II diabetic patients were in excellent glycemic control and their mean LDL glycosylation was increased to a lesser extent (1.2-fold) over the control value than in the type I diabetic patient group.

From these studies, we concluded that LDL from diabetic patients, compared to that from nondiabetic control subjects, is poorly recognized by the classic LDL receptor, perhaps contributing to hyperlipidemia in diabetes. In human monocyte-derived macrophages, glycosylated LDL may stimulate more rapid foam cell formation, and thereby accelerate the atherosclerotic process. Furthermore, we concluded that these effects were dependent on the increased glycosylation of apo B-100 in diabetes, because no other alteration in the particle was detected.

Interactions of In Vitro–Glycosylated LDL with Human Macrophages

These conclusions were supported by further experiments in our laboratory using LDL glycosylated in vitro under antioxidant conditions.[33] The levels of glycosylation obtained (approximately a fourfold increase) were greater than those previously found in vivo,[31] and a proportionately greater effect on macrophage metabolism was observed (Figure 10.2B). The highly glycosylated LDL stimulated much more cholesteryl ester synthesis and accumulation in macrophages, and receptor-mediated intracellular degradation was also increased.

Because recognition of highly glycosylated LDL by the classic LDL receptor in macrophages, as in fibroblasts, was diminished, the increased uptake and degradation of the particle was considered to be mediated through a different pathway. Competition studies using acetyl-LDL clearly showed that the scavenger receptor pathway was not involved (Figure 10.3). To exclude the possibility that the increased uptake, degradation, and accumulation of the glycosylated LDL might be a nonspecific effect of glycosylation, the interaction of the macrophages with control and glycosylated albumin (native albumin is nonspecifically taken up by macrophages) and thyroglobulin (whose molecular weight is similar to that of apo B) was investigated. In these experiments, degradation of the glycosylated forms of the proteins was, if anything, decreased. To exclude the possibility that the macrophage glycoprotein receptor might be implicated, the lipoprotein degradation experiments were performed in the presence of increasing concentrations of yeast mannan, which is known to block this receptor. The mannan had no effect on the degradation of either control or glycosylated LDL. A separate low-affinity, high-capacity receptor pathway, by which glycosylated LDL gains entry into the macrophage, was therefore proposed.

Recent studies in our laboratory, as yet unpublished, further support the enhanced atherogenicity of glycosylated LDL in diabetes. In these studies, we isolated two fractions of intact LDL using boronate affinity chromatography as described by Jack et al.[34] The boronate affinity column binds fructose–lysine adducts on the intact lipoprotein particle. Whereas the method was described as a convenient means to measure lipoprotein glycosylation, we have used it simply to isolate "bound" and "nonbound" (ie, more and less glycosylated) LDL fractions, which can then be used in lipoprotein–cell interaction studies. We isolated these two LDL fractions from both type I diabetic patients and nondiabetic control subjects. The diabetic group had a mean HbA$_{1c}$ of 9.1% and had mild, but not significant, increases in mean plasma triglycerides and cholesterol. Glycosylation of the nonbound fractions was low, and almost identical between

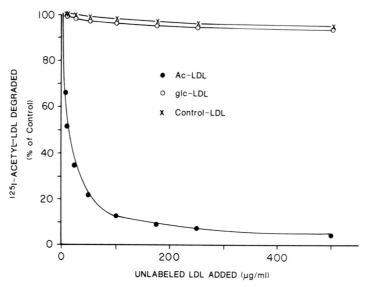

Figure 10.3 Inability of unlabeled control (×) and glycosylated (○) low-density lipoproteins (LDL) to inhibit the degradation of ^{125}I-labeled acetyl-LDL. They are not recognized by the scavenger receptor, which does recognize acetyl-LDL, and therefore have no effect. Unlabeled acetyl-LDL (●) competes successfully for the scavenger receptor. (*Reprinted, by permission, from Lopes-Virella MF, Klein RL, Lyons TJ, et al: Glycosylation of low-density lipoprotein enhances cholesteryl ester synthesis in human monocyte-derived macrophages. Diabetes 1988;37:554.*)

control and diabetic samples. In the bound fractions, glycosylation was increased compared to nonbound fractions in both control subjects (twofold increase) and diabetic patients (threefold increase). The fact that the increase in glycosylation, effectively per LDL particle, was greater in the diabetic patients suggests that a higher proportion of the lysine residues in each particle had been glycosylated. This may imply that lysine residues other than those that primarily determine binding to the affinity column were glycosylated in the high ambient glucose concentrations present in diabetes.

We studied the metabolic behavior of the fractions, isolated as described above, again using human fibroblasts and human monocyte-derived macrophages. With fibroblasts and LDL from nondiabetic control subjects, LDL receptor-mediated degradation of the bound fraction was impaired compared to the nonbound LDL fraction. Non-LDL receptor-mediated degradation was low in both bound and nonbound fractions, and did not differ significantly between them. Similar observations were made for fibroblasts with LDL from diabetic patients. LDL receptor-mediated degradation was markedly depressed for the bound LDL. This confirms previous studies wherein impaired recognition of glycosylated LDL by LDL receptors on fibroblasts was observed, and again the impairment was directly related to the degree of glycosylation of the particle. Non-LDL receptor-mediated degradation was low, and similar, in the bound and nonbound fractions.

In human monocyte-derived macrophages, in contrast to what happened in fibroblasts, LDL receptor-mediated degradation of the bound and nonbound LDL fractions isolated from nondiabetic control subjects was similar, confirming previous work showing that a mild degree of glycosylation will not impair the recognition of LDL by the LDL receptor in these cells.[32] However, non-LDL receptor-mediated degradation was increased twofold for the bound, compared to the nonbound, fraction. LDL receptor-mediated degradation of the bound LDL isolated from diabetic patients was mildly impaired, although not to the same extent as was seen with fibroblasts. Again, with LDL from diabetic patients, non-LDL receptor-mediated degradation was significantly increased in the bound compared to the nonbound fractions, as expected. Thus the high levels of glycosylation in the bound LDL particles from diabetic patients seemed both to impair their recognition by the macrophage LDL receptor and to stimulate their recognition by non-LDL receptor-mediated mechanisms. Again, therefore, it appears that in humans, although glycosylated LDL is poorly recognized by the classic LDL receptor on fibroblasts, it is recognized by another high-capacity, low-affinity pathway on monocyte-derived macrophages, enhancing uptake by these cells and thereby enhancing foam cell formation.

Lipoprotein Glycosylation and Oxidation

Lipoproteins, containing unsaturated fatty acids in their cores, are particularly vulnerable to oxidative damage, and the role of oxidized lipoproteins in the pathogenesis of atherosclerosis in diabetes has been reviewed recently by one of us.[35] Oxidized LDL is a potent stimulator of foam cell formation by macrophages. There are theoretical reasons to believe that the processes of oxidation and glycosylation may be linked. Both simple monosaccharides and fructose–lysine "auto-oxidize" under physiologic conditions, in the presence of traces of metal ions, generating superoxide radicals.[18,36] Thus, it is thought that glycosylation of lipoproteins may enhance the likelihood of oxidative damage. Despite this, there is little evidence to suggest that oxidation of plasma lipoproteins is increased in uncomplicated diabetes, whereas glycosylation clearly is. Also, there are no studies demonstrating a correlation between lipoprotein oxidation and glycemic control in diabetic patients. Nevertheless, the situation may well be different for lipoproteins that have become extravasated and are sequestered in the vessel wall. Here the processes of glycosylation, oxidation, and browning may be closely interwoven, causing vicious cycles of vascular injury. As discussed below, glycosylation and browning of vascular connective tissue proteins may increase covalent, glucose-mediated binding of lipoproteins, trapping them in the vessel wall and allowing greater degrees of glycosylation and oxidation than could otherwise occur. This covalent binding may also be enhanced by glycosylation of the lipoproteins themselves.

Lipoprotein Glycosylation and Platelet Function

Studies have recently been performed to assess the effect of LDL glycosylation on platelet aggregation. In our laboratory, Watanabe et al[37] isolated LDL from young type I diabetic patients in good or fair glycemic control, and also from a group of age- and sex-matched nondiabetic control subjects. Glycosylation of LDL from the diabetic patients was increased, although LDL composition was similar in the two groups. Throughout the study, ethylenediaminetetra-acetic acid (EDTA) was used to prevent LDL oxidation. Compared to LDL from control subjects, LDL from diabetic patients was a more potent stimulator of thromboxane B_2 release and thrombin-induced platelet aggregation. In addition, LDL was glycosylated in vitro in the presence of EDTA to prevent oxidation. This glycosylated LDL also caused a marked enhancement in thrombin-, collagen-, and ADP-induced platelet aggregation. However, it was noted that, in general, the enhancement was seen irrespective of the concentration of glucose used in the incubation, the lowest concentration of glucose (10 mmol/L) being almost as effective as the highest (150 mmol/L). Thus it appeared that the effect was not linearly related to the extent of LDL glycosylation. We proposed that subtle alterations in the composition of platelet membranes induced by interaction with glycosylated LDL may underlie the effects on platelet behavior. Finally, when LDL from type I diabetic patients was subfractionated by affinity chromatography into bound and nonbound fractions, using the method of Jack et al[34] as previously described, platelet aggregation was enhanced to a significantly greater extent by the bound (highly glycosylated) fraction.[38]

Glycosylation of Other Lipoproteins

Increased glycosylation affects other apolipoproteins apart from apo B-100 in LDL. Elevated levels in VLDL and HDL apoproteins have been demonstrated by Curtiss and Witztum,[39] and are thought to affect the cellular interactions, function, and metabolism of these particles. Recently, VLDL isolated from normolipemic patients with both type I and type II diabetes was found to interact abnormally with cultured human monocyte-derived macrophages,[32,40] stimulating increased cholesteryl ester synthesis and accumulation. However, the effect was not as marked as with LDL. Also, subtle alterations in lipid and apoprotein composition were observed in the VLDL from diabetic patients, and these may have accounted for some of the findings. Nevertheless, increased glycosylation of the apoproteins of VLDL may be important. Investigation of this problem is hampered by the difficulty of measuring the extent of glycosylation of the various apoproteins on the VLDL particle.

Glycosylation of HDL was first studied by Witztum et al.[41] HDL was glycosylated in vitro, and clearance from the circulation in guinea pigs was accelerated. This finding was in contrast to the effect on glycosylated LDL, whose catabolic rate was reduced. The effect was seen even with mild degrees of glycosylation, and was proposed as a possible cause of low plasma levels of HDL in diabetic patients, and thus as another contributing factor to the increased risk for atherosclerotic disease in diabetic patients. More recently, Duell et al[42] have shown that high-affinity binding of glycosylated HDL to fibroblasts is impaired, and that this reduces its capacity to remove cholesterol from peripheral cells.

Lipoprotein Glycosylation and the Immune System

Modification of proteins, as by glycosylation and oxidation, may alter their structure sufficiently to render them immunogenic. Curtiss and Witztum[43] performed studies to investigate the possible immunogenic properties of glycosylated lipoproteins. They injected guinea pigs with homologous LDL that had been subjected to in vitro glycosylation in the presence and absence of cyanoborohydride, producing heavily (60% of lysine residues glycosylated) and mildly (6% of lysine residues glycosylated) modified particles, respectively. The heavily modified particles were potent immunogens, stimulating the production of antibodies that did not interact with unmodified LDL but did interact with other "reductively glycosylated" proteins (ie, those that had undergone glycosylation in the presence of cyanoborohydride). Glucitol–lysine, the product of cyano-borohydride reduction of Schiff base (Figure 10.1), was shown to be an important part of the epitope. In vivo, however, glucitol–lysine does not exist, and the initial stable product of glycosylation that is formed, fructose–lysine, was not recognized by the antibody raised against reductively glycosylated LDL. When the in vitro glycosylation was performed in the absence of cyanoborohydride, resulting in the formation of fructose–lysine as would occur in vivo, the more mildly modified LDL was a much less potent immunogen. Control LDL, which inevitably contains some glycosylated LDL, and, to a greater extent, in vitro-glycosylated LDL both competed for this antibody.

The presence of antibodies against reductively glycosylated LDL leads to accelerated clearance of these particles from guinea pig plasma, but antibodies against nonreductively glycosylated LDL had no effect on its rate of clearance.[44] It appears that the difference in antibody response and subsequent clearance rates may be in part the result of different degrees of apolipoprotein modification and in part the result of epitope differences. However, the existence of even low levels of antibodies against the less modified, fructose–lysine–containing, gly-cosylated LDL may have pathophysiologic relevance, because it may imply the presence of circulating antigen–antibody complexes, which, as discussed below, have been found to be potentially atherogenic. In addition, the more severely modified ("glycoxidized") lipoproteins that may be present in vessel walls may behave as much more potent antigens than the less modified particles found in the plasma, stimulating the in situ formation of immune complexes.[22]

It has been shown by us[45,46] and by others[47] that LDL/anti-LDL immune complexes (LDL-ICs) are potent inducers of foam cell formation. The transformation of human monocyte-derived macrophages into foam cells can be induced either by insoluble LDL-ICs, presented to the macrophages as large aggregates, or by soluble LDL-ICs, presented to the macrophages adsorbed to red blood cells (RBCs). Both types of LDL-ICs may be formed in vivo. Subendothelial LDL deposits are likely to include LDL-ICs formed in situ, and these are probably large, insoluble aggregates. Soluble LDL-ICs present in circulation, however, are likely to be formed in antigen excess, and they will tend to be adsorbed to RBCs via C3b receptors and other nonspecific interactions. Once absorbed to RBCs, LDL-ICs are transported to organs rich in tissue macrophages (eg, the liver), where the LDL-ICs can be transferred to phagocytic cells and catabolized. The transfer of LDL-ICs takes place without obvious damage to the RBCs, probably for a variety of reasons. First, the binding of LDL-ICs to the CR1 receptor on RBCs is followed by degradation of C3b, and binding affinity to the RBCs consequently decreases. Also, LDL-ICs may be adsorbed to RBCs through very-low-affinity interactions, not involving any defined receptor. In either case, the LDL-ICs are easily transferred to phagocytic cells expressing Fc receptors of higher affinity.[48] In vitro, both insoluble and soluble (RBC-adsorbed) LDL-ICs induce profound alterations in lipoprotein metabolism and cholesterol homeostasis of monocyte-derived macrophages.[45,46]

The rapid transformation of human monocyte-derived macrophages into foam cells is one of the most striking abnormalities induced by either insoluble or RBC-bound LDL-ICs. Relatively low concentrations of LDL-ICs can induce this response, particularly when RBC-bound LDL-ICs are involved: they are 15-fold more potent than insoluble LDL-ICs. Surprisingly, while inducing foam cell formation, the LDL-IC also stimulates a considerable increase (approximately 20-fold) in LDL receptor activity. The uptake of the LDL-ICs by macrophages also leads to activation of the cells, and to the release of interleukin-1 (IL-1) and tumor necrosis factor α (TNF-α). The pathogenic potential of this phenomenon to accelerate the development of atherosclerosis is enormous. Both IL-1 and TNF-α can enhance the expression of vascular cell adherence molecules on endothelial cells.[49] IL-1 has been shown to induce synthesis and cell surface expression of procoagulant activity in endothelial cells,[50] to increase vascular permeability,[51] to induce IL-1 release from endothelial cells by a positive feedback mechanism,[52] to promote the release of an increased amount of platelet activating factor by endothelial cells,[53] and to increase neutrophil adherence.[54,55] Also, IL-1 may be indirectly responsible for fibroblast and smooth muscle cell proliferation, by inducing production of platelet-derived growth factor AA by these cells, activating what appears to be an autocrine growth-regulating mechanism.[56] However, IL-1 also induces secretion of prostaglandins by smooth muscle cells.[57] Prostaglandins are known to have growth-inhibiting properties, and therefore the in vivo effect of IL-1 release in the arterial wall is unclear. TNF-α, which can be produced not only by macrophages but also by smooth muscle cells, induces some responses similar to those of IL-1, including cell surface expression of procoagulant activity[50] and production of IL-1 by endothelial cells.[58]

Glycosylation and Antithrombin III Activity

Brownlee et al[59] showed that increased glycosylation of antithrombin III impairs its thrombin-inhibiting activity, and suggested that a resulting defect in inhibition of the coagulation cascade could contribute to the accumulation of fibrin in diabetic tissues. The glycosylation-induced inhibition of antithrombin III activity is completely reversible by an excess of sodium heparin. Later, Ceriello et al[60] described an inverse correlation between antithrombin III activity and both HbA_{1c} and plasma glucose independent of plasma concentrations of antithrombin III. They proposed that antithrombin III activity was probably influenced by glycosylation. In contrast, in vitro glycosylation of fibrinogen was not found to influence its function, and therefore does not appear to promote thrombosis.[61]

Conclusions: Atherogenic Consequences of the Initial Glycosylation Reaction

It is clear that increased glycosylation of lipoproteins has significant effects on lipoprotein metabolism. Increased glycosylation occurs from the time of onset of diabetes, and therefore, although the effects are not as dramatic as are seen with other more severely modified lipoproteins (eg, oxidized LDL), over a period of years they may have significant pathologic effects. Impaired recognition of glycosylated LDL by the classic LDL receptor may delay clearance of the particles, and thus contribute to hyperlipidemia and to greater degrees of lipoprotein modification. Similarly, sequestration and covalent binding in the vessel walls, enhanced by increased glycosylation of both the lipoproteins themselves and the vessel wall structural proteins, may facilitate degrees of in situ modification (both glycosylation and oxidation) greater than those occurring in the plasma. Also in vessel walls, enhanced uptake of glycosylated LDL by human macrophages may accelerate foam cell formation. In this respect, the human monocyte-derived macrophage behaves differently from its murine peritoneal counterpart. Glycosylation of LDL enhances platelet aggregation in vitro, and may increase the susceptibility of both its lipid and protein components to oxidative damage, further increasing atherogenicity. Glycosylation of VLDL and HDL may also contribute to the acceleration of atherosclerosis. Glycosylation and glycoxidation of lipoproteins may stimulate immune complex formation, resulting in stimulation of foam cell formation and cytokine release. Glycosylation of antithrombin III may promote thrombosis but glycosylation of fibrinogen appears to have no effect.

Browning of Vascular Structural Proteins

The first section of this chapter was concerned with the consequences of glycosylation of circulating proteins, especially lipoproteins, and discussed the evidence that they contribute to the acceleration of atherosclerosis in diabetes. In this section, we consider the evidence that glycosylation and browning of vascular wall structural proteins may also be important, and that these processes not only alter the characteristics of the vessel wall itself, but also influence its interaction with circulating plasma constituents.

Collagen: Effects of Aging and Diabetes

Among the long-lived structural proteins of the body, collagen in its various forms has been the most widely studied. In diabetes, most studies have utilized skin and tendon collagen, but the nonenzymatic nature of the glycosylation and browning reactions make it reasonable to extrapolate the physicochemical alterations observed in these collagens to those in other sites, including those in the arterial wall.

Changes in the Physical Properties of Collagens With Aging: Relationship with Glycosylation and Browning

With advancing age, collagen becomes increasingly insoluble, thermally stable, and resistant to enzymatic attack.[62] Some of these changes are sufficiently predictable to allow determination of the age of the donor of a collagen sample with considerable accuracy.[63] The changes are accompanied by, and are thought to be caused by, the formation of stable cross-links. Evidence is accumulating that many of the cross-links are derived from glucose via the browning process, in which case the changes in physical properties of collagen with age should be exaggerated in the presence of diabetes. Studies over the past 20 years have demonstrated that this is indeed so. In 1975, Hamlin et al[64] found that their ability to predict the age of a patient by measuring collagen digestibility failed in the presence of diabetes: three diabetic patients whose true ages were 33, 41, and 44 years were found to have collagen digestibility ages of 84, 103, and 106 years, respectively.

To determine whether increased glycosylation and/or browning of collagen might be responsible for the changes in its physical properties, experiments were performed in which collagen was glycosylated in vitro. Short-term (1-week) incubations did not confer any increased resistance to enzymatic digestion[65] but did increase the stability of rat tail tendons.[66] Longer term incubations using lens crystallin (another very long-lived protein) produced spectrophotometric changes similar to those occurring with age,[14] and incubations using basement membrane collagens caused enhanced thermal stability.[67]

Glycosylation and Browning of Structural Proteins in Diabetes

Rosenberg et al,[68] in 1979, were the first to measure collagen glycosylation (fructose–lysine content) in diabetic and control environments. They found that glycosylation of aortic collagen in diabetic rats was significantly increased, and suggested this might be relevant to the accelerated development of atherosclerosis. Subsequently, increased glycosylation of collagen in diabetes was confirmed in rat glomerular basement membranes,[69] human tendon and skin,[70–73] and human aorta, glomerular basement membrane, and tendon.[74,75]

In diabetes, glycosylation (fructose–lysine content) of insoluble skin collagen correlates closely with HbA_1,[72] and falls promptly after a relatively short (4-month) period of improved glycemic control.[76] In nondiabetic subjects, collagen glycosylation increases only very slightly between the ages of 20 and 80 years.[1] These findings suggest that collagen glycosylation is in a steady state relationship with ambient glucose concentrations.

In contrast to fructose–lysine, glycoxidation (browning) products in insoluble collagen accumulate continuously from birth to death.[1,7] In diabetic patients, the rate of accumulation is accelerated.[64,77,78] Thus middle-aged or even young diabetic patients may develop levels of these products higher than those seen even in the oldest nondiabetic subject.[79] The degree of excess accumulation in diabetes may depend on duration of diabetes, average glycemic control, and individual susceptibility to oxidative damage. The accumulation of glycoxidation products in collagen, like rust on a car, appears to be an irreversible process.[76]

Relationship of Collagen Glycosylation and Browning to Diabetic Complications

No study has shown a significant relationship between collagen glycosylation (fructose–lysine content) and the presence or severity of diabetic complications. However, Monnier and co-workers found an association between both collagen-linked fluorescence (in insoluble skin collagen)[77] and pentosidine content[80] and the severity of diabetic retinopathy, joint stiffness, and arterial stiffness. Recently, we have shown that CML, pentosidine, and total collagen fluorescence levels all correlate closely with one another,[76] and that they are related to various diabetic complications (unpublished observations). A relationship between collagen browning and diabetic nephropathy was also found in a recent study by Makita et al.[81] These results are consistent with, but do not prove, a role for the glycoxidation process in the pathogenesis of complications. Cumulative "glycosylative" stress may be a function of duration of diabetes and average glycemic control; oxidative stress may be more a function of individual variation, independent of the presence or absence of diabetes. Mechanisms by which glycosylation and browning of vascular wall structural proteins may contribute to atherogenesis are considered below; some have substantial supporting evidence, whereas others are more speculative.

Abnormal Vascular Rigidity and Tone

Monnier et al[77] showed that increased collagen fluorescence is associated with increased arterial stiffness (assessed in vivo) and with elevated systolic and diastolic blood pressures. Increased aortic stiffness in autopsy studies of patients with type I diabetes was confirmed by Oxlund et al,[82] but the level of glycoxidation products was not determined. It is probable that loss of the normal elasticity and compliance of arteries and arterioles in diabetes is at least partially due to increased glucose-mediated cross-linking. This may contribute directly to the development of hypertension, whereas arterial stiffness and hypertension together may result in abnormal shear stresses on the endothelium, predisposing it to injury and the development of atherosclerosis.

Recent evidence suggests that the presence of collagen glycoxidation products quenches the activity of nitric oxide (endothelium-derived relaxing factor) both in vitro and in vivo.[83] This quenching leads to an impairment of endothelium-mediated vasodilation, and therefore may cause abnormalities in vascular tone. It is possible that local abnormalities of flow, perfusion, and blood pressure may result, and these may be injurious to arteries and arterioles.

Covalent Binding of Plasma Constituents

Endothelial injury allows increased permeation of plasma constituents into the vessel wall, where they come into contact with elevated levels of connective tissue glycoxidation products. Brownlee et al[84] demonstrated increased LDL–collagen cross-linking when the lipoprotein was exposed to modified collagen (containing browning products) compared to control collagen. In diabetic compared to nondiabetic animals, cross-linking of LDL to aortic collagen was increased 2.5-fold. Trapped in a high-glucose environment in the vessel wall, the LDL particles will undergo extensive glycative and oxidative modification, with further increases in particle atherogenicity. Free radical chain reactions in the trapped LDL may damage not only the lipids within the particle but also neighboring structural proteins and cells. It has been shown, for instance, that products of lipid peroxidation stimulate cross-linking of collagen.[85] In diabetes, these interrelated mechanisms are likely to result in various vicious cycles, leading to damage of the arterial wall and in situ formation of lipoprotein immune complexes,[22] further accelerating foam cell formation.

The Macrophage "AGE Receptor"

As discussed earlier in this chapter, monocyte-derived macrophages are intimately involved in the development of atherosclerotic lesions. It is now established that these cells possess a specific receptor that recognizes glycoxidation products; this has been termed the "AGE receptor," and has been shown to be distinct from other scavenger receptors.[86] Macrophages expressing this receptor are capable of engulfing not just protein molecules but also entire cells that have glycoxidation products on their surfaces.[87] The presence of glycoxidation products (or AGE) in vessel walls is chemotactic to circulating monocyte-derived macrophages, inducing them to migrate through the vascular endothelium.[88] Also, the interaction of AGE proteins with the AGE receptor has been shown to be accompanied by release of cytokines, TNF-α, and IL-1,[89] which are known to mediate growth and remodeling processes and which, as previously discussed, may accelerate the atherosclerotic process.

Renal Impairment

Accumulating glycoxidation products may contribute to the development of renal impairment in diabetes.[77,81] Recently a correlation between skin collagen browning and microalbuminuria, the earliest manifestation of renal disease, was found (unpublished observations). This suggests that a generalized collagen abnormality may underlie the development of microalbuminuria, and this may partly explain the identification of microalbuminuria as a risk factor for macrovascular disease. The mild hypertension and lipid abnormalities associated with renal impairment may further contribute to the development of atherosclerosis.

Is It Possible To Inhibit the Glycosylation and Browning of Vascular Structural Proteins?

If the gradual, and irreversible, accumulation of glycoxidation products in vascular structural proteins is indeed harmful, it would clearly be desirable to inhibit the process, particularly in diabetic patients. Ways to inhibit the "glycosylative" and "oxidative" arms of the process may be considered separately.

Reducing Glycosylative Stress

The most obvious measure is to optimize glycemic control in order to minimize fructose–lysine formation. Also, the existing levels of fructose–lysine may be reduced: even a short-term improvement in glycemic control can reduce the fructose–lysine content of insoluble skin collagen,[76] and presumably that of arterial collagens as well. This should decrease the subsequent formation of glycoxidation products. In the future, pharmacologic intervention may be possible. Aminoguanidine, a hydrazine that binds to reactive carbonyl groups, has been the subject of intensive study by Brownlee et al.[90] It is thought to act by blocking the open-chain form of glucose and/or reactive dicarbonyl browning intermediates that are derived from the dissociation of fructose–lysine.[91] Aminoguanidine has been successful in preventing the browning process both in vitro and in vivo.[90]

Reducing Oxidative Stress

Currently there is little evidence concerning the efficacy of any treatment aimed to reduce oxidative damage to proteins in diabetes. Probucol may be effective in reducing lipid peroxidation,[92] and may therefore have a protective effect in the vessel wall. Another approach involves the supplementation of free radical scavengers. Of these, ascorbate is believed to be the most important,[93] and plasma levels of this and platelet levels of vitamin E, another free radical scavenger, tend to be abnormally low in diabetic patients.[94,95] However, no studies exist to demonstrate that supplementation of these vitamins will affect the progress of atherosclerosis in diabetic patients.

Conclusion

The processes of glycosylation and browning, or "glycoxidation," are thought to play a significant role in the acceleration of atherosclerosis in diabetes. The initial glycosylation reaction increases the atherogenicity of lipoproteins and diminishes the activity of antithrombin III. Glycosylation is also thought to enhance the propensity of vessel wall structural proteins to bind extravasated plasma proteins, including lipoproteins. In the longer lived vascular structural proteins, and in trapped, extravasated plasma proteins, browning, or "glycoxidation," reactions ensue. These involve free radical–mediated oxidation, and multiple vicious cycles of damage to the vessel wall may be set in motion: protein cross-linking, lipid peroxidation, foam cell formation, and free radical–mediated cytotoxicity are all interrelated. Finally, the generation of severely modified proteins and lipoproteins may stimulate immune complex formation. All of these factors combine to accelerate the atherosclerotic process in diabetes.

References

1. Dunn JA, McCance DR, Thorpe SR, et al: Age-dependent accumulation of N^{ϵ}-(carboxymethyl)lysine and N^{ϵ}-(carboxymethyl)hydroxylysine in human skin collagen. *Biochemistry* 1991;30:1205–1210.
2. Ledl F, Schleicher E: New aspects of the Maillard reaction in foods and in the human body. *Angew Chem (Int Ed Engl)* 1990;29:565–594.
3. Njoroge FG, Monnier VM: The chemistry of the Maillard reaction under physiological conditions: A review. *Prog Clin Biol Res* 1989;304:85–107.
4. Baynes JW, Monnier VM (eds): *The Maillard Reaction in Aging, Diabetes and Nutrition.* New York, Alan R Liss, Inc, 1989.
5. Ahmed MU, Thorpe SR, Baynes JW: Identification of carboxymethyllysine as a degradation product of fructose-lysine in glycosylated protein. *J Biol Chem* 1986;261: 4889–4994.
6. Ahmed MU, Dunn JA, Walla MD, et al: Oxidative degradation of glucose adducts to protein. Formation of 3-(N epsilon-lysino)-lactic acid from model compounds and glycosylated proteins. *J Biol Chem* 1988;263:8816–8821.
7. Sell DR, Monnier VM: Structure elucidation of a senescence cross-link from human extracellular matrix. Implication of pentoses in the aging process. *J Biol Chem* 1989; 264:21597–21602.
8. Dunn JA, Ahmed MU, Murtiashaw MH, et al: Reaction of ascorbate with lysine and protein under autoxidizing conditions: Formation of N^{ϵ}-(carboxymethyl)lysine by reaction between lysine and products of autoxidation of ascorbate. *Biochemistry* 1990; 29:10964–10970.
9. Grandhee SK, Monnier VM: Mechanism of formation of the Maillard protein cross-link pentosidine. Glucose, fructose and ascorbate as pentosidine precursors. *J Biol Chem* 1991;266:11649–11653.
10. Sell DR, Monnier VM: End-stage renal disease and diabetes catalyze the formation of a pentose-derived crosslink from aging human collagen. *J Clin Invest* 1990;85:380–384.
11. Dyer DG, Blackledge JA, Thorpe SR, et al: Formation of pentosidine during nonenzymatic browning of proteins by glucose. Identification of glucose and other carbohydrates as possible precursors of pentosidine *in vivo. J Biol Chem* 1991;266: 11654–11660.
12. Fu M-X, Knecht KJ, Thorpe SR, et al: Role of oxygen in the cross-linking and chemical modification of collagen by glucose. Proceedings of IDF Satellite Symposium. *Diabetes,* to be published.
13. Baynes JW: Role of oxidative stress in development of complications in diabetes. *Diabetes* 1991;40:405–412.
14. Monnier VM, Cerami A: Non-enzymatic browning *in vivo.* Possible process for aging of long-lived proteins. *Science* 1981;211:491–493.

15. Cerami A, Vlassara H, Brownlee M: Glucose and aging. *Sci Am* 1987;256:90–96.
16. Monnier VM: Toward a Maillard reaction theory of aging. *Prog Clin Biol Res* 1989; 304:1–22.
17. Harman D: The ageing process. *Proc Natl Acad Sci USA* 1981;78:7124–7128.
18. Wolff SP, Dean RT: Glucose autoxidation and protein modification: The potential role of "autoxidative glycosylation" in diabetes mellitus. *Biochem J* 1987;245:243–250.
19. Kennedy L, Baynes JW: Non-enzymatic glycosylation and the chronic complications of diabetes: An overview. *Diabetologia* 1984;26:93–98.
20. Witztum JL, Steinbrecher UP, Kesaniemi YA, et al: Autoantibodies to glucosylated proteins in the plasma of patients with diabetes mellitus. *Proc Natl Acad Sci USA* 1984;81:3204–3208.
21. Palinski W, Rosenfeld ME, Yla-Herttuala S, et al: Low density lipoprotein undergoes oxidative modification *in vivo. Proc Natl Acad Sci USA* 1989;86:1372–1376.
22. Brownlee M, Pongor S, Cerami A: Covalent attachment of soluble proteins by non-enzymatically glycosylated collagen: Role in the *in situ* formation of immune complexes. *J Exp Med* 1983;158:1739–1744.
23. Stamler J: Epidemiology, established major risk factors, and the primary prevention of coronary heart disease, in Parmley W, Chatterjee K (eds): *Cardiology.* Philadelphia, JB Lippincott, 1987, pp 1–41.
24. Schleicher E, Deufel T, Wieland OH: Non-enzymatic glycosylation of human serum lipoproteins. *FEBS Lett* 1981;129:1–4.
25. Gonen B, Baenziger J, Schonfeld G, et al: Non-enzymatic glycosylation of low-density lipoproteins *in vitro. Diabetes* 1981;30:875–878.
26. Witztum JL, Mahony EM, Branks MJ, et al: Nonenzymatic glucosylation of low-density lipoprotein alters its biologic activity. *Diabetes* 1982;31:283–291.
27. Sasaki J, Cottam GL: Glycosylation of LDL decreases its ability to interact with high-affinity receptors of human fibroblasts *in vitro* and decreases its clearance from rabbit plasma *in vivo. Biochim Biophys Acta* 1982;713:199–207.
28. Steinbrecher UP, Witztum JL: Glucosylation of low density lipoproteins to an exent comparable to that seen in diabetes slows their catabolism. *Diabetes* 1984;33:130–134.
29. Lyons TJ, Patrick JS, Baynes JW, et al: Glycosylation of low density lipoprotein in patients with type 1 diabetes: Correlations with other parameters of glycaemic control. *Diabetologia* 1986;29:685–689.
30. Lopes-Virella MF, Sherer GK, Lees AM, et al: Surface binding, internalization and degradation by cultured human fibroblasts of low density lipoproteins isolated from type I (insulin-dependent) diabetic patients: Changes with metabolic control. *Diabetologia* 1982;22:430–436.
31. Lyons TJ, Klein RL, Baynes JW, et al: Stimulation of cholesteryl ester synthesis in human monocyte-derived macrophages by low-density lipoproteins from type I (insulin-dependent) diabetic patients: The influence of non-enzymatic glycosylation of low-density lipoprotein. *Diabetologia* 1987;30:916–923.
32. Klein RL, Lyons TJ, Lopes-Virella MF: Metabolism of very low- and low density lipoproteins isolated from normolipidaemic type 2 (non-insulin-dependent) diabetic patients by human monocyte-derived macrophages. *Diabetologia* 1990;33:299–305.
33. Lopes-Virella MF, Klein RL, Lyons TJ, et al: Glycosylation of low-density lipoprotein enhances cholesteryl ester synthesis in human monocyte-derived macrophages. *Diabetes* 1988;37:550–557.
34. Jack CM, Sheridan B, Kennedy L, et al: Non-enzymatic glycosylation of low-density lipoprotein. Results of an affinity chromatography method. *Diabetologia* 1988;31:126–128.
35. Lyons TJ: Oxidized low density lipoproteins—a role in the pathogenesis of atherosclerosis in diabetes? *Diabetic Med* 1991;8:411–419.
36. Mullarkey CJ, Edelstein D, Brownlee M: Free radical generation by early glycation

products: A mechanism for accelerated atherogenesis in diabetes. *Biochem Biophys Res Commun* 1990;173:932–939.

37. Watanabe J, Wohltmann HJ, Klein RL, et al: Enhancement of platelet aggregation by low density lipoproteins from IDDM patients. *Diabetes* 1988;37:1652–1657.

38. Klein RL, Lopes-Virella MF, Colwell JA: Enhancement of platelet aggregation by the glycosylated subfraction of low density lipoprotein (LDL) isolated from patients with insulin-dependent diabetes mellitus (IDDM). *Diabetes* 1990;39(suppl 1):173a.

39. Curtiss LK, Witztum JL: Plasma apo-lipoproteins A-I, A-II, B, C-I and E are glucosylated in hyperglycemic diabetic subjects. *Diabetes* 1985;34:452–461.

40. Klein RL, Lyons TJ, Lopes-Virella MF: Interaction of very-low-density lipoprotein isolated from type 1 (insulin-dependent) diabetic subjects with human monocyte-derived macrophages. *Metabolism* 1989;38:1108–1114.

41. Witztum JL, Fisher M, Pietro T, et al: Nonenzymatic glucosylation of high-density lipoprotein accelerates its catabolism in guinea pigs. *Diabetes* 1982;31:1029–1032.

42. Duell PB, Oram JF, Bierman EL: Nonenzymatic glycosylation of HDL and impaired HDL-receptor-mediated cholesterol efflux. *Diabetes* 1991;40:377–384.

43. Curtiss LK, Witztum JL: A novel method of generating region-specific monoclonal antibodies to modified proteins. Application to the identification of human glucosylated low density lipoproteins. *J Clin Invest* 1983;72:1427–1438.

44. Witztum JL, Steinbrecher UP, Fisher M, et al: Nonenzymatic glucosylation of homologous low density lipoprotein and albumin renders them immunogenic in the guinea pig. *Proc Natl Acad Sci USA* 1983;80:2757–2761.

45. Griffith RL, Virella GT, Stevenson HC, et al: LDL metabolism by macrophages activated with LDL immune complexes: A possible mechanism of foam cell formation. *J Exp Med* 1988;168:1041–1059.

46. Gisinger C, Virella GT, Lopes-Virella MF: Erythrocyte-bound low density lipoprotein (LDL) immune comlexes lead to cholesteryl ester accumulation in human monocyte derived macrophages. *Clin Immunol Immunopathol* 1991;59:37–52.

47. Klimov AN, Denisenko AD, Popov AV, et al: Lipoprotein-antibody immune complexes: Their catabolism and role in foam cell formation. *Atherosclerosis* 1985;58:1–15.

48. Cornacoff JB, Hebert LA, Smead WL, et al: Primate erythrocyte-immune complex-clearing mechanism. *J Clin Invest* 1983;71:236–247.

49. Luscinskas FW, Brock AF, Arnaout MA, et al: Endothelial-leukocyte adhesion molecule-1-dependent and leukocyte (CD11/CD18)-dependent mechanisms contribute to polymorphonuclear leukocyte adhesion to cytokine-activated human vascular endothelium. *J Immunol* 1989;142:2257–2263.

50. Bevilacqua MP, Pober JS, Majeau GR, et al: Interleukin-1 induces biosynthesis and cell surface expression of procoagulant activity in human vascular endothelial cells. *J Exp Med* 1984;160:618–622.

51. Martin S, Maruta K, Burkart V, et al: IL-1 and INF-g increase vascular permeability. *Immunology* 1988;64:301–305.

52. Warner SJC, Auger KR, Libby P: Interleukin-1 induces interleukin-1. II. Recombinant human interleukin-1 induces interleukin-1 production by adult human vascular endothelial cells. *J Immunol* 1987;139:1911–1917.

53. Breviario F, Bertocchi F, Dejana E, et al: IL-1 induced adhesion of polymorphonuclear leukocytes to cultured human endothelial cells. Role of platelet-activating factor. *J Immunol* 1988;141:3391–3397.

54. Pohlman TH, Staness KA, Beatty PG, et al: An endothelial cell surface factor(s) induced *in vitro* by lipopolysaccharide, interleukin-1 and tumor necrosis factor α increases neutrophil adherence by a CDw18-dependent mechanism. *J Immunol* 1986; 136:4548–4553.

55. Kilpatrick JM, Hyman B, Virella G: Human endothelial cell damage induced by interactions between polymorphonuclear leukocytes and immune complex-coated erythrocytes. *Clin Immunol Immunopathol*, 1987;44:335–347.

56. Raines EW, Dower SK, Ross R: Interleukin-1 mitogenic activity for fibroblasts and smooth muscle cells is due to PDGF-AA. *Science* 1989;243:393–396.

57. Libby P, Warner SJC, Friedman GB: IL1: A mitogen for human vascular msooth muscle cells that induces the release of growth inhibitory prostanoids. *J Clin Invest* 1988;81: 487–498.

58. Nawroth PP, Bank I, Hadley D, et al: Tumor necrosis factor/cachectin interacts with endothelial cell receptors to induce release of interleukin-1. *J Exp Med* 1986;165: 1363–1375.

59. Brownlee M, Vlassara H, Cerami A: Inhibition of heparin-catalyzed antithrombin III activity by non-enzymatic glycosylation: Possible role in fibrin deposition in diabetes. *Diabetes* 1984;33:532–535.

60. Ceriello A, Guigliano D, Quatraro A, et al: Daily rapid blood glucose variations may condition antithrombin biological activity but not its plasma concentration in insulin dependent diabetes: A possible role for labile non-enzymatic glycation. *Diabete Metab* 1987;13:16–19.

61. McVerry VA, Thorpe S, Gaffney JP, et al: Non-enzymatic glycosylation of fibrinogen. *Haemostasis* 1981;10:261–270.

62. Hamlin CR, Kohn RR: Evidence for progressive, age-related structural changes in post-mature human collagen. *Biochim Biophys Acta* 1971;236:458–467.

63. Hamlin CR, Kohn RR: Determination of human chronological age by study of a collagen sample. *Exp Gerontol* 1972;7:377–379.

64. Hamlin CR, Kohn RR, Luschin JH: Apparent accelerated aging of human collagen in diabetes mellitus. *Diabetes* 1975;24:902–904.

65. Lyons TJ, Kennedy L: Effect of in vitro non-enzymatic glycosylation of human skin collagen on susceptibility to collagenase digestion. *Eur J Clin Invest* 1985;15:128–131.

66. Yue DK, McLennan S, Delbridge L, et al: The thermal stability of collagen in diabetic rats: Correlation with severity of diabetes and non-enzymatic glycosylation. *Diabetologia* 1983;24:282–285.

67. Bailey AJ, Kent MJC. Non-enzymatic glycosylation of fibrous and basement membrane collagens, in Baynes JW, Monnier VM (eds): *The Maillard Reaction in Aging, Diabetes and Nutrition*. New York, Alan R Liss, Inc, 1989, pp 109–122.

68. Rosenberg H, Modrak JB, Hassing JM, et al: Glycosylated collagen. *Biochem Biophys Res Commun* 1979;91:498–501.

69. Cohen MP, Urdanivia E, Surma M, et al: Increased glycosylation of glomerular basement membrane collagen in diabetes. *Biochem Biophys Res Commun* 1980;95:765–769.

70. Schneider SL, Kohn RR: Glycosylation of human collagen in aging and diabetes mellitus. *J Clin Invest* 1980;66:1179–1181.

71. Schnider SL, Kohn RR: Effects of age and diabetes mellitus on the solubility and non-enzymatic glucosylation of human skin collagen. *J Clin Invest* 1981;67:1630–1635.

72. Lyons TJ, Kennedy L: Non-enzymatic glycosylation of skin collagen in patients with limited joint mobility. *Diabetologia* 1985;28:2–5.

73. Vishwanath V, Frank KE, Elmets CA, et al: Glycosylation of skin collagen in type I diabetes mellitus: Correlations with long-term complications. *Diabetes* 1986;35:916–921.

74. Vogt BW, Schleicher ED, Wieland OH: α-amino-lysine-bound glucose in human tissues obtained at autopsy. *Diabetes* 1982;31:1123–1127.

75. Garlick RL, Bunn HF, Spiro RG: Non-enzymatic glycosylation of basement membranes from human glomeruli and bovine sources. *Diabetes* 1988;37:1144–1150.

76. Lyons TJ, Bailie K, Dunn JA, et al: Decrease in skin collagen glycosylation with improved glycemic control in patients with insulin-dependent diabetes mellitus. *J Clin Invest* 1991;87:1910–1915.

77. Monnier VM, Vishwanath V, Frank KE, et al: Relations between complications to type I diabetes mellitus and collagen-linked fluorescence. *N Engl J Med* 1986;314:403–408.

78. Monnier VM, Sell DR, Abdul-Karim FW, et al: Collagen browning and cross-linking are increased in chronic experimental hyperglycemia. Relevance to diabetes and aging. *Diabetes* 1988;37:867–872.

79. Baynes JW, Dyer DG, Dunn JA, et al: Accumulation of Maillard reaction products in skin collagen in diabetes and aging. *Diabetologia* 1991;34(suppl 2):A7.

80. Sell DR, Lapolla A, Monnie VM: Relationship between pentosidine and the complications of long-standing type 1 diabetes. *Diabetes* 1991;40:302A.

81. Makita Z, Radoff S, Rayfield EJ, et al: Advanced glycosylation end products in patients with diabetic nephropathy. *N Engl J Med* 1991;325:836–842.

82. Oxlund H, Rasmussen LM, Andreassen TT, et al: Increased aortic stiffness in patients with type 1 (insulin-dependent) diabetes mellitus. *Diabetologia* 1989;32:748–752.

82. Bucala R, Tracey KJ, Cerami A: Advanced glycosylation products quench nitric oxide and mediate defective endothelium-dependent vasodilatation in experimental diabetes. *J Clin Invest* 1991;87:432–438.

84. Brownlee M, Vlassara H, Cerami A: Nonenzymactic glycosylation products on collagen covalently trap low-density lipoprotein. *Diabetes* 1985;34:938–941.

85. Hicks M, Delbridge L, Yue DK, et al: Increase in crosslinking of nonenzymatically glycosylated collagen induced by products of lipid peroxidation. *Arch Biochem Biophys* 1989;268:249–254.

86. Vlassara H, Brownlee M, Cerami A: Novel macrophage receptor for glucose-modified proteins is distinct from previously described scavenger receptors. *J Exp Med* 1986; 164:1301–1309.

87. Vlassara H, Valinsky J, Brownlee M, et al: Advanced glycosylation end products on erythrocyte cell surface induce receptor-mediated phagocytosis by macrophages. A model for turnover of aging cells. *J Exp Med* 1987;166:539–549.

88. Kirstein M, Brett J, Radoff S, et al: Advanced protein glycosylation induces transendothelial human monocyte chemotaxis and secretion of platelet-derived growth factor: Role in vascular disease of diabetes and aging. *Proc Natl Acad Sci USA* 1990;87: 9010–9014.

89. Vlassara H, Brownlee M, Manogue KR, et al: Cachectin/TNF and IL-1 induced by glucose-modified proteins: Role in normal tissue remodeling. *Science* 1988;240:1546–1548.

90. Brownlee M, Vlassara H, Kooney A, et al: Aminoguanidine prevents diabetes-induced arterial wall protein cross-linking. *Science* 1986;232:1629–1632.

91. Requena JR: The main mechanism of action of aminoguanidine. *Diabetologia* 1991; 34(suppl 2):A162.

92. Parthasarathy S, Young SG, Witztum JL, et al: Probucol inhibits oxidative modification of low density lipoprotein. *J Clin Invest* 1986;77:641–644.

93. Frei B, England L, Ames BN: Ascorbate is an outstanding antioxidant in human plasma. *Proc Natl Acad Sci USA* 1989;86:6377–6381.

94. Jennings PE, Chirico S, Jones AF, et al: Vitamin C metabolites and microangiopathy in diabetes mellitus. *Diabetes Res* 1987;6:151–154.

95. Karpen CW, Cataland S, O'Dorisio TM, et al: Production of 12 HETE and vitamin E status in platelets from type 1 human diabetic subjects. *Diabetes* 1985;34:526–531.

Chapter 11

Endothelial Cell Abnormalities in Diabetes

George L. King, MD, Nirmal K. Banskota, MD,
Teruo Shiba, MD, PhD, F. Javier Oliver, PhD,
Toyoshi Inoguchi, MD, PhD, and Ching Fai Kwok, MD

Endothelium is one of the largest organs of the body, composed of a single type of cell, the endothelial cell. Recent studies have documented that endothelial cells can perform an incredible array of actions that are regulated in order to ensure that the vasculature can carry out its main function of providing adequate nutrients to various parts of the body. To accomplish this important goal, the endothelium must regulate coagulation, monitor flow and contractility, establish levels of permeability, and regenerate when injured. These functions of endothelial cells can be influenced by other vascular cells, tissue metabolism, and hematologic elements. A discussion of the regulation of endothelial cell function by these various factors is beyond the scope of this review. Therefore, this discussion focuses on the abnormalities in endothelial cells that have been described in diabetes in vivo or induced by the diabetic melieu in vitro.

Endothelial Abnormalities In Vivo

A wide range of vascular abnormalities have been described in diabetic patients and animals involving all blood vessels at both the micro- and macrovascular levels. Clinically, these pathologic changes affect the functions of retina, renal glomeruli, and certain areas of large vessels such as lower extremities, heart, and neural circulation.[1-5] Pathologic changes in these micro- and macrovessels are numerous, with both common characteristics and those specific for individual vascular tissues.

Abnormalities of Basement Membrane

One common hallmark of diabetic angiopathy is basement membrane thickening, which is a generalized phenomenon that occurs in the basement membranes of vascular tissues.[1-3] However, thickening also occurs in nonvascular tissues such as mammary ducts,[6] testes,[7] sweat glands[8] as well as sarcoplasmic

191

and perineural basement membrane[9] and alveolar epithelium.[10] Most of these sites have been defined by light microscopy, but ultrastructural studies also confirm the increase in some tissues. Because of the relative clinical insignificance of basement membrane thickening in nonvascular tissues, they have been studied less extensively. Retinal and renal basement membrane lesions have been studied most often because of their clinical importance. The basement membrane separates the cell from the interstitial space except in the glomerulus of kidney, where the basement membrane is between the endothelial cells of the capillary and the epithelial cells of Bowman's capsule, and in the central nervous system, where it is between the endothelial cells and the glial cells or the pericytes. The glomerular basement membrane is continuous with the tubular basement membrane via Bowman's capsule. Ultrastructurally defined, the capillary basement membrane is composed of fine filaments embedded in a homogeneous matrix, with two clear zones (inner and outer) separated from a dense middle zone (the laminae interna and externa and lamina pensa, respectively). In the capillaries, the endothelial cell lining is enriched with a variable number of pericytes. The thickening of the basement membrane is usually found between the endothelial cells and the pericytes. This thickening often correlates with the intracapillary pressures.

The chemical components of basement membrane are now well recognized and include collagens (mainly type IV), proteoglycans, chondroitin and heparin sulfates, and various glycoproteins such as laminin.[10,11] In normal tissues, basement membranes form boundaries between endothelial cells and other cell types. They function to provide structural support, maintain architecture, modify cellular functions such as cellular proliferation, and provide a filtration barrier. Alterations in basement membrane morphology can thus easily be envisaged to have functional consequences, and vice versa.

The retinal capillary basement membrane thickens with aging.[12] In the diabetic patient as well as in animal models of the disease, basement membrane thickening is a consistent feature.[13-15] In the retina of diabetic rats, capillary thickening is more prominent in the inner capillary bed (nerve and ganglion layer) compared to the inner and outer plexiform layers.[14,15] Experimentally, basement membrane thickening of retinal capillaries similar to that seen in diabetic rats is seen in galactose-fed rats.[16]

The glomerular capillary basement membrane thickening in diabetes mellitus has long been recognized as a prominent morphologic feature of diabetic nephropathy following the initial description of diabetic renal glomerular capillary by Kimmelstiel and Wilson.[17] The basement membrane thickening in diabetes has classically been described as a slow process occurring over a long time. It is now recognized that an acute glomerular hypertrophy occurs early in the course of diabetes mellitus, but it is uncertain whether this phenomenon is a sequela or a precursor of the classic renal lesions of diabetes mellitus as described by Osterby in newly diagnosed diabetic patients.[18] Similar structural changes have been described in streptozotocin-diabetic rats.[19] The expansion of the mesangium is the other major lesion that is observed in diabetic glomerulopathy, and this expansion is thought to be the main factor leading to decreased renal function. Progressive thickening of the basement membrane occurs over the duration of diabetes.[20,21] The clinical significance of progressive increase in the mesangial matrix is that capillary surface area (filtration area) is lost.[22] Increases in mesangial volume fraction (mesangial volume/glomerular volume) has strong clinical correlation with declining glomerular filtration rate (GFR) and albuminuria. Such a functional correlation is not shown with increases in glomerular basement membrane thickness.[22] Along with changes in the composition of the basement membrane, this leads to altered permeability and eventually to glomerular occlusion and decreased filtering capacity.

Functional changes also occur in early diabetes.[23-32] Glomerular filtration rate and filtration fraction (GFR/renal plasma flow) increase early in diabetes and can be corrected by intensive insulin treatment and, in experimental animals, with insulin treatment or islet transplantation.[30-32] Permeability of the capillaries is altered such that excretion of proteins with molecular weights of 44,000 to 150,000 are increased.[26] This initial alteration in permeability does not seem to be due to simply increased glomerular porosity.[27] Alteration of charge selection and permeability barrier also may be involved (such as reduction in sialic acid and heparin sulfates content in diabetic glomeruli), allowing the increased leakage of plasma proteins seen in glomerular basement membrane of established diabetic nephropathy.

Vascular Cell Changes

Besides generalized changes in the basement membrane, specific and clear changes in the vascular cells are also documented. Figure 11.1 depicts in schematic fashion the sequence of histologic changes that are observed in the retinal

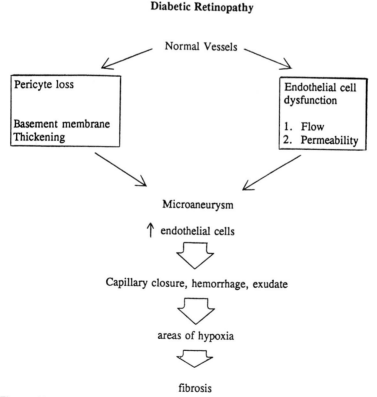

Figure 11.1 Schematic drawing of the progression of diabetic retinopathy.

microvessels of diabetic patients and probably dogs as well.[4,29,30] In background diabetic retinopathy, the earliest histologic change is the loss of the retinal pericytes.[29,30] Normally the retinal capillaries have a comparable number of endothelial cells and pericytes (ratio of 1:1), which is very different from peripheral capillaries, which have many more endothelial cells than pericytes. In diabetic patients, Kuwabara and Cogan showed that the pericyte–endothelial cell ratio in a trypsin digest preparation of retinal microvessels increased to 1:4 after several years of diabetes.[29] The ratio will expand to 1:10 with longer duration of the disease. In parallel with the loss of the pericytes, several other histologic changes appear to follow, including increased capillary diameter, basement membrane thickening, changes in retinal flow, and formation of microaneurysms.[4,29,30] It has been postulated that many of these changes are consequences of the loss of pericytes. In vitro pericytes cause inhibition of endothelial proliferation and migration mediated by transforming growth factor β (TGF-β).[31,32] As in retinopathy, the main site of abnormality in the kidney is located in the microvessels of the glomeruli, involving basement membrane thickening and, more significantly, the expansion of the mesangial matrix and altered intrarenal hemodynamics.[20,21] Significant differences between the two tissues exist (Figure 11.2). In glomeruli endothelial cells are lost, not increased in number as in the retina. The mesangial cell, a contractile cell like pericytes, will expand in size and probably number, unlike the pericytes, which are lost.[33–35] In diabetic macroangiopathy, the cellular changes are characterized by injury to the endothelial cells and excessive proliferation of the smooth muscle cells, which do not occur in retinopathy and nephropathy.

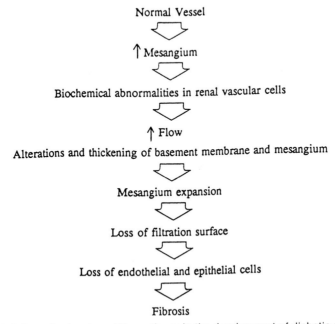

Figure 11.2 Schematic drawing of the pathway in the development of diabetic nephropathy.

Coagulation Abnormalities

The abnormalities found in the endothelial cells from diabetic patients or animals can be separated generally into four functional categories: coagulation, flow and contractility, permeability, and regeneration. In the area of coagulation, multiple alterations have been reported. This review focuses on the metabolic products and changes in the endothelial cells from diabetic tissues and does not discuss the abnormalities that have been reported in platelets, other hematopoietic cells, and the plasma of diabetic patients or animals.

In the endothelium, abnormalities have been found in the levels of factor VIII, prostaglandin, and fibrinolysis activities and others.[36,37] The levels of tissue plasminogen activator (t-PA) and tissue plasminogen activator inhibitor 1 (PAI-1) have been evaluated in several studies. Some of the studies have found that t-PA activity is decreased or there is an absence of response by type II diabetes only when stimulated by desmopressin, although this correlated with obesity rather than diabetes per se.[38] However, other studies have reported no change or an increase in t-PA levels. A decrease in t-PA would support the finding of diminished fibrinolysis activity in diabetic patients, because plasminogen activity, secreted by the endothelial cells, converts plasminogen to plasmin, which is involved in fibrinolysis. The activities of t-PA can be inhibited by PAI-1.[39] Thus, it is possible that the decrease in t-PA activities reported previously could be due to PAI-1, which has been reported to be increased in diabetic patients.[40]

Another parameter for assessing the coagulation state is von Willebrand factor (vWF), which complexes with factor VIII to form factor VIII–related antigen (F.VIIIR:Ag), which is produced by endothelial cells and is involved in platelet adhesion to the subendothelium and in thrombus formation.[41] In general, most studies have reported that the vWF level is increased in both insulin-dependent and insulin-independent diabetic patients.[42,43] Similarly, vWF level is also increased in animals with chemically induced diabetes. Glycemic control normalizes vWF levels in patients whether it is achieved by diet, sulfonylurea, or insulin treatment,[42,43] although some studies have not found this to be so.[44] The duration of the diabetic state seems to correlate with the level of vWF,[45] although other studies show that it may be elevated in young patients with diabetes without vascular disease[46] and early in the diabetic state of streptozotocin-diabetic rats.[47] This may simply reflect early endothelial cell injury or dysfunction secondary to the hyperglycemia.

Diabetes and hyperglycemia have been reported to affect the metabolism of prostaglandins (PGs), which are also potent metabolites of endothelial cells that affect platelet aggregation and vascular thrombosis. Specifically, PGI_2 production in endothelial cells has been evaluated extensively because PGI_2 is an inhibitor of platelet aggregation and adhesion to the endothelium and a strong vasodilator as well.[48,49] These properties have suggested that reduction of PGI_2 level may increase thrombosis and contractility, which has been reported in diabetic patients and animals. PGI_2 production has been reported to be reduced in the serum of diabetic animals and patients, and this decrease may be due to changes in its production because the exposure of human umbilical endothelial cells to sera from diabetic patients inhibits PGI_2 production. However, elevated glucose level alone did not have any inhibitory activities. In vivo treatment of diabetic rats with insulin was able to reverse the sera's inhibitory effect. Interestingly, vitamin E treatment also reversed the inhibitory effect of diabetic sera, suggesting a possible role for antioxidant in the treatment of vascular complications.

Alteration in Vascular Permeability

Increase in vascular permeability is another hallmark of vascular abnormality in diabetic patients and animals. The most clinically obvious sites of vascular permeability are in the retina and renal glomeruli. In the latter, the abnormality in the early stages is probably located in the basement matrix, as described earlier. Thus, the diabetic melieu is affecting the ability of either glomerular endothelial or epithelial cells to regulate the synthesis or degradation of the basement membrane. In the retina, fluorescein leakage can easily be detected in areas of clinical pathology, such as microaneurysms and exudate. Because fluorescein has a very small molecular weight (less than 300), some reports have found fluorescein leakage in vessels before any clinical pathology has been observed.[50–52] In diabetic animals, increased permeability to labeled albumin has been reported after 4 to 6 weeks of chemically induced diabetes.[51] Because the vascular barrier in the retinal capillary is formed predominantly by tight junctions between the capillary endothelial cells, the increase in permeability is probably due to abnormality in the endothelial cells. However, this increase in permeability has been described in many vascular tissues and in nonvascular tissues such as skin as well. Because peripheral microvessels contain mostly endothelial cells with very few vascular supporting cells such as pericytes, the effect of diabetes is again likely dysfunction in the endothelial cells.

Abnormalities in Contractility and Flow

The third general area of endothelial cell function that has been found to be abnormal in diabetes is that of contractility and flow. Increased blood flow in the renal glomeruli has been documented in diabetic patients and animals.[53–56] This increase in renal blood flow appears to precede any pathologic changes, and the mechanisms responsible for it are not clear at this time. However, one interesting report has suggested that a vasoactive substance may be involved. Atrial natriuretic peptide (ANP) has been shown to increase renal blood flow and filtration rate.[53] In addition, the infusion of antibodies to ANP normalized renal blood flow, which further supported a role for ANP increasing renal blood flow in the diabetic state.[53] Other growth factors, such as growth hormone and insulin-like growth factor 1 (IGF-1) have also been implicated, because they can cause renal enlargement and increases in GFR when infused.[57] However, transgenic mice with increased expression of either IGF-1 or growth hormone did not develop nephropathy exactly like that found in diabetes, although they did have glomerular sclerosis[57] (Table 11.1).

Not all vascular beds experience increased flow at the initiation of the disease. In the retina, the retinal blood flow in the first 2 to 5 years of disease appears to be decreased. When background retinopathy is present, the retinal blood flow will be increased. However, in advanced stages of proliferative retinopathy, retinal blood flow appears to decrease again, which could lead to hypoxia and induce proliferation.[58–63] Thus, the effect of diabetes on vascular flow may vary according to vascular tissues and duration of disease. In animal

Table 11.1 Some Vasoactive Hormones Evaluated in Diabetic Patients

Hormone	Effect on Renal Blood Flow
Renin + angiotensin	$\downarrow \rightarrow$
Vasopressin	$\uparrow$ (when stimulated)
Histamine	$\uparrow$
Endothelin	$\uparrow$
Atrial naturietic peptide	$\uparrow \rightarrow$
Aldosterone	$\uparrow \rightarrow$
Catecholamines	$\uparrow$ (poorly controlled) $\rightarrow$

studies involving large vessels, multiple and conflicting results regarding vascular contractility have been reported. In general, there appears to be a delay in the relaxation phase, which is usually mediated by the release of endothelium-dependent releasing factor (EDRF).[53–57] In the aorta of chemically induced diabetic rats or rabbits, the EDRF response to acetylcholine and Ca^{2+} ionosphore is decreased. This attenuated response is observed mainly in the presence of endothelium and is not observed with nitroprusside or adenosine, which would suggest the secretion of EDRF could be reduced or that of vasoconstrictor increased. Evidence is available to support both of these possibilities. Either the effect of EDRF could be reduced by decreases in production or the EDRF produced could be quenched by glycosylated proteins. The latter has been reported to occur in in vitro studies in which glycosylated proteins have been shown to reduce the effectiveness of nitric oxide, a major component of EDRF.

The attenuated vasodilatory response when exposed to acetylcholine is also observed in the microvascular circulation. These observations have been reported in the small mesenteric arteries of diabetic rats studied in situ.[64] Another classic example is the microvessel of isolated penile corpora cavernosa, which will dilate when activated by acetylcholine.[65] In tissue from diabetic patients with impotence, the EDRF response to acetylcholine was reported to be decreased, although the response to sodium nitroprusside and papaverine was not diminished. These data again support an abnormality in the endothelium.

Abnormalities in vascular contractility could also be present as a result of changes in the levels or actions of vasoactive hormones. Increased sensitivity in diabetics to renin and angiotensin has been postulated, although very little evidence is available to support this postulate. Recently, interesting results have shown a possible relationship between diabetes and endothelin (ET-1), a potent vasoconstrictor that can cause prolonged hypertension in vivo.[66–68] In diabetic patients on insulin therapy, the plasma level of ET-1 was higher than that in nondiabetic patients.[69] One possible reason for the elevation of ET-1 is the effect of glucose, which has been reported to increase ET-1 production in cultured aortic endothelial cells.[70] Another reason could be the effect of insulin on endothelial cells, which we have reported to enhance the transcription rate of ET-1 mRNA[71] (this is described later in the discussion of growth factors). These alterations in this vasoactive hormone could be the reason for the abnormality in contractility and the high incidence of hypertension in the diabetic and insulin-resistant populations.[72]

Abnormalities in Regeneration

Both cellular proliferation and loss are also prominent features of diabetic vascular disease. Endothelial cells in micro- and macrovessels react differently to diabetic conditions. In macrovessels, endothelial cells are believed to be injured, which could lead to many of the vascular dysfunctions noted above. In the microvessels, the evidence seems to suggest that there is an increase of endothelial cell proliferation, as demonstrated by the propensity to form microaneurysms and neovascularization.

The appearance of capillary microaneurysms has also been attributed to the loss of pericytes. It has been reported that the growth of retinal endothelial cells can be inhibited by co-culturing with pericytes.[31,32] The inhibitory effect of pericytes can only be observed if the two types of cells are in physical contact. Further studies have suggested that, although these cells are in contact, endothelial cells are able to release active forms of TGF-β, which has been shown to inhibit the growth of endothelial cells.[31,32] Therefore, in the retina of diabetic patients, the loss of pericytes as a result of hyperglycemia will prevent the expression of active TGF-β by the endothelial cells, which are then prone to proliferate, resulting in the formation of microaneurysms, which histologically are a group or cluster of endothelial cells lacking in pericytes.

Hyperglycemia can also directly enhance retinal endothelial cell proliferation as well as playing an indirect role by contributing to the loss of pericytes. Recently, we have shown that the exposure of cultured retinal microvascular endothelial cells to elevated levels of glucose (400 mg/dL or 20 mmol/L versus 100 mg/dL or 5.6 mmol/L) will increase protein kinase C (PKC) activities in the cellular membrane, which represents the active pool of PKC.[73,74] Metabolic labeling studies have shown that the activation of the PKC activities is probably due to an increased level of diacylglycerol, a physiologic activator of PKC, along with Ca^{2+} and phospholipids.[74,75] (The mechanism of PKC and diacylglycerol changes in diabetes is discussed further later in this chapter.) Recently, we and others have shown that PKC activities are also elevated in the retina, aorta, heart, and renal glomeruli of diabetic rats. Preliminary studies have shown that not only are PKC activities increased, but these changes can be documented as an increase of PKC protein in the membrane by using Western blot analysis and antibodies to various specific isoenzymes of PKC. The finding of PKC activities in the retina and the vasculature in general could potentially be very important for the enhancement of cellular proliferation because the activation of PKC has been implicated in the mechanism of many growth factors, such as platelet-derived growth factor (PDGF),[76] epidermal growth factor (EGF),[77] and the IGFs.[78] In addition, a regulatory role for PKC has been suggested for basement membrane synthesis, vascular contractility, and permeability as well.[76] Many of these changes will biochemically enhance the likelihood that the retinal vasculature will proliferate when the balance between growth inhibitors and promoters is shifted to the latter.

Not much is known about growth inhibitors, but it has been shown that vitreous from normal eyes will inhibit angiogenesis in various in vivo assays.[79] Taylor and Weiss have partially purified an inhibitor of angiogenesis from the vitreous that is a glycoprotein of 5,700 daltons.[80] Others have reported that the lyophilized vitreous and its guanidinium chloride extract will also contain inhibitory activities.[81] Table 11.2 lists some of the reported growth inhibitors that

Table 11.2 Growth Modulations of Endothelial Cells

Identified in the Retina	Measured in the Eyes of Diabetic Animals	
Fibroblast growth factors (FGF)	aFGF + bFGF	↑ ↔
Epidermal growth factor (EGF)	EGF	↔
Transforming growth factor β (TGF-β)	TGF-β	↑
Platelet-derived growth factor (PDGF)		?
Insulin	Insulin	↔
Insulin-like growth factor 1 (IGF-1)	IGF-1	↑ ↔
Insulin-like growth factor 2 (IGF-2)	IGF-2	↑ ↔
Growth hormone (GH)	GH	↑
Endothelial cell–stimulating angiogenesis factor (ECAF)		?
Tumor necrosis factor α (TNF-α)	TNF-α	↔
Vascular endothelial cell growth factor (VEGF)		?

are expressed in the retina or vitreous and have been shown to inhibit either angiogenesis or endothelial cell proliferation in vitro. Interestingly, both TGF-β and tumor necrosis factor α (TNF-α) have the paradoxical effects of inhibiting endothelial cell proliferation in vitro yet apparently being angiogenic in vivo.[82]

With the combination of local growth factors, probably activated by hypoxia and the availability of plasma growth factor as a result of leaky vasculatures, new retinal capillaries will begin to develop. The resultant new capillaries are very fragile and tend to hemorrhage. Fibrin will form with the resolution of the hemorrhage.

The exact identity of the growth factor or factors that are responsible for the development of neovascularization and fibrosis in the diabetic retina has not been determined. However, numerous types of growth factors have been identified in the retina. They are listed in Table 11.2. In general, they can be classified as local and systemic growth factors, with the latter acting as enhancing factors rather than being initiators of proliferative changes. Because only specific vascular beds such as the retina are involved in diabetes, local growth factors probably play a major role in the initiation of proliferative changes.

The fibroblast-derived growth factor (FGF) family of polypeptides has been shown to be responsible for a large part of the mitogenic activities from the retina and vitreous fluid aspirated from eyes suffering from proliferative disease. Two types of FGF have been found in the retina cells—acidic FGF (aFGF) and basic FGF (bFGF); both are 17-kD proteins that bind to heparin.[83] They are not secreted from the cells because they lack a leader sequence, but could be released by the disruption of cells. Once released, they are found bound to basement matrix and are presumed to be activated by basement membrane turnover or degradation.[84] The FGFs are angiogenic but can stimulate the growth of many types of cells besides endothelial cells.[85] Their role in proliferative diabetic retinopathy is not clear. Several studies involving a small number of patients and controls have provided conflicting results. The most recent studies by Sivalingam et al using an immunoassay for bFGF reported that patients with proliferative diabetic retinopathy are prone to have a higher level of bFGF than those patients without diabetes or proliferative disease. However, no means or actual levels of bFGF were provided.[86] Thus, it clearly has not been established whether the elevation of FGFs plays a role in diabetic proliferative retinopathy.

TGF-β has also been found in the retina and could also be synthesized by retinal pigmented epithelial cells.[87] As described earlier, it has an inhibitory effect on endothelial cell proliferation but can be angiogenic in vivo, probably via its chemotatic properties in recruiting monocytes. Connor et al have recently reported that total TGF-β levels in the vitreous, as measured by radioreceptor assay, were three times greater in patients with proliferative vitreoretinopathy (PVR) than in those who have retinal detachment without PVR.[88] Because PVR occurs in a significant percentage of patients with late stages of diabetic proliferative disease, TGF-β may play a role both in early stages in the formation of microaneurysms, and late stages in the formation of fibrosis.

Another growth factor that has been specifically studied with respect to retinal proliferative disease is the endothelial cell–stimulating angiogenesis factor (ESAF), which was reported by Taylor et al to be a low-molecular-weight (400) compound,[89] isolated from the retina and vitreous that is angiogenic and can activate procollagenase activities.[90] It is different from other growth factors because it is not a protein and may be specific for microvascular endothelial cells. Bioassays have suggested that ESAF levels may be increased in retina and vitreous from kittens with oxygen-induced retrolental fibroplasia, which includes neovascularization in its pathologies. In a preliminary report, purified ESAF activities from vitreous aspirates of patients with neovascularization appeared to be elevated when compared to those from normal eyes taken from autopsy specimens. These findings are intriguing, especially because ESAF has an additive effect with FGF in biologic activities.

The last group of growth factors to be discussed includes growth hormone and IGF-1 and -2. Growth hormone was postulated to play a significant role in diabetic proliferative retinopathy when it was discovered that diabetic patients who are also made growth hormone deficient by surgery or radiation will have amelioration of their proliferative retinopathy.[91,92] However, levels of serum growth hormone were not predictive of the development or the severity of diabetic retinopathy. Because growth hormone mediates most of its growth effects by increasing the levels of IGF-1, Merrimee measured IGF-1 levels in the serum and vitreous.[91] His group reported that IGF-1 levels were increased in only a small group of patients who suffered from very aggressive diabetic proliferative retinopathy. In vitro studies from our laboratory and others have demonstrated that retinal endothelial cells have receptors for IGF-1 and are responsive to it for growth.[93] Grant et al indicated that IGF-1 demonstrates chemotactic and angiogenic activities as well.[94] Unfortunately, other reports with larger patient numbers demonstrated no correlation between plasma IGF-1 and the presence of proliferative retinopathy in general.[95]

Endothelial Abnormalities In Vitro

Studies of insulin and IGF-1 receptors and actions on vascular cells in culture have stimulated a great deal of interest because of the possible involvement of these receptors in the development of hypertension, atherosclerosis, and other vascular complications that are prevalent in the diabetic population. Numerous publications have suggested that hyperinsulinemia or insulin resistance may be a risk factor for the development of hypertension and the acceleration of atherosclerosis, which clearly occur in diabetic patients.[96]

Endothelial Cell Insulin Receptor Function

Insulin and IGF-1 receptors have been described on all vascular cells studied. These included cells from different vascular sites such as retina, aorta, fat, renal glomeruli, and umbilical vein.[97-100] In addition, insulin receptors have also been detected on vascular cells from different species, including humans, pigs, cows, rats, and rabbits. In general, insulin receptors on the vascular cells are structurally very similar to those expressed on the "classic" insulin-sensitive tissues such as fat and liver.[100] A summary of insulin and IGF receptors is presented in Table 11.3.

These receptors have high affinity for insulin and are very specific, although IGF-1 and IGF-2 can also bind to the insulin receptors at affinities 50 to 100 times less than insulin (Table 11.3). On addition of insulin, autophosphorylation of the receptors occur immediately at both the tyrosine and the serine. So far all the findings in endothelial cells are comparable to the findings in other types of cells. However, there are many major differences between endothelial cells and peripheral tissues with regard to location, processing, and actions.

Endothelial cells, unlike other cells, are polarized, with an apical surface that faces the intraluminal side of the blood vessel. The basolateral surface is attached to the basement membrane. We have shown that most if not all of the insulin receptors are located on the apical surface.[101] This finding is very important for functions of insulin receptors on endothelial cells.

The processing and internalization of insulin receptors in endothelial cells have been demonstrated to be unusual and possibly physiologically important.[102] We have shown that the insulin receptors on the apical surface of the cell will bind and internalize insulin for transport across the cells without significant degradation. This process is called receptor-mediated transcytosis of insulin, and probably also applies to IGF-1[103] but not to IGF-2.

Direct measurement of the transport of ^{125}I-labeled insulin by aortic endothelial cells in vitro using a two-compartment system confirms that insulin

Table 11.3 Characterization of Receptors and Actions of Insulin and IGF-1 and -2 in Endothelial Cells

Receptor	Size in Endothelial Cells (kD)		Biologic Activities
	Microvascular	Macrovascular	
Insulin			Metabolic (glycogen incorporation, amino acid transport, glucose transport): 10^{-9} M
α subunit	135–140	135–140	
β subunit	95	95	
	(tyrosine kinase)		
IGF-1			Growth (thymidine incorporation, protein synthesis cell replication): 10^{-8} M
α subunit	140	140	
β subunit	95	95	
	(tyrosine kinase)		
IGF-2	220	220 (nonreduced)	
	260	260 (reduced)	

can be rapidly and unidirectionally transported by receptor-mediated transcytosis. The transport observed was inhibited by an excess of unlabeled insulin[103] and by specific antibodies to the insulin receptor, but not by an excess of unrelated polypeptide, such as nerve growth factor.

Collectively, these studies show that insulin receptors on endothelial cells may also function as transporters of insulin across the vascular barrier. In the continuously lined capillaries of muscle and adipose tissue, where endothelial cells are the principal obstacle to the free diffusion of insulin from blood to tissue, receptor-mediated transcytosis most likely provides an efficient and highly regulated system of insulin delivery. An example of a physiologic role for receptor-mediated transcytosis is the special case of insulin transport across the blood–brain barrier. This scheme has been convincingly demonstrated in vivo.[102] Both brain and retinal microvessel endothelial cells have insulin receptors with the same structural and functional properties as those found in nonneuronal tissues. Peripheral intravenous infusion of insulin into human subjects raised plasma insulin levels from 12 ± 1.2 to 268 ± 35 mU/mL, and concomitantly raised cerebrospinal fluid insulin levels from 0.9 ± 0.1 to 2.8 ± 0.4 μU/mL.[102] The authors interpreted these data as suggesting a potential mechanism by which peripheral insulin could provide a feedback signal to the central nervous system to regulate food intake.

In addition to the ability to transport insulin in a receptor-mediated pathway, insulin receptors on endothelial cells can also mediate "classic" effects of insulin. Interestingly, there is a differential responsiveness to insulin between endothelial cells of macro- and microvessels, although no difference in binding affinity or receptor number has been found.[104] Capillary endothelial cells isolated from normal rats are responsive to both the metabolic and growth effects of insulin.[100] In contrast, the same cells isolated from capillaries of diabetic rats have been reported to have a decreased number of insulin receptors and actions as measured by receptor autophosphorylation and glucose incorporation into glycogen. The mRNA and the protein structure of the insulin receptors from the endothelial cells of diabetic and control rats did not demonstrate any differences as determined by Northern blot and trypsin digest analysis, respectively. It is possible that the decreased number of insulin receptors in cells from diabetic rats may be due to alterations in receptor processing or degradation. It is postulated that such alteration in the processing could be due to PKC activation because it has been shown that increased serine phosphorylation of the insulin receptor can enhance its internalization rate in the endothelial cell.[78]

Although macrovascular endothelial cells are rather insensitive to insulin with respect to its classic actions, we have recently found that they are sensitive to insulin's effect on expression of the mRNA of ET-1, which is a potent vasoconstrictor synthesized in large quantities by endothelial cells. The transcription rate of ET-1 can be enhanced by three- to fourfold by insulin at physiologic concentrations within 30 minutes.[70]

Effects of Hyperglycemia

One of the major causes of vascular dysfunction is hyperglycemia, but the exact mechanism of its detrimental effect is not clear. It is very possible that hyperglycemia is mediating its adverse effects via multiple mechanisms because glucose and its metabolites are utilized by numerous pathways. Over the last several

Table 11.4 Possible Mechanisms of the Adverse Effect of Hyperglycemia on Vascular Complications

Aldose reductase, polyol pathway
Nonenzymatic glycation hypothesis
Alteration of redox potential
Diacylglycerol-PKC pathway

years several hypotheses have been proposed to explain hyperglycemia's adverse effects. They are listed in Table 11.4.

Sorbitol Polyol Hypothesis

The sorbitol polyol hypothesis has been the most studied, a postulate based on the finding that glucose can be converted to sorbitol in most cells by aldose reductase.[105–107] Subsequent metabolism of sorbitol is relatively slow, which will result in the accumulation of sorbitol. Initially, it was thought that the increase in osmolarity from the accumulation of sorbitol could lead to cellular dysfunction. This could be the explanation for the increase in cataract formation, which can be prevented by inhibitors to aldose reductase.[108] However, the amount of sorbitol accumulation differs greatly from tissue to tissue. Therefore, small increases in osmolarities from the sorbitol may not be significant in vascular cells. In neurologic tissue of diabetic animals, the accumulation of sorbitol could lead to a reduction of cellular myoinositol levels and Na^+/K^+ adenosine triphosphatase (ATPase) activities, both of which could lead to cellular dysfunction. In vascular endothelial cells, the reports so far have shown that the sorbitol increase is small, and no decreases in total myoinositol levels have been reported.[105] However, Na^+/K^+-ATPase activities may be decreased.[105]

Thus, the results are not clear as to the role of sorbitol and aldose reductase activity in diabetic vascular disease. Initial trials of aldose reductase inhibitor (ARI) have shown some promising results in neurologic dysfunction and possibly normalization of renal GFRs. However, clinical studies of ARI have not demonstrated remarkable efficacy in neuropathy or retinopathy.[109,110] Some of the possible problems in the lack of effect of ARI could be due to the inability of the specific ARI compound tested to react on the intended tissues, or the need to initiate the treatment at the very onset of the disease. It is also possible that no one single type of inhibitor will abolish all vascular complications, which are clearly multifactorial disease or diseases.

Nonenzymatic Glycosylation Hypothesis

The nonenzymatic glycosylation of proteins and possibly DNA has been postulated to be another mechanism that can cause vascular dysfunctions. This hypothesis is based on the observation that glucose can attach to the amino groups of proteins and possibly DNA using a nonenzymatic process that forms a Schiff base compound. This Schiff base adduct will convert to form stable glycosylation products such as glycosylated albumin or hemoglobins. After several days and weeks of increased formation of glycosylated products, such as found in diabetes, these products will proceed to oxidize, which can generate free radicals that could cause more protein cross-linking and degradation. This process is accelerated when there is an increased amount of glucose present either intracellular or extracellularly. The effect of nonenzymatic glycosylation obviously will be more important in extracellular proteins, which have prolonged half-lives, than in intracellular proteins, which tend to have a more rapid turnover time.

Some of the glycosylated products that have been shown to accumulate intravascularly are albumin, hemoglobin, low-density lipoproteins, and other basement membrane components.[111-113] In addition, in in vitro conditions it has been shown that DNA and other compounds with long half-lives can also form these glycated products, which have been termed the advanced glycation end products (AGE). A detailed summary of this theory is not presented here because it has recently been reviewed elsewhere.[111-113] In vitro glycosylated low-density lipoproteins have been shown to bind less well as compared to their nonglycosylated counterparts. In addition, basement membrane components such as collagen have also been shown to be glycosylated.[114] These glycosylated basement membrane components are more resistant to digestion by proteases. Therefore, their turnover will be decreased. This could explain the accumulation of basement membrane components in microvascular tissues found in diabetic patients. In addition, these AGE proteins can bind to possible specific receptors on monocytes, which can then stimulate the release of cytokines, such as TNF or interleukin 1, which in turn could cause a series of metabolic actions on vascular endothelium, such as increased permeability, neovascularization, and other inflammatory types of action.[115]

If the primary amine groups of the nucleotides can be nonenzymatically glycosylated, then a long and persistent action of hyperglycemia can be translated into genetic changes that will be difficult to reverse, as found in the diabetic population who have been treated with insulin in a well-monitored, normoglycemic manner. Recent studies in animals using inhibitors to nonenzymatic glycosylation have shown some promising results. These inhibitors were shown to decrease in the thickness of renal glomeruli and in addition possibly prevent the onset of some early retinal microvascular changes in diabetic rats.[114,116] However, these data are very preliminary. More studies are needed to ascertain the pathophysiologic role of the AGE products.

Diacylglycerol/PKC Hypothesis

Studies regarding the effects of elevated levels of glucose and hyperglycemia on diacylglycerol levels and PKC activities have suggested another hypothesis of how hyperglycemia may cause vascular dysfunctions (Figure 11.3). It has been shown that, with elevation of glucose levels and in diabetic states, the vascular endothelial cell and its vascular supporting cells in both micro- and macrovessels will have an increased level of diacylglycerol and PKC activities in the membraneous pool.[73-75] These phospholipids and enzyme systems have been shown to be important regulators of vascular cell function, such as modulation of vascular permeability, contractility, basement membrane composition, neovascularization, and synthesis of various cytokines. All of these functions have been shown to be abnormal in diabetics with vascular complications. Therefore, finding increases in diacylglycerol and PKC clearly presented suggestive evidence that this pathway may be providing a role for elevated glucose to cause

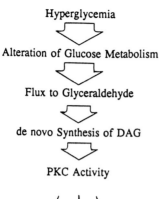

Hyperglycemia

Alteration of Glucose Metabolism

Flux to Glyceraldehyde

de novo Synthesis of DAG

PKC Activity

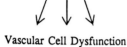

Vascular Cell Dysfunction

Figure 11.3 Schematic drawing of the effect of hyperglycemia on diacylglycerol (DAG) synthesis and PKC activation.

complications. In vivo studies have shown that increased diacylglycerol and PKC are found in the retina, renal glomeruli, heart, and aorta. Interestingly, no change was found in the brain, suggesting that this effect of elevated glucose may not be generalized to all tissues. Functionally, the increasing of PKC may be involved in the regulation of vascular contractility, as shown by the ability of inhibitors to PKC to normalize the increase in aortic ring contractility found in diabetic rabbits.[55] In addition, inhibitors of PKC can also normalize retinal blood flow as well as blood flow in granulation tissue models of diabetes.[117]

The mechanism by which elevated glucose is increasing diacylglycerol and PKC appears to involve the ability of glucose to increase the synthesis of total diacylglycerol, which in turn will activate PKC from the cytosol to its membraneous location.[76] This effect of glucose does not appear to affect the usual synthesis of diacylglycerol, which occurs via the phosphoinositol turnover pathway. In vitro studies have shown this pathway of glucose to increase diacylglycerol and PKC in multiple vascular cells in culture, such as in retinal microvascular endothelial cells, aortic endothelial cells, and rat capillary endothelial cells and aortic smooth muscle cells.[74,75]

Redox Potential Change Hypothesis

The last of the hypotheses regarding the adverse effects of hyperglycemia deals with possible changes in redox potential caused by elevation of glucose. Multiple pathways of glucose utilization affect the levels of NADP/NADPH in diabetes. The postulate is that the metabolism of glucose via glycolysis or the polyol pathway will cause an increase in NADPH.[118] This increase in NADPH levels can cause changes such as increased glycation of proteins as well as increased synthesis of diacylglycerol. In vivo studies in animals suggest that the administration of pyruvate, which restores the NADPH levels, can reverse some of the effects of hyperglycemia on vascular dysfunctions.[118]

Summary

These hypotheses have shown that elevation of glucose levels can affect many important pathways in the cell. These changes can easily affect vascular cell functions, which can then lead to the complications described above in diabetic patients and animals. It is not clear at this time, however, which of these theories has a predominant role in causing cellular dysfunctions. It is likely that more than one of these pathways is responsible, and the predominance of one pathway may not apply to all vascular tissues.

Conclusion

This review has attempted to describe some of the present knowledge on the vascular dysfunctions as found both in vivo and in vitro with regard to diabetes. In addition, the theories of how elevated glucose may cause these changes have been described. From these discussions it is obvious that the basics of the pathogenic mechanism of diabetic vascular complications are not well explained but are actively being studied from multiple perspectives. It is also clear that the causes of the variety of pathologies will also be multiple.

Acknowledgments.   The authors wish to thank Leslie Balmat and Nikki Russell for their excellent secretarial assistance. This paper was supported by National Institutes of Health grants EY05110, EY09178, and NIDDK 36433, the Massachusetts Lions Eye Research, and National Institutes of Health grant DERC 36836.

References

1. Bergstrand A, Bucht H: The glomerular lesions of diabetes mellitus and their electron microscopic appearance. *J Pathol Bacteriol* 1959;77:231–242.
2. Mogensen CE, Østerby R, Gundersen HJG: Early functional and morphologic vascular renal consequences of the diabetic state. *Diabetologia* 1979;17:71–76.
3. Williamson JR, Kilo C: Extracellular matrix changes in diabetes mellitus, in Scarpelli DG, Migaki G (eds), *Comparative Pathobiology of Major Age-Related Disease.* New York, Alan R. Liss Inc., 1984, p 269.
4. Cogan DG, Toussaint D, Kuwabara T: Retinal vascular patterns IV: Diabetic retinopathy. *Arch Ophthalmol* 1961;60:100–112.
5. Colwell JA, Lopes-Virella M, Halushka PV: Pathogenesis of atherosclerosis in diabetes mellitus. *Diabetes Care* 1981;4:121–133.
6. Merriam JC, Sommers SC: Mammary periductal hylin in diabetic women. *Lab Invest* 1957;6:412–420.
7. Schoffling K, Federlin K, Kitschuneit H, et al: Disorder of sexual function in male diabetic patients. *Diabetes* 1963;12:519–527.
8. Durand M, Durand A: Les altération vasculires dermal-hypodermic des diabetiques: Étude aux microscopic optique et electromicroscopie. *Pathol Biol* 1966;14:1005–1019.
9. Johnson PC: Non-vascular basement membrane thickening in diabetes mellitus. *Lancet* 1981;2:932–933.
10. Vracko R, Thorning D, Huang TW: Basal lamina of alveolar epithelium and capillaries: Quantitational changes with aging and in diabetes mellitus. *Annu Rev Resp Dis* 1979;120:973–983.
11. Farquhar MG: The glomerular basement membrane. A selective macromolecular filter, in Hay ED (ed): *Cell Biology of Extracellular Matrix.* New York, Plenum, 1981, pp 335–378.
12. Nagata M, Katz M, Robison Jr WG: Age-related thickening of retinal capillary basement membranes. *Invest Ophthalmol Vis Sci* 1986;27:437–440.
13. Robison WG Jr, Kador PF, Akagi Y, et al: Prevention of basement membrane thick-

ening in retinal capillaries by a novel inhibitor of aldose reductase, tolrestat. *Diabetes* 1986;35:295–299.

14. Waber S, Meiser V, Rossi GL, et al: Studies on retinal microangiopathy and coronary macroangiopathy in rats with streptozotocin-induced diabetes. *Virchows Arch B (Cell Pathol)* 1981;37:1–10.

15. Fischer F, Gaertner J: Morphometric analysis of basal laminae in rats with long-term streptozotocin diabetes. *Exp Eye Res* 1983;37:55–64.

16. Robison WG Jr, Nagata M, Kinoshita JH: Aldose reductase and retinal capillary basement membrane thickening. *Exp Eye Res* 1988;46:343–348.

17. Kimmelsteil P, Wilson C: Intercapillary lesions in the glomeruli of the kidney. *Am J Pathol* 1936;12:83–98.

18. Østerby R, Gundersen HJG: Glomerular size and structure in diabetes mellitus. I. Early abnormalities. *Diabetologia* 1975;11:225–229.

19. Østerby R, Gundersen HJG: Fast accumulation of basement membrane material and the rate of morphological changes in acute experimental diabetic glomerular hypertrophy. *Diabetologia* 1980;18:493–500.

20. Østerby R: Early phases in the development of diabetic glomerulosclerosis. *Acta Med Scand* 1975;574:1–80.

21. Mauer SM, Steffes MW, Ellis EN, et al: Structural-functional relationships in diabetic nephropathy. *J Clin Invest* 1984;74:1143–1155.

22. Steffes MW, Mauer SM: Diabetic glomerulopathy: A morphological approach to monitoring development, progression and reversibility. *Diabetic Nephrop* 1985;4:114–117.

23. Wiseman MJ, Saunders AJ, Keen H, et al: Effect of blood glucose control on increased glomerular filtration rate and kidney size in insulin-dependent diabetes. *N Engl J Med* 1985;312:617–621.

24. Rasch R: Prevention of diabetic glomerulopathy in streptozotocin diabetic rats by insulin treatment. *Diabetologia* 1980;18:413–416.

25. Steffes MW, Brown DM, Bagsen JM, et al: Amelioration of mesangial volume and surface alterations following islet transplantation in diabetic rats. *Diabetes* 1980;29:509–515.

26. Schnider S, Aronoff SL, Tchou P, et al: Urinary protein excretion in prediabetic (PD), normal (N), and diabetic (D) Pima Indians and normal Caucasians (NC). *Diabetes* 1977;26(suppl 1):362.

27. Myers BD, Winetz JA, Chui F, et al: Mechanism of proteinuria in diabetic nephropathy: A study of glomerular barrier function. *Kidney Int* 1982;21:633–641.

28. Tilton RG, Miller EJ, Kilo C, et al: Pericyte form and distribution in rat retinal and uveal capillaries. *Invest Ophthalmol Vis Sci* 1985;26:60–73.

29. Kuwabara T, Cogan DG: Retinal vascular patterns VI. Mural cells at the retinal capillaries. *Arch Ophthalmol* 1963;69:492–502a.

30. Ashton N: Injection of the retinal vascular system in enucleated eyes in diabetic retinopathy. *Br J Ophthalmol* 1950;54:38–44.

31. Antonelli-Orlidge A, Saunders KB, Smith SR, et al: An activated form of transforming growth factor B is produced by cocultures of endothelial cells and pericytes. *Proc Natl Acad Sci USA* 1989;86:4544–4548.

32. Sato Y, Rifkin DB: Inhibition of endothelial cell movement by pericytes and smooth muscle cells: Activation of a latent transforming growth factor B1-like molecule by plasmin during co-culture. *J Cell Biol* 1989;109:309–315.

33. Arnqvist HJ, Ballerman BJ, King GL: Receptors for and effects of insulin and IGF-1 in rat glomerular mesangial cells. *Am J Physiol* 1988;254:C411–C416.

34. Striker GE, Killen P, Farim FM: Human glomerular cells in vitro: Isolation and characterization. *Transplant Proc* 1980;12:88–89.

35. Kriesberg JI, Karnovsky MJ: Glomerular cells in culture. *Kidney Int* 1983;23:439–447.

36. Ishii H, Umeda F, Nawata H: Platelet function in diabetes. *Diabetes Metab Rev* 1992;8:53–66.

37. Ostermann H, van de Loo J: Factors of the haemostatic system in diabetic patients: A survey of controlled studies. *Haemostasis* 1986;16:386–416.

38. Grant MB, Fitzgerald C, Guay C, et al: Fibrinolytic capacity following stimulation with desmopressin acetate in patients with diabetes. *Metabolism* 1989;38:901–907.

39. Kruithof EKO: Plasminogen activator inhibitor type 1: Biochemical, biological and clinical aspects. *Fibrinolysis* 1988;2:59–70.

40. Small M, Kluft C, MacCuish AC, et al: Tissue plasminogen activator inhibition in diabetes mellitus. *Diabetes Care* 1989;12:655–658.

41. Moroose R, Hoyer LW: Van Willebrand factor and platelet function. Ann Rev Med 1986;37:157–163.

42. Gonzalez J, Colwell JA, Sarji KE, et al: Effect of metabolic control with insulin on plasma von Willebrand factor activity (VIIIR:WF) in diabetes mellitus. *Thromb Res* 180;17:261–266.

43. Paton RC, Kernoff PBA, Wales JK, et al: Effects of diet and glicazide on the haemostatic system of non-insulin dependent diabetics. *Br Med J* 1981;283:1018–1020.

44. Coller BS, Frank RN, Milton RC, et al: Plasma cofactors of platelet function: Correlation with diabetic retinopathy and hemoglobin Ala-c. Studies in diabetic patients and normal persons. *Ann Intern Med* 1978;88:311–316.

45. Porta M, Maneschi F, White MC, et al: Twenty-four hour variations of von Willebrand factor and factor VIII-related antigen in diabetic retinopathy. *Metabolism* 1981;30:695–699.

46. Muntean WE, Borkenstein MH, Haas J: Elevation of factor VIII coagulant activity over factor VIII coagulant antigen in diabetic children without vascular disease. A sign of the factor VIII coagulant moiety during poor diabetes control. *Diabetes* 1985;34:140–144.

47. Winocour PD, Lopes-Virella M, Laimins M, et al: Effect of insulin treatment in streptozotocin-induced diabetic rats on in vitro platelet function and plasma von Willebrand activity and factor VIII-related antigen. *J Lab Clin Med* 1985;106:319–325.

48. Aanderud S, Krane H, Nordoy A: Influence of glucose, insulin and sera from diabetic patients on the prostacyclin synthesis in vitro in cultured human endothelial cells. *Diabetologia* 1985;28:641–644.

49. Umeda F, Inoguchi T, Nawata H: Reduced stimulatory activity on prostacyclin production by cultured endothelial cells in serum from aged and diabetic patients. *Atherosclerosis* 1989;75:61–66.

50. Wallow IHL, Engerman RL: Permeability and patency of retinal blood vessels in experimental diabetes. *Invest Ophthalmol Vis Sci* 1977;16:447–454.

51. Williamson JR, Chang K, Rowold E, et al: Sorbinil prevents diabetes-induced increases in vascular permeability but does not alter collagen cross-linking. *Diabetes* 1985;34:703–705.

52. Cunha-Vaz J, De Abrew JRF, Campose AJ: Early breakdown of the retinal barrier in diabetes. *Br J Ophthalmol* 1975;59:649–656.

53. Ortola FV, Ballermann BJ, Anderson S, et al: Elevated plasma atrial naturietic peptide levels in diabetic rats: Potential mediator of hyperfiltration. *J Clin Invest* 1987;80:670–674.

54. Gebremedhin D, Koltai MZ, Pogasta G, et al: Differential contractile responsiveness of femoral arteries from healthy and diabetic dogs: Role of endothelium. *Arch Int Pharmacodyn* 1987;288:100–108.

55. Tesfamariam B, Brown ML, Cohen RA: Elevated glucose impairs endothelium-dependent relaxation by activating protein kinase C. *J Clin Invest* 1991;87:1643–1648.

56. Tanz RD, Chang KSK, Weller TS: Histamine relaxation of aortic rings from diabetic rats. *Agents Actions* 1989;28:1–8.

57. Doi T, Striker LJ, Quaife C, et al: Progressive glomerulosclerosis develops in transgenic mice chronically expressing growth hormone and growth hormone releasing factor but not in those expressing insulin-like growth factor I. *Am J Pathol* 1988;131:398–403.

58. Bussell SE, Clermont AC, Shiba T, et al: Evaluating retinal circulation using video fluorecein angiography in control and diabetic rats. *Curr Eye Res* 1992;11:295.

59. Grunwald JE, Riva CE, Martin DB, et al: Effect of an insulin-induced decrease in blood glucose on the human diabetic retinal circulation. *Ophthalmology* 1987;94: 1614–1620.

60. Ditzel J, Standl E: The problem of tissue oxygenation in diabetes mellitus. I. Its relation to the early functional changes in the microcirculation of diabetic subjects. *Acta Med Scand* 1975;578(suppl):49–58.

61. Yoshida A, Feke GT, Moralles-Stoppello J, et al: Retinal blood flow alteration during progression of diabetic retinopathy. *Arch Ophthalmol* 1983;101:225–227.

62. Hickam JB, Frayser R: A photographic method for measuring mean retinal circulation time using fluorescein. *Invest Ophthalmol Vis Sci* 1965;4:876–884.

63. Kohner EM, Hamilton AM, Saunders RH, et al: The retinal blood flow in diabetes. *Diabetologia* 1975;11:27–33.

64. Fortes ZB, Leme JG, Scivoletto R: Vascular reactivity in diabetes mellitus. Possible role of insulin on the endothelial cell. *Br J Pharmacol* 1984;83:635–643.

65. de Tejada IS, Goldstein I, Azadzoi K, et al: Impaired neurogenic and endothelium-mediated relaxation of penile smooth muscle from diabetic men with impotence. *N Engl J Med* 1989;320:1025–1030.

66. Yanagisawa M, Kurlihara H, Kimur S, et al: A novel potent vasoconstrictor peptide produced by vascular endothelial cells. *Nature* 1988;332:411–415.

67. Takahashi K, Brooks RA, Kanse SM, et al: Production of endothelin-1 by cultured bovine retinal endothelial cells and presence of endothelin receptors and associated pericytes. *Diabetes* 1989;38:1200–1202.

68. Marsden PA, Danthuruli NR, Brenner BM, et al: Endothelin action on vascular smooth muscle involves inositol biphosphate and calcium mobilization. *Biochem Biophys Res Commun* 1989;158:86–93.

69. Takahashi K, Ghatei MA, Lam HC, et al: Elevated plasma endothelin in patients with diabetes mellitus. *Diabetologia* 1990;33:306–310.

70. Yamauchi T, Ohnaka K, Takayanagi R: Enhanced secretion of endothelin-1 by elevated glucose levels from cultured bovine aortic endothelial cells. *FEBS Lett* 1990; 267:16–18.

71. Oliver FJ, de la Rubia G, Feener EP, et al: Stimulation of endothelin-1 gene expression by insulin in endothelial cells. *J Biol Chem* 1991;266:23251–23256.

72. Simonson DC: Etiology and prevalence of hypertension in diabetic patients. *Diabetes Care* 1988;11:821–827.

73. King GL, Johnson S, Wu G: Possible growth modulators involved in the pathogenesis of diabetic proliferative retinopathy, in Westermark B, Betsholtz C, Hokfelt B (eds): *Growth Factors in Health and Disease*. Amsterdam, Elsevier Science, 1990, pp 303–317.

74. Inoguchi T, Battan R, Handler E, et al: Preferential activation of protein kinase C isoform βII and diacylglycerol levels in the aorta and heart of diabetic rats. *Proc Natl Acad Sci USA* 1992 (November).

75. Craven PA, Davidson CM, De Rubertis FR: Increase in diacyglycerol mass in isolated glomeruli by glucose from de novo synthesis of glycerolipids. *Diabetes* 1990;39:667–674.

76. Kikkawa U, Nishizuka Y: The role of protein kinase C in transmembrane signalling. *Annu Rev Cell Biol* 1986;2:149–178.

77. Schlessinger J: Allosteric regulation of the epidermal growth factor receptor kinase. *J Cell Biol* 1986;103:2067–2072.

78. Backer JM, King GL: Regulation of receptor-mediated endocytosis by phorbol esters. *Biochem Pharmacol* 1991;41:1267–1297.

79. Raymond L, Jacobson B: Isolation and identification of stimulatory and inhibitory cell growth factors in bovine vitreous. *Exp Eye Res* 1982;34:267–286.

80. Taylor CM, Weiss JB: Partial purification of a 5.7 kb glycoprotein from bovine vitreous. *Biochem Biophys Res Commun* 1985;133:911–916.

81. Lutty GA, Thompson DC, Gallup J, et al: Vitreous: An inhibitor of retinal extract-induced neovascularization. *Invest Ophthalmol Vis Sci* 1983;24:52–56.

82. Frater-Schroder M, Risau W, Hallmann R, et al: Tumor necrosis factor type alpha, a potent inhibitor of endothelial cell growth in vitro, is angiogenic in vivo. *Proc Natl Acad Sci USA* 1987;84:5277–5281.

83. Jaye M, Howk R, Burgess W, et al: Human endothelial cell growth factor: Cloning, nucleotide sequence, and chromosome localization. *Science* 1986;233:541–545.

84. Klagsbrun M, Baird A: A dual receptor system is required for basic fibroblast growth factor activity. *Cell* 1991;67:229–231.

85. Sprugel KH, McPherson JM, Clowes AW, et al: Effects of growth factors in vivo. I. Cell ingrowth into porous subcutaneous chambers. *Am J Pathol* 1987;129:601–613.

86. Sivalingham A, Kenny J, Brown GC, et al: Basic fibroblast growth factor leads in the vitreous of patients with proliferative diabetic retinopathy. *Arch Ophthalmol* 1990; 108:869–872.

87. Glaser BM: Extracellular modulating factors and the control of intraocular neovascularization. An overview. *Arch Ophthalmol* 1988;106:603–607.

88. Connor TB Jr, Roberts AB, Sporn MB, et al: Correlation of fibrosis and transforming growth factor-beta type 2 levels in the eye. *J Clin Invest* 1989;83:1661–1666.

89. Taylor CM, Kessin RD, Schor AN, et al: Endothelial cell-stimulating angiogensis factor in vitreous form extraretinal neovascularization. *Invest Ophthalmol Vis Sci* 1989;30: 2174–2178.

90. Taylor CM, Weiss JB, McLaughlin B, et al: Increased procollagenase activating angiogenic factor in the vitreous humour of oxygen treated kittens. *Br J Ophthalmol* 1988;72:2.

91. Merimee TJ: Diabetic retinopathy: A synthesis of perspectives. *N Engl J Med* 1990; 322:978–983.

92. Balodimos MC, Rees SB, Aiello LM, et al: in Goldberg MF, Fine SI (eds): *Symposium on the Treatment of Diabetic Retinopathy.* Public Health Service publication No. 1890. Washington, DC, Government Printing Office, 1968, p 153.

93. King GL, Goodman AD, Buzney S, et al: Receptors and growth promoting effects of insulin and insulin like growth factors on cells from bovine retinal capillaries and aorta. *J Clin Invest* 1985;75:1028–1036.

94. Grant M, Russell B, Fitzgerald C, et al: Insulin-like growth factors in vitreous. *Diabetes* 1986;35:416–420.

95. Lamberton RP, Goodman AD, Kassoff A, et al: Von Willebrand factor, fibronectin and insulin-like growth factor I and II in diabetic retinopathy and nephropathy. *Diabetes* 1984;33:125–129.

96. Pyorala K, Laakso M, Vvsitupa M: Diabetes and atherosclerosis: An epidemiologic view. *Diabetes Metab Rev* 1987;3:464–524.

97. King GL, Buzney S, Kahn CR, et al: Differential responsiveness to insulin of endothelial and support cells from micro- and macrovessels. *J Clin Invest* 1983;71:974–977.

98. Jialal I, Crettaz M, Hachiya HL, et al: Characterization of the receptors for insulin and the insulin-like growth factors on micro- and macrovascular tissues. *Endocrinology* 1984;117:1222–1229.

99. Bar RS, Boes M: Distinct receptors for IGF-I, IGF-II, and insulin are present on bovine capillary endothelial cells and large vessel endothelial cells. *Biochem Biophys Res Commun* 1984;124:203–209.

100. Kwok CF, Goldstein BJ, Muller-Wieland D, et al: Identification of persistent defects in insulin receptor structure and function in capillary endothelial cells from diabetic rats. *J Clin Invest* 1989;83:127–136.

101. Bottaro DP, Bonner-Weir S, King GL: Insulin receptor recycling in vascular endothelial cells. *J Biol Chem* 1989;264:5916–5923.

102. Wallum BJ, Taborsky GJ, Porte D, et al: Cerebrospinal fluid insulin levels increase during intravenous insulin infusions in man. *J Clin Endocrinol Metab* 1987;64:190–194.

103. King GL, Johnson SM: Receptor-mediated transport of insulin across endothelial cells. *Science* 1985;227:1583–1586.

104. King GL, Goldman AD, Buzney S, et al: Receptors and growth promoting effects of insulin and insulin like growth factors on cells from bovine retinal capillaries and aorta. *J Clin Invest* 1985;75:1028–1036.

105. Greene DA, Lattimer SA, Sima AAF, et al: Sorbitol, phosphoinositides, and sodium-potassium ATP-ase in the pathogenesis of diabetic complications. *N Engl J Med* 1987;316:559–606.

106. MacGregor LC, Matschinsky FM: Treatment with aldose reductase inhibitor of my-oinositol arrests deterioration of the electroretinogram of diabetic rats. *J Clin Invest* 1985;24:1250–1258.

107. Gabbay KH: The sorbitol pathway and the complications of diabetes. *N Engl J Med* 1973;288:831–836.

108. Kador PF, Robison WG, Kinoshita JH: Pharmacology of aldose reductase inhibitors. *Annu Rev Pharmacol Toxicol* 1985;25:691–714.

109. Frank RN: Aldose reductase inhibition. The chemical key to the control of diabetic retinopathy? *Arch Ophthalmol* 1990;108:1229–1231.

110. Dyck PJ, Zimmerman BR, Vilen TH, et al: Nerve glucose, fructose, sorbitol, myo-inositol, and fiber degeneration and regeneration in diabetic neuropathy. *N Engl J Med* 1988;319:542–548.

111. Brownlee M, Cerami A, Vlassara H: Advanced glycosylation end products in tissue and the biochemical basis of diabetic complications. *N Engl J Med* 1988;318:1315–1321.

112. Brownlee M, Vlassara H, Cerami A: Nonenzymatic glycosylation and the pathogenesis of diabetic complications. *Ann Intern Med* 1984;101:527–537.

113. Brownlee M: Glycosylation products as toxic mediators of diabetic complications. *Annu Rev Med* 1991;42:159–166.

114. Brownlee M, Vlassara H, Kooney A, et al: Aminoguanidine prevents diabetes-induced arterial wall protein cross-linking. *Science* 1986;232:1629–1632.

115. Vlassara H, Esposito C, Gerlach H, et al: Receptor-mediated binding of glycosylated albumin to endothelium induces tissue necrosis factor and acts synergistically with TNF procoagulant activity. *Diabetes* 1989;38(suppl 2):32A.

116. Hammes HP, Martin S, Federlin K, et al: Aminoguanidine treatment inhibits the development of experimental diabetic retinopathy. *Proc Natl Acad Sci USA* 1991;88:11555–11558.

117. Wolf BA, Williamson JR, Easom RA, et al: Diacylglycerol accumulation and micro-vascular abnormalities induced by elevated glucose levels. *J Clin Invest* 1991;87:31–38.

118. Pugliese G, Tilton RG, Williamson JR: Glucose-induced metabolic imbalances in the pathogenesis of diabetic vascular disease. *Diabetes Metab Rev* 1991;7:35–59.

Chapter 12

Thrombosis and Atherogenesis in Diabetes

Peter D. Winocour, PhD, and Mary Richardson, PhD

Diabetes mellitus is associated with enhanced development of atherosclerosis and its thrombotic complications. Theories about the development of atherosclerosis in diabetes have come mainly from schemes proposed for the nondiabetic population, and any mechanism(s) that are uniquely associated with diabetes have not been defined. The morphologic appearance of atherosclerosis in diabetic patients is similar to that in nondiabetic subjects, although it develops earlier and with greater severity. Diabetes is associated with the established risk factors for cardiovascular disease, hypercholesterolemia, and dyslipoproteinemia, as well as raised blood glucose concentrations.[1-4] It is also probable that injury to the arterial endothelium in a diabetic setting, either directly by the metabolic imbalance associated with hyperglycemia or by insulin, is involved in the pathogenesis of diabetes-related atherosclerosis.[4,5] The increased thrombogenic diathesis in diabetes not only heightens the tendency for thrombotic complications to occur in association with established lesions but may also further promote atherogenesis.[6]

Thrombosis in Diabetes

Arterial thrombi, composed mainly of platelets and fibrin, predominantly form at sites of atherosclerosis at vessel branches and bifurcations. The risk for thrombosis represents an imbalance in the prothrombotic, antithrombotic, and thrombolytic processes. The factors involved in these processes include plasma- or vessel wall–derived activators and inhibitors of coagulation, fibrinolysis, and platelets and alterations in the sensitivity of platelets to stimuli, as well as in the reactivity of the vessel wall, especially involving endothelial responses to stimulation. There is evidence that all of these features are altered in diabetes, resulting in an increased tendency toward thrombosis.

It has been suggested that a "hypercoagulable state" exists in diabetes. The effect is increased formation of fibrin. Fibrin deposits have been identified in diabetic microvascular lesions and could be a contributing factor to these lesions.[1,7] A hypercoagulable state could result from alterations in concentrations and/or activities of factors involved in the activation or inhibition of coagulation and fibrinolysis.

Altered Coagulation in Diabetes

Early studies showed a shortened clotting time in coagulation tests in diabetes. More recently, alterations in specific coagulation factors in diabetes have been described, including higher plasma concentrations of factors V, VII, VIII, and X and fibrinogen.[8]

Altered Factor VIII Complex in Diabetes

Part of the factor VIII complex (F.VIII:vWF) consists of a von Willebrand factor (vWF) component, which is produced by the endothelium and megakaryocytes and is involved in platelet adherence to the subendothelium under conditions of high shear. vWF is a multimeric glycoprotein, and in its smaller polymeric form it possesses antigenic activity, which is known as factor VIII–related antigen (F.VIIIR:Ag). In the plasma, vWF circulates in association with the other component of the factor VIII complex, coagulant factor VIII (F.VIII:C), which is synthesized by the liver.

Numerous studies have observed elevated plasma concentrations of vWF, either as F.VIII:vWF or F.VIIIR:Ag, in diabetic patients, and this correlated with the presence and severity of vascular disease.[8] Other studies reported raised vWF concentrations in diabetic children and in diabetic adults without detectable vascular complications.[2,3] Also, concentrations of vWF were notably higher during diabetic ketoacidosis and were reduced following treatment.[7] However, high vWF concentrations have been found in nondiabetic subjects with vascular disease, and it is unclear whether the concentrations are increased more in diabetic patients with a similar degree of vascular disease. Plasma F.VIII:C concentrations also have been found to be increased in diabetic patients with or without vascular complications, although in some studies normal concentrations were reported.[8]

An elevated plasma concentration of vWF in diabetic patients may reflect endothelial stimulation consequent on the metabolic imbalance, rather than clinical vascular disease. It is likely, however, that it will enhance platelet adhesion under conditions of high shear, such as in the smaller arteries and microcirculation, and thereby contribute to microvascular disease.

Altered Fibrinogen Concentrations in Diabetes

Fibrinogen concentrations have often been found to be increased in diabetes, particularly in the presence of clinical vascular disease. Metabolic control of the diabetic subjects reduced the elevated fibrinogen concentration.[9] However, as with vWF, high fibrinogen concentrations also have been found in nondiabetic patients with vascular complications, and it is unclear if the elevated concentrations in diabetic patients are a cause or a result of enhanced thrombotic disease. Increased fibrinogen turnover has also been found in diabetic individuals, and this returned to normal during euglycemia. Infusion of heparin also returned the impaired fibrinogen clearance toward normal, whereas aspirin or dipyridamole administration had no effect. This indicated that the increased fibrinogen turnover involved enhanced thrombin activity.[9] Plasma and urinary concentrations of fibrinopeptide A have been found to be elevated in types I and II diabetic patients and correlated with plasma glucose concentrations, and correlated in type I diabetic patients with duration of diabetes.[10]

Alterations in Inhibitors of Coagulation in Diabetes

There are several physiologic inhibitors of coagulation. Decreased plasma concentrations of these inhibitors have been associated with increased risk for venous thrombosis in nondiabetic subjects, but their relationship to arterial thrombosis is unclear. Alternatively, decreased concentrations of these inhibitors may reflect increased consumption.

Antithrombin III (AT-III) inactivates thrombin and a number of other coagulation factors, including factors Xa, XIa, and XIIa. AT-III also inactivates plasmin and has heparin cofactor activity. In general, the activity of AT-III and the presence of thrombin–AT-III complexes have been found to be reduced in the plasma from both types I and II diabetic patients, whereas the concentrations of AT-III have been reported to be either normal or increased.[11,12] The decreased activity of AT-III in diabetic patients was restored with more effective insulin therapy.[12] The discrepancies between results of activities and concentrations may indicate that AT-III continues to circulate at normal or increased concentrations in diabetes, but its ability to complex with thrombin is impaired.[9] Consistent with this, in vitro glycation of AT-III caused impaired antithrombin activity, and AT-III isolated from diabetic patients was glycated more extensively than that from control subjects and the extent of glycation correlated with the degree of metabolic control.[11]

Protein C and its cofactor, protein S, inhibit several coagulation factors, including factors V and VII. Thrombomodulin is an endothelial membrane protein also found in plasma and is a cofactor for thrombin-induced activation of protein C. Plasma protein C, protein S, and thrombomodulin concentrations all have been described as being increased in diabetic patients.[13–15]

Heparin cofactor II (HcII) is a protease inhibitor of thrombin. HcII activity has been found to be reduced in type I diabetic patients and inversely correlated with plasma glucose concentrations, whereas circulating concentrations of HcII were normal or increased.[16,17] This discrepancy may result from an effect of increased glycation of HcII. In vitro glycation of HcII has been shown to inhibit its antithrombin activity in a way similar to the observations for AT-III.[18]

α_2-Macroglobulin is another physiologic inhibitor of coagulation. The concentrations of α_2-macroglobulin were reported to be increased in type II diabetes and correlated with the presence and severity of clinical vascular disease and with the degree of metabolic control.[19]

Altered Fibrinolysis in Diabetes

Fibrinolytic activity is a limiting factor in the growth and dissolution of thrombi. Depressed fibrinolysis has been associated with a number of diseases in which there is a high incidence of thrombosis. Early studies of the fibrinolytic activity of blood or blood components from diabetic patients using a variety of assays yielded inconsistent results. Fibrinolytic activity was found to be decreased, increased, or unchanged in diabetic patients compared to normal subjects.[3,20] Part of the inconsistency in results may have arisen from the fact that many of the assays that were used measured the balance between activities of activators and inhibitors of fibrinolysis, the presence of which in the samples may depend on the manner in which the sample is prepared. For example, the preparation of a euglobulin precipitate of plasma removes most of the inhibitors of fibrinolysis. More recently, greater information about mechanisms of normal fibrinolysis has enabled the development of more specifically defined assays to examine the different components of fibrinolysis. An additional problem in interpreting earlier studies is that the type of diabetes, degree of vascular disease, and sex and age of subjects, all of which have been shown to influence fibrinolysis, were not clearly identified.

In recent studies there has been greater emphasis on investigating in diabetes the production of tissue plasminogen activator (t-PA) and plasminogen activator inhibitor (PAI) by the vascular endothelium, and the fibrinolytic response to endothelial stimulation either by venous occlusion or by drugs. Almer and his colleagues[20a] were one of the earliest groups to observe reduced t-PA activity in veins taken at biopsy from types I and II diabetic patients and less stimulation of fibrinolytic activity in the blood in response to venous occlusion in diabetic patients with retinopathy, compared to control subjects; this was interpreted as decreased plasminogen activator release in the diabetic patients. However, diabetic patients with autonomic neuropathy appeared to be protected from the impaired fibrinolytic activity.[20b] The importance of PAI activity in the regulation of fibrinolysis has been emphasized. Fibrinolytic activity was reported to be decreased in types I and II diabetic patients in the presence of high t-PA antigen and PAI activity.[21] This was explained on the basis of increased t-PA–PAI complex formation, resulting in reduced free t-PA levels.

Insulin-induced hypoglycemia in both control and type I diabetic subjects led to an increase in fibrinolytic activity, but the increase was less extensive in the diabetic subjects.[22] Type I diabetic patients in whom normoglycemia was established with an artificial pancreas showed increased plasma insulin levels and decreased fibrinolytic activity.[23] Also, higher levels of plasma insulin in the presence of hyperglycemia in type II diabetic patients was associated with increased PAI activity and impaired fibrinolysis.[24] The increased fibrinolytic activity observed previously in response to insulin-induced hypoglycemia[22] may have resulted from hypoglycemia, rather than from insulin per se. Insulin therapy may impair fibrinolysis and provide a mechanism for the suggested link between hyperinsulinism and atherosclerosis.[4] Other inhibitors of fibrinolysis—α_2-antiplasmin, α_2-macroglobulin, and α_1-antitrypsin—have been found in increased concentrations in most diabetic patients in whom they have been sought.[20]

Impaired plasmin formation has been reported using t-PA and/or plasminogen from poorly controlled diabetic patients, and this improved with metabolic control of the diabetes.[25] A similar impairment of plasmin formation was observed following in vitro glycation of plasminogen, although the impairment was less pronounced than when using plasminogen glycated in vivo in poorly controlled diabetic subjects.[25] Because the glucose concentrations used in in vitro studies were considerably higher than would be encountered in vivo in a diabetic patient, additional factors, such as altered metabolism of glycated compared with nonglycated plasminogen, were suggested. In support of this the half-life of glycated plasminogen in rabbits was 10 hours compared with 24 hours for nonglycated plasminogen.[25]

Thus, the different effects of glycemia, plasma insulin concentration, and type of diabetes on t-PA, PAI, and plasminogen concentrations or activities may explain many of the discrepancies in the literature regarding fibrinolytic activity in diabetic patients.

Role of Platelets in Diabetic Vascular Disease

Platelets can contribute to vascular disease by releasing factors that can modify the vessel wall and by forming thrombi. In response to vessel injury, platelets adhere to the exposed subendothelial constituents, particularly collagen, which leads to the release of the granule contents from adherent platelets. These contents include factors that can stimulate proliferation and migration of smooth muscle cells within the vessel wall, which is an important component of atherogenesis, and other released contents can cause aggregation and release from platelets not directly adherent to collagen. Hypersensitivity of platelets to collagen exposed in injured vessels and/or to agonists generated at the site of vessel damage could therefore contribute to enhanced vascular disease in diabetic subjects.

Evidence for Enhanced Platelet Adhesion in Diabetes

Early studies indicated enhanced retention on glass bead columns of platelets from diabetic individuals; this was interpreted as enhanced platelet adhesion.[1,3,20,26] However, this test involves platelet aggregation as well as adhesion. The responses of platelets from diabetic patients to collagen in the aggregometer have been reported to be increased[1,3,20,26] but, as in the observations of greater retention on glass bead columns, enhanced aggregation in response to materials released from adherent platelets may be responsible. More recently, when specific tests of adhesion have been used, platelets from diabetic humans or animals did not adhere more than control platelets. The adherence of platelets from diabetic humans or rats to a collagen-coated glass surface examined using a rotating probe device was similar to that of platelets from control subjects.[3,27,27a] In addition, Nievelstein and his colleagues found no difference in the adherence of platelets from diabetic patients to extracellular matrix from control endothelial cells compared to platelets from control subjects.[28] In diabetic rats, platelet adherence to aortas during the first 30 minutes following balloon catheter de-endothelialization was not different from that in control rats (P. D. Winocour, M. Richardson, R. L. Kinlough-Rathbone, unpublished data). Thus, platelet adhesion may not be altered in diabetes, and the enhanced adhesion reported in earlier studies may reflect rather a raised sensitivity for aggregation. It is still possible, however, that diabetes causes an increase in the amount and/or potency of materials released from granules from adherent platelets, which could lead to greater effects in modifying the vessel wall and promoting thrombosis; this has not been systematically addressed.

Evidence for Enhanced Platelet Aggregation and Release of Granule Contents in Diabetes

Platelets from patients with type I or type II diabetes have been found to be hypersensitive to aggregating agents in most studies.[1,20,26,27] These studies have been carried out mainly in citrated plasma, and platelets from diabetic patients showed increased sensitivity to secondary aggregation in response to adenosine diphosphate (ADP), collagen, arachidonic acid, platelet activating factor (PAF), and thrombin. The relationship between the hypersensitivity of platelets from diabetic patients and the degree of metabolic control of the diabetes or the type of therapy remains uncertain. It is also unclear whether the hypersensitivity of platelets from diabetic subjects is primary or secondary to established vascular disease, since a similar hypersensitivity occurs with platelets from nondiabetic patients with clinical vascular disease. However, diabetic patients free from detectable vascular disease and diabetic children also have been reported to have hypersensitive platelets,[27] which supports the concept that platelet changes occur before and therefore could contribute to vascular changes in diabetes. It is likely that, once vascular disease is established in diabetic patients, hypersensitivity of their platelets would be more readily detected.

Studies with platelets from diabetic animals, mainly rats, in general support the data from diabetic humans. Washed platelets from rats with streptozotocin-induced or genetically determined diabetes have been shown to be hypersensitive to ADP or thrombin; results with collagen have been less consistent.[27] The increased ADP-induced aggregation of platelets from diabetic rats occurred without activation of the arachidonate pathway or release of granule contents, which indicates enhanced primary aggregation. The hypersensitivity of platelets from diabetic rats preceded vessel wall changes, as detected by a rise in the plasma vWF concentration.[3,27] Results of studies in diabetic rats therefore support those in diabetic humans in indicating that platelet hypersensitivity occurs before detectable vascular changes.

It is unclear if platelets from diabetic subjects are more sensitive to release of their granule contents in vitro in response to release-inducing agents. Release of amine storage granule contents from platelets from diabetic individuals with or without retinopathy was similar to that in control subjects.[27] In contrast, washed platelets from diabetic rats released more serotonin from their amine storage granules in response to thrombin or collagen.[27] There is evidence for increased release of the contents of the α-granules by platelets from diabetic subjects in vivo. Greater plasma concentrations of the platelet-specific proteins, platelet factor 4 and β-thromboglobulin contained in platelet α-granules, have been found in diabetic subjects; this indicates increased release of these proteins by platelets in vivo.[27] Also, platelet extracts from type I diabetic patients in poor metabolic control have been shown to have greater growth-promoting potential for vascular smooth muscle cells in culture; this returned to normal with intensive insulin therapy.[27] The platelet-derived growth factor and serotonin contents of platelets from diabetic patients were reported to be less than in control subjects; this may further indicate increased release in vivo of the contents of α- and amine storage granules, respectively.[29,30]

Mechanisms of Platelet Hypersensitivity in Diabetes

Platelet Arachidonate Pathway

Enhanced activity of the arachidonate pathway and increased prostaglandin and thromboxane A_2 formation by platelets from diabetic patients in response to a number of agonists have been reported in many studies.[3,27] Increased plasma or urinary concentrations of thromboxane B_2 have also been found in diabetic subjects in some, although not all, studies[27,31,32]; this indicates activation of the arachidonate pathway in platelets from these subjects in vivo.

Platelets from diabetic rats also formed more thromboxane A_2 in response to thrombin in vitro.[3,27] Because enhanced arachidonate mobilization from membrane phospholipids has also been found in platelets from diabetic rats,[3] this may be responsible for the increased thromboxane A_2 formation, rather than altered activities of the enzymes involved in the conversion of arachidonate to thromboxane A_2. Furthermore, increased arachidonate mobilization may reflect altered earlier mechanisms involved in platelet activation.

Fibrinogen Binding to Platelets

When platelets are stimulated by agonists, the glycoprotein IIb/IIIa complex, which is the receptor for fibrinogen, is expressed on the platelet surface and binds fibrinogen that helps to hold platelets together during aggregation. Fibrinogen binding to platelets from diabetic patients with retinopathy has been found to be greater than that to platelets from control subjects, although in one study this was not found.[27] An increased number of glycoprotein IIb/IIIa molecules has been reported on unstimulated platelets from diabetic patients and attributed to the larger volume of these platelets.[33] Platelets from rats with streptozotocin-induced or genetically determined diabetes also bound more fibrinogen 10 seconds after addition of ADP and in the absence of activation of the arachidonate pathway or release of amine storage granule contents.[34] Enhanced fibrinogen binding therefore appears to be related to early events involved in aggregation and not to result from effects of thromboxane A_2/endoperoxides formed or materials released from platelet granules.

Alterations in Nonarachidonate Pathways of Platelet Activation

Platelets from diabetic subjects with retinopathy or diabetic rats have been found to be hypersensitive to thrombin through a mechanism(s) independent of activation of the arachidonate pathway or effects of released ADP.[3,27] The amount of thrombin that bound to its receptor on platelets from diabetic rats was similar to that in control rats[35]; this has not been examined in diabetic humans. Postreceptor mechanisms involved in platelet activation may be responsible, therefore, for the hypersensitivity to thrombin of diabetic platelets. In a recent study, thrombin induced greater phosphoinositide hydrolysis, intracellular Ca^{2+} mobilization, and myosin light chain kinase–mediated P20 phosphorylation in hypersensitive washed platelets from type II diabetic patients compared with control subjects.[36] Other studies have also found increased collagen- or thrombin-induced Ca^{2+} influx and internal Ca^{2+} mobilization in platelets from types I and II diabetic patients.[37–39] However, in contrast, decreased phosphoinositide hydrolysis in response to thrombin has been reported in platelet-rich plasma from type I diabetic patients.[40] Increased thrombin-induced inositol triphosphate formation also has been found with washed platelets from rats with genetically determined diabetes.[41] It is of interest that platelets from type II diabetic patients recently were shown to have impaired expression of inhibitory G proteins for adenylate cyclase associated with depressed stimulated adenylate cyclase activity; this was suggested as contributing to the hypersensitivity of platelets from diabetic subjects.[42]

Platelet Membrane Lipid Fluidity

Membrane lipid fluidity modulates cell function. Alterations in the sensitivity of platelets from diabetic subjects could result from changes in membrane lipid fluidity. Erythrocytes from diabetic patients had a reduced membrane lipid fluidity, which inversely correlated with increases in the cholesterol-to-phospho-lipid molar ratio and in the extent of glycation of membrane proteins. Hyper-sensitive platelets from poorly controlled types I and II diabetic patients had a decreased membrane lipid fluidity.[43] Isolated platelet membranes from diabetic patients also had a reduced membrane lipid fluidity, which inversely correlated with increases in the extent of glycation of membrane proteins, but the cho-lesterol-to-phospholipid molar ratio was not increased in these membranes.[44] When isolated platelet membranes from nondiabetic subjects were incubated in a medium containing a glucose concentration often found in poorly controlled diabetic subjects, the membrane lipid fluidity was decreased in association with an increase in the extent of glycation of membrane proteins.[44a] A role for in-creased glycation of membrane proteins has been proposed for the hypersen-sitivity of platelets from diabetic patients, although in one study increases in the extent of glycation of membrane proteins of platelets from diabetic patients were not associated with increases in the sensitivity of these platelets to agonists.[27]

Evidence for Enhanced Thrombosis In Vivo in Diabetes

Although there are a number of changes in both coagulation and platelet sen-sitivity in diabetes that could indicate a prothrombic state, only relatively few studies have examined evidence for enhanced thrombosis in vivo in diabetic humans or animals, and these studies have mainly involved the microcirculation. Platelet microthrombi were reported to occur in the microvasculature of sural nerves from diabetic patients with neuropathy[45,46] and in the cerebral circulation of patients with diabetic ketoacidosis.[47] Platelet aggregates have been found in the retinal and endoneurial vessels of diabetic humans and animals.[48–50] There is also some evidence that thrombosis in large vessels will occur more readily in response to vessel injury in diabetes. In diabetic rabbits, increased ADP-induced platelet thrombus formation was observed in response to electrical injury to pial arteries.[51] The presence of platelets and microthrombi was re-ported at sites of endothelial cell loss in aortas of diabetic rats.[52] Greater platelet accumulation occurred on aortas repeatedly damaged for 4 days with indwelling catheters in rats with genetically determined diabetes, although macroscopic thrombi did not form in either control or diabetic rats.[53] In contrast, platelets did not accumulate more on the subendothelium exposed after mechanical in-jury to the ear artery in diabetic rabbits.[54] Therefore, in general, there is evidence to indicate a greater tendency for thrombi to form in vivo in large vessels and the microcirculation in diabetes, but clearly more work is needed in this area. The greater thrombotic tendency and the hypersensitivity of platelets also may play an important role in the enhanced development of atherosclerosis in diabetes.

Atherogenesis in Diabetes

Atherogenesis is associated with raised plasma cholesterol concentrations and also with the response to intimal injury.[55,56] Denuding endothelial injury exposes the subendothelium and results in the interaction of platelets, white blood cells, and fibrin(ogen) with the exposed connective tissues. Such injury can lead to the development of lipid-containing atherosclerotic lesions in both normo- and hyperlipidemic experimental animals.

Atherosclerotic vascular disease is prevalent in humans with either type I or type II diabetes[1-4] even though the lipoprotein profiles associated with each form of the disease are different.[5] It is considered that some form of acute or chronic endothelial injury or stimulation, which leads to an alteration in endothelial function, is an integral component of atherogenesis associated with diabetes mellitus.

Experimental Atherosclerosis in Diabetes

Recent experimental observations on the development of atherosclerosis in diabetic animals are consistent with clinical evidence for diabetes being an important risk factor in atherogenesis. The results of older experimental studies on atherosclerosis in the diabetic animal were unclear and sometimes confusing. This is in part because some of the evidence was obtained in strains of rats, which are relatively resistant to atherosclerosis,[52,57-59] and also because of the original observations made by Duff and McMillan in 1949 that diabetes exerted a protective effect on diet-induced atherosclerosis in rabbits.[60] The identification in diabetic rabbits with severe diet-induced hypercholesterolemia of an abnormal lipoprotein profile, including a very large amount of very-low-density lipoprotein, which is not atherogenic,[61] has provided a possible explanation for these observations. Wilson et al[62] showed that, in cholesterol-fed diabetic rabbits, dietary manipulation to maintain the same plasma concentrations of cholesterol as in the nondiabetic controls resulted in a similar degree of atherosclerosis in both groups. However, in this study the animals were hypercholesterolemic before the induction of diabetes. It is possible that diabetes results in an increased susceptibility to atherogenesis, and this would have been masked in these earlier studies.[60,62] When a diet that does not induce gross alterations in plasma cholesterol concentrations or lipid profiles is fed to alloxan-treated rabbits, the diabetic animals develop enhanced aortic atherosclerosis compared to the nondiabetic animals fed the same diet.[63]

The use of appropriate strains of rats has confirmed that diabetes will enhance the development of experimental atherosclerosis. An insulin-resistant, diabetes-prone rat, the JCR corpulent rat, has recently been described that develops severe spontaneous atherosclerosis that is associated with intimal injury.[64] In obese Zucker rats, with a metabolic profile similar to that of non-insulin-dependent diabetic humans, the lesions that developed following denuding endothelial injury were more extensive than in lean control animals.[65]

Evidence for Endothelial Injury in Diabetes

In humans, denuding endothelial injury may occur during certain surgical procedures, but there is recent evidence that such injury is unlikely to occur spontaneously in vivo. Injury or stimulation of the endothelium that does not result in frank endothelial cell loss (ie, nondenuding injury) has been implicated in atherogenesis and has been demonstrated in the initial stages of diet-induced experimental atherosclerosis. Nondenuding endothelial injury has been considered to have occurred in vivo whenever increased synthesis of endothelial DNA is seen in the absence of morphologic evidence of endothelial cell loss.

There is considerable evidence from in vitro and in vivo studies to indicate endothelial dysfunction in both human and experimental diabetes, but the need for a better understanding of the pathobiology of endothelium in diabetes has recently been emphasized.[66] There are alterations in the thrombogenicity of the endothelium associated with diabetes. Diabetic endothelium in vitro showed a reduced capacity to secrete prostaglandin (PG) I_2, whereas thromboxane A_2 synthesis was increased.[67] Endothelial cells cultured in media containing high concentrations of glucose produce increased amounts of F.VIIR:Ag[27] and are induced to overexpress t-PA and PAI activity.[66] These observations are consistent with in vivo data. Altered circulating levels of PAI-1[24] as well as increased loss of vWF and decreased production of PGI_2[67] and t-PA[21] have been described in both types of human diabetes as well as in experimental diabetes and further indicate endothelial dysfunction.

Other studies of endothelium cultured in a glucose-enriched medium have demonstrated alterations in functions that are relevant to atherogenesis, including impaired histamine metabolism,[68] increased low-density lipoprotein (LDL) uptake and metabolism,[69] and increased endothelial cell replication rate.[66] From in vivo studies, diabetes is known to be associated with a reduced capacity for vascular relaxation. In experimental diabetes, this has been attributed to alterations in sensitivity to catecholamines[67] and also directly to an impaired endothelial ability to produce endothelial-derived relaxing factor (EDRF)[70] and an increased production of endothelin.[71] In diabetic patients, the vascular dilation response to ischemia was reduced compared to that in age-matched healthy controls.[72]

There is morphologic evidence for endothelial injury in diabetic experimental animals. We have defined morphologic alterations in the aortic endothelium, consistent with a progressive nondenuding injury, during the first 6 months of alloxan-induced diabetes in rabbits.[73] The alterations included an increase in the endothelial cell thymidine index, increased accumulation of white blood cells and platelets, and increased deposition of fibrin-like material on the endothelial surface. At no stage was frank endothelial cell denudation observed. There was intimal proliferation, resulting in an increase in the numbers of smooth muscle cells and in the amount of connective tissue, including proteoglycan. These alterations are similar to the diffuse intimal thickening that is regarded as an initiating state of atherogenesis. We also observed that the mild hyperlipidemia that developed in some of the diabetic rabbits was associated with enhanced intimal proliferation but not with increased severity of endothelial injury. Other studies have reported morphologic alterations in the arterial endothelium of diabetic rabbits[74] or rats in vivo.[52,59] Morphologic alterations were correlated with an impaired production of EDRF in the genetically determined diabetic rat. Some studies evaluated only one time interval after induction of diabetes,[52,59,74] but all studies reported evidence of endothelial injury, including fibrin on the endothelial surface, consistent with our observations in rabbits.[73]

Various mechanisms have been proposed for injury to the endothelium in diabetes, including effects of insulin,[5] dyslipoproteinemia,[1–4] nonenzymatic glycation of proteins such as LDL and collagen,[1] and the formation of advanced glycosylation end products (AGE).[75] It is also possible that the increase in the thrombotic potential and the interaction by formed elements of the blood with the endothelial surface may be involved in the progression of atherogenesis in diabetes.

Intimal Proteoglycan in Diabetes and Atherogenesis

Proteoglycan, synthesized by endothelial and smooth muscle cells, is the principal constituent of nonfibrous connective tissue. The association of proteoglycan with atherosclerosis has been mainly related to the formation of insoluble proteoglycan-LDL complexes. Increased amounts of abnormal proteoglycan have been identified in human, experimental diet–induced, and denuding endothelial injury–induced atherosclerosis.[76] Macrophages produce proteoglycan in vitro and express a receptor-mediated pathway for the metabolism of the proteoglycan-LDL complex.[76] Endothelial stimulation and increased interaction with formed elements is likely to affect intimal proteoglycan. Accumulation of proteoglycan in the thickened intima may increase the potential for extracellular lipid to be deposited.

In diabetes, the available data support the concept that there is an alteration of proteoglycan in the arterial wall, although the loss of heparan sulfate from the glomerular basement membrane and the associated increase in permeability have been the focus of most studies.[77] In diabetic rabbits, an increase in aortic proteoglycan was described.[55] In diabetic dogs, the glycosaminoglycan content of the coronary artery wall showed a 29% increase, with variable changes in chondroitin sulfate and hyaluronic acid and a decrease in dermatan sulfate, chondroitin sulfate, and heparan sulfate in the aorta.[55] From our preliminary data, the distribution of the proteoglycan in the arterial intima in diabetic rabbits is similar to the alterations that were observed previously in the aortas of aged rabbits.

Thrombosis and Atherogenesis in Diabetes

The increased tendency for thrombosis in diabetes may be strongly associated with the enhanced risk of atherosclerosis.[9] The relationship among endothelial cell activation, coagulation, and atherosclerosis has long been recognized.[6] Elevated plasma concentrations of factor VII and fibrinogen[78] have been suggested as being risk factors for coronary thrombosis in the nondiabetic subject, and fibrinogen and factor VIII are involved under some conditions in platelet activation.[7] A lower fibrinolytic activity has been found in types I and II diabetic patients and would support fibrin formation. It is also possible that increased interaction of white blood cells with stimulated endothelium, such as we observed on the endothelium of diabetic rabbits,[73] is a stimulus for fibrin formation. Macrophages become procoagulant when stimulated by PAF and in response to an atherogenic diet, and in atherosclerotic lesions macrophages express mRNA for tissue factor. Endothelium has the potential to respond to stimulation by interaction with formed blood elements, especially white blood cells, promoting thrombosis and stimulating repair of the damaged vessel wall. Normally this response ensures homeostasis, but in a situation of chronic stimulation, such as hyperlipidemia or hyperglycemia, the hyperresponsiveness of endothelial cells to formed blood elements may be the initiating stage of atherogenesis.

There are a number of mechanisms by which fibrin could influence the initiation of endothelial injury and the progression to atherosclerosis. Endothelial permeability is increased in the presence of fibrin-derived peptides, produced by the action of both thrombin and plasmin.[79] This increased permeability is related to the cell retraction[79] or disorganization of cell shape, and increased pinocytotic transport. Fibrin(ogen) degradation products have been identified in the normal rabbit arterial intima, and in increased amounts in the diabetic rabbit aorta,[80] following balloon de-endothelialization of nondiabetic rabbit aortas,[80] in the thickened intima in humans,[78] and in atherosclerotic lesions,[78] where they will associate with hyaluronic acid and are implicated in the sequestration of LDL.[78] Fibrinogen is chemotactic to smooth muscle cells and stimulates and is mitogenic to macrophages. The interaction of fibrin(ogen) with endothelial cells is mediated through the expression of integrins. The fibrin(ogen) then may interact with red blood cells and platelets. Increased fibrinogen binding to diabetic platelets has been described,[27] and there is an increased accumulation of red blood cells on diabetic endothelium.[1] The precise mechanism(s) that result in the accumulation of red blood cells and possibly platelets on diabetic endothelium have not been defined, but it is likely that fibrinogen may be involved. Fibrin interaction with endothelium may be self-limiting by stimulating the release of antithrombotic factors PGI_2 and t-PA, and the response by endothelium to fibrin is consistent with promoting wound healing. Under abnormal conditions, however, fibrin(ogen) has the potential to promote atherogenesis.

It should also be noted, however, that, although Kannel et al[81] recently found from analysis of the Framingham data that elevated concentrations of fibrinogen were associated with a higher risk for cardiovascular disease in diabetic patients, there was no reduction in the risk for cardiovascular disease when the data were adjusted for fibrinogen concentrations, indicating that other factors are involved.

The role of thrombosis, including increased plasma fibrinogen concentrations and fibrin formation, in enhanced atherosclerotic disease in diabetes remains to be clearly defined.

Conclusions

Although it is well recognized that diabetes mellitus is a major risk factor for atherosclerosis, no single parameter which can totally account for the increased susceptibility has been identified. Theories about the development of atherosclerosis in diabetes have come mainly from schemes proposed for the nondiabetic population. In both settings atherosclerosis is associated with an increased thrombotic tendency and this represents an imbalance in the prothrombotic, antithrombotic and thrombolytic processes. There is evidence for alterations in all of these processes in diabetes which would favor an increased thrombogenic risk, although relatively few studies have examined thrombosis in vivo. Increased thrombosis is both a complication of atherosclerosis and a contributory factor to the development of atherosclerosis. Endothelial injury and platelet hypersensitivity have both been associated with diabetes-related metabolic alterations and are highly likely to be crucial factors in the heightened susceptibility to atherosclerosis and thrombosis in diabetic subjects.

Further examination of these various processes involved in hemostasis in a diabetic setting will lead to a better understanding of the mechanisms involved in the vascular complications in diabetes and lead to the design of more effective approaches to treatment.

References

1. Brownlee M, Cerami A: The biochemistry of the complications of diabetes mellitus. *Annu Rev Biochem* 1981;50:385–432.
2. Banga JD, Sixma JJ: Diabetes mellitus, vascular disease and thrombosis. *Clin Haematol* 1986;15:465–492.
3. Colwell JA, Lopes-Virella MF, Winocour PD, et al: New concepts about the pathogenesis of atherosclerosis in diabetes mellitus, in Levin ME, O'Neal LW (eds): St. Louis, CV Mosby, 1988, pp 51–70.
4. Ruderman NB, Haudenschild C: Diabetes as an atherogenic factor. *Prog Cardiovasc Dis* 1981;24:373–412.
5. Stehbens WE, Wierzbicki E: The relationship of hypercholesterolemia to atherosclerosis with particular emphasis on familial hypercholesterolemia, diabetes mellitus, obstructive jaundice, myxedema, and the nephrotic syndrome. *Prog Cardiovasc Dis* 1988;30:289–306.
6. Moore S: Thrombosis and atherosclerosis—the chicken and the egg. Contribution of platelets in atherogenesis. *Ann N Y Acad Sci* 1985;454:146–153.
7. Greaves M, Preston FE: Haemostatic abnormalities in diabetes, in Jarrett RJ (ed): *Diabetes and Heart Disease.* Amsterdam, Elsevier Science Publishers BV, 1984, pp 47–80.
8. Breddin K: Detection of prethrombotic states in patients with atherosclerotic lesions. *Semin Thromb Hemost* 1986;12:110–123.
9. Jones RL, Peterson CM: Hematologic alterations in diabetes mellitus. *Am J Med* 1981;70:339–352.
10. Jones RL: Fibrinopeptide-A in diabetes mellitus. Relation to levels of blood glucose, fibrinogen disappearance, and hemodynamic changes. *Diabetes* 1985;34:836–843.
11. Villanueva GB, Allen N: Demonstration of altered antithrombin III activity due to nonenzymatic glycosylation at glucose concentrations expected to be encountered in severely diabetic patients. *Diabetes* 1988;37:1103–1107.
12. Ceriello A, Giugliano D, Quatraro A, et al: Evidence for a hyperglycaemia-dependent decrease of antithrombin III-thrombin complex formation in humans. *Diabetologia* 1990;33:163–167.
13. Conrad J, Samama MM: Inhibitors of coagulation, atherosclerosis, and arterial thrombosis. *Semin Thromb Hemost* 1986;12:87–90.
14. Takahashi H, Tatewaki W, Wada K, et al: Plasma protein S in disseminated intravascular coagulation, liver disease, collagen disease, diabetes mellitus, and under oral anticoagulant therapy. *Clin Chim Acta* 1989;182:195–208.
15. Oida K, Takai H, Maeda H, et al: Plasma thrombomodulin concentration in diabetes mellitus. *Diabetes Res Clin Pract* 1990;10:193–196.
16. Ceriello A, Quatraro A, Russo PD, et al: Evidence for a reduced heparin cofactor II biological activity in diabetes. *Haemostasis* 1990;20:357–361.
17. Gram J, Jespersen J: Increased concentrations of heparin cofactor II in diabetic patients, and possible effects on thrombin inhibition assay of antithrombin III. *Clin Chem* 1989;35:52–55.
18. Ceriello A, Marchi E, Barbanti M, et al: Non-enzymatic glycation reduces heparin cofactor II anti-thrombin activity. *Diabetologia* 1990;33:205–207.
19. Ceriello A, Giugliano D, Quatraro A, et al: Increased alpha$_2$-macroglobulin in diabetes: A hyperglycemia related phenomenon associated with reduced antithrombin III activity. *Acta Diabetol Lat* 1989;26:147–154.

20. Ostermann H, van de Loo J: Factors of the hemostatic system in diabetic patients: A survey of controlled studies. *Haemostasis* 1986;16:386–416.

20a.Almer L-O, Nilsson IM: On fibrinolysis in diabetes mellitus. *Acta Med Scand* 1975; 198:101–106.

20b.Almer L-O, Sundkvist G, Liya B: Fibrinolytic activity, autonomic neuropathy, and circulation in diabetes mellitus. *Diabetes* 1983;32(suppl 2): 4–7.

21. Auwerx J, Bouillon R, Collen D, et al: Tissue-type plasminogen activator antigen and plasminogen activator inhibitor in diabetes mellitus. *Arteriosclerosis* 1988;8:68–72.

22. Dalsgaard-Nielsen J, Madsbad S, Hilsted J: Changes in platelet function, blood coagulation and fibrinolysis during insulin-induced hypoglycemia in juvenile diabetics and normal subjects. *Thromb Haemost* 1982;47:254–258.

23. Juhan-Vague I, Vague P, Poisson C, et al: Effect of 24 hours of normoglycaemia on tissue-type plasminogen activator plasma levels in insulin-dependent diabetes. *Thromb Haemost* 1984;51:97–98.

24. Juhan-Vague I, Roul C, Alessi MC, et al: Increased plasminogen activator inhibitor activity in noninsulin dependent diabetic patients—relationship with plasma insulin. *Thromb Haemost* 1989;61:370–373.

25. Geiger M, Binder BR: Plasminogen activation in diabetes mellitus. Kinetics of plasminogen formation with tissue plasminogen activator and plasminogen from individual diabetic donors and with in vitro glucosylated plasminogen. *Enzyme* 1988;40: 149–157.

26. Hendra T, Betteridge DJ: Platelet function, platelet prostanoids and vascular prostacyclin in diabetes mellitus. *Prostaglandins Leukot Essent Fatty Acids* 1989;35:197–212.

27. Colwell JA, Winocour PD, Lopes-Virella MF: Platelet function and platelet-plasma interactions in atherosclerosis and diabetes mellitus, in Rifkin H, Porte D (eds): *Ellenberg and Rifkin's Diabetes Mellitus, Theory and Practice*, ed 4. Amsterdam, Elsevier Science Publishers BV, 1990, pp 249–256.

27a.Winocour PD, Watala C, Kinlough-Rathbone RL: Reduced membrane fluid and increased glycation of membrane proteins of platelets from diabetic subjects are not associated with increased platelet adherence to glycated collagen. *J Lab Clin Med* 1992, in press.

28. Nievelstein PFEM, Sixma JJ, Ottenhof-Rovers M, et al: Platelet adhesion and aggregate formation in Type 1 diabetes under flow conditions. *Diabetes* 1991;40:1410–1417.

29. Guillausseau PJ, Dupuy E, Bryckaert MC, et al: Platelet-derived growth factor (PDGF) in type I diabetes mellitus. *Eur J Clin Invest* 1989;19:172–175.

30. Barradas MA, Gill DS, Fonseca VA, et al: Intraplatelet serotonin in patients with diabetes mellitus and peripheral vascular disease. *Eur J Clin Invest* 1988;18:399–404.

31. Davi G, Catalano I, Averna M, et al: Thromboxane biosynthesis and platelet function in type II diabetes mellitus. *N Engl J Med* 1990;322:1769–1774.

32. Alessandrini P, McRae J, Feman S, et al: Thromboxane biosynthesis and platelet function in type I diabetes mellitus. *N Engl J Med* 1988;319:208–212.

33. Tschöpe D, Rösen P, Kaufmann L, et al: Evidence for abnormal platelet glycoprotein expression in diabetes mellitus. *Eur J Clin Invest* 1990;20:166–170.

34. Winocour PD, Perry DW, Kinlough-Rathbone RL: Hypersensitivity to ADP of platelets from diabetic rats associated with enhanced fibrinogen binding. *Eur J Clin Invest* 1992;22:19–23.

35. Winocour PD, Perry DW, Hatton MWC, et al: The hypersensitivity to thrombin of platelets from diabetic rats is not due to increased thrombin binding. *Thromb Res* 1991;61:469–475.

36. Ishii H, Umeda F, Hashimoto T, et al: Changes in phosphoinositide turnover, Ca^{2+} mobilization of protein phosphorylation in platelets from NIDDM patients. *Diabetes* 1990;39:1561–1568.

37. Bergh CH, Hjalmarson H, Holm G, et al: Studies on calcium exchange and uptake in human diabetes. *Eur J Clin Invest* 1988;18:92–97.

38. Tschöpe D, Rösen P, Gries FA: Increase in the cytosolic concentration of calcium in platelets of diabetics type II. *Thromb Res* 1991;62:421–428.

39. Ishii H, Umeda F, Hashimoto T, et al: Increased intracellular calcium mobilization in platelets from patients with type 2 non-insulin-dependent diabetes mellitus. *Diabetologia* 1991;34:332–336.

40. Bastyr EJ, Kadrofske MM, Dershimer RC, et al: Decreased platelet phosphoinositide turnover and enhanced platelet activation in IDDM. *Diabetes* 1989;38:1097–1102.

41. Winocour PD, Vickers JD, Kinlough-Rathbone RL, et al: Enhanced thrombin-induced inositol triphosphate formation by platelets from spontaneously diabetic rats [abstract]. *Diabetes* 1989;38(suppl 2):A214.

42. Livingstone C, McLellan AR, McGregor M-A, et al: Altered G-protein expression and adenylate cyclase activity in platelets of non-insulin-dependent diabetic (NIDDM) male subjects. *Biochim Biophys Acta* 1991;1096:127–133.

43. Winocour PD, Bryszewska M, Watala C, et al: Reduced membrane fluidity in platelets from diabetic patients. *Diabetes* 1990;39:241–244.

44. Winocour PD, Watala C, Kinlough-Rathbone RL: Membrane fluidity is related to the extent of glycation of proteins, but not to alterations in the cholesterol to phospholipid molar ratio in isolated platelet membranes from diabetic and control subjects. *Thromb Haemost* 1991;67:567–571.

44a.Winocour PD, Watala C, Perry DW, et al: Decreased platelet membrane fluidity due to glycation or acetylation of membrane proteins. *Thromb Haemost* 1992, in press.

45. Timperley WR, Ward JD, Preston FE, et al: Clinical and histological studies in diabetic neuropathy. *Diabetologia* 1976;12:237–243.

46. Williams E, Timperley WR, Ward JD, et al: Electron microscopical studies of vessels in diabetic peripheral neuropathy. *J Clin Pathol* 1980;33:462–470.

47. Timperley WR, Preston FE, Ward JD: Cerebral intravascular coagulation in diabetic ketoacidosis. *Lancet* 1974;1:952–956.

48. Bloodworth JMB, Molitor DL: Ultrastructural aspects of human and canine diabetic retinopathy. *Invest Ophthalmol* 1965;4:1037–1048.

49. Ishibashi T, Tanaka K, Taniguchi Y: Platelet aggregation and coagulation in the pathogenesis of diabetic retinopathy in rats. *Diabetes* 1981;30:601–606.

50. Sima AAF, Thibert P: Proximal motor neuropathy in the BB-Wistar rat. *Diabetes* 1982; 31:784–788.

51. Honour AJ, Hockaday TDR: Increased sensitivity of in vivo platelet aggregation in rabbits after alloxan or streptozotocin. *Br J Exp Pathol* 1976;57:1–10.

52. Arbogast BW, Berry DL, Newell CL: Injury of arterial endothelial cells in diabetic, sucrose-fed and aged rats. *Atherosclerosis* 1984;51:31–45.

53. Winocour PD, Kinlough-Rathbone RL, Mustard JF: Platelet survival in rats with spontaneous diabetes mellitus. *J Lab Clin Med* 1987;109:464–468.

54. Ingerman-Wojenski CM, Smith M, Silver MJ: Alloxan-induced hyperglycemia in rabbits and the response of platelets to aggregating agents *in vitro* and to exposed subendothelium *in vivo*. *Thromb Res* 1987;46:635–647.

55. Moore S: Pathogenesis of atherosclerosis. *Metabolism* 1985;34:13–16.

56. Ross R: The pathogenesis of atherosclerosis—an update. *N Engl J Med* 1986;314: 488–500,

57. Moore SA, Bohlen HG, Miller BG, et al: Cellular and vessel wall morphology of cerebral cortical arterioles after short-term diabetes in adult rats. *Blood Vessels* 1985;22:265–277.

58. Wu JX, Maes L, Andries R, et al: Early morphologic changes in coronary arteries of experimental diabetic rats. *Acta Diabetol Lat* 1985;22:317–326.

59. Reinila A: Long-term effects of untreated diabetes on the arterial wall in rat. An ultrastructural study. *Diabetologia* 1981;20:205–212.

60. Duff GL, McMillan GC: The effect of alloxan diabetes on experimental cholesterol atherosclerosis in the rabbit. I. The inhibition of cholesterol atherosclerosis in alloxan diabetes. *J Exp Med* 1949;89:611–630.

61. Nordestgaard BG, Stender S, Kjeldsen K: Reduced atherogenesis in cholesterol-fed diabetic rabbits. Giant lipoproteins do not enter the arterial wall. *Arteriosclerosis* 1988;8:421–428.

62. Wilson RB, Martin JM, Hartroft WS: Evaluation of the relative pathogenic roles of diabetes and serum cholesterol levels in the development of cardiovascular lesions in rats. *Diabetes* 1967;16:71–82.

63. Miller RA, Wilson RB: Atherosclerosis and myocardial ischaemic lesions in alloxan-diabetic rabbits fed a low cholesterol diet. *Arteriosclerosis* 1984;4:586–591.

64. Russell JC, Ahuja SK, Manickavel V, et al: Insulin resistance and impaired glucose tolerance in the atherosclerosis-prone LA/N corpulent rat. *Arteriosclerosis* 1987;7: 620–626.

65. Haudenschild CC, Van Sickle W, Chobanian AV: Response of the obese Zucker rat to injury. *Arteriosclerosis* 1981;1:186–191.

66. Lorenzi M, Cagliero E: Pathobiology of endothelial and other vascular cells in diabetes mellitus. Call for data. *Diabetes* 1991;40:653–659.

67. Koltai MZ, Rosen P, Hadhazy P, et al: Relationship between vascular adrenergic receptors and prostaglandin biosynthesis in canine diabetic coronary arteries. *Diabetologia* 1988;31:681–686.

68. Orlidge A, Hollis TM: Aortic endothelial and smooth muscle histamine metabolism in experimental diabetes. *Arteriosclerosis* 1982;2:142–150.

69. Grunwald J, Hesz A, Robenek H, et al: Proliferation, morphology and low-density lipoprotein metabolism of arterial endothelial cells cultured from normal and diabetic minipigs. *Exp Mol Pathol* 1985;42:60–70.

70. Altan VM, Karasu C, Ozuari A: The effects of type-1 and type-2 diabetes on endothelium-dependent relaxation in the rat aorta. *Pharmacol Biochem Behav* 1989;33: 519–522.

71. Hattori Y, Kasai K, Nakamura T, et al: Effects of glucose and insulin on immunoreactive endothelin-1 release from cultured porcine aortic endothelial cells. *Metabolism* 1991;40:165–169.

72. Jorgensen RG, Russo L, Mattiolo L, et al: Early detection of vascular dysfunction in type 1 diabetes. *Diabetes* 1988;37:292–296.

73. Hadcock SJ, Richardson M, Winocour PD, et al: Intimal alterations in the first six months of alloxan-induced diabetes. *Arterioscler Thromb* 1991;11:517–529.

74. Dolgov VV, Zaikina OE, Bondarenko MF, et al: Aortic endothelium of alloxan diabetic rabbits: A quantitative study using scanning electron microscopy. *Diabetologia* 1982; 22:338–343.

75. Esposito C, Gerlach H, Brett J, et al: Endothelial receptor-mediated binding of glucose-modified albumin is associated with increased monolayer permeability and modulation of cell surface coagulant properties. *J Exp Med* 1989;170:1387–1407.

76. Wight TN: Cell biology of arterial proteoglycans. *Arteriosclerosis* 1989;9:1–20.

77. Shimomura H, Spiro R: Studies of macromolecular components of human glomerular basement membrane and alterations in diabetes. Decreased levels of heparan sulphate proteoglycan and laminin. *Diabetes* 1987;36:374–381.

78. Smith EB: Interactions of lipoproteins with vascular intima in atherosclerosis. *Biochem Soc Trans* 1991;19:235–241.

79. Rowland FN, Donovan MJ, Picciano PT, et al: Fibrin-mediated vascular injury. Identification of fibrin peptides that mediate endothelial cell retraction. *Am J Pathol* 1984; 117:418–428.

80. Witmer MR, Hadcock SJ, Peltier S, et al: Altered levels of antithrombin III and fibrinogen in the aortic wall of the alloxan-induced diabetic rabbit: Evidence of a prothrombotic state. *J Lab Clin Med* 1992;119:221–230.

81. Kannel WB, D'Agostino RB, Wilson PWF, et al: Diabetes, fibrinogen, and risk of cardiovascular disease: The Framingham experience. *Am Heart J* 1990;120:672–676.

Chapter 13

Diabetes and Atherosclerosis: Epidemiological Considerations

Steven M. Haffner, MD, Michael P. Stern, MD, and Marian Rewers, MD

Cardiovascular disease is a major cause of morbidity and mortality in subjects with diabetes mellitus. According to the National Hospital Discharge Survey, 77% of hospitalizations attributable to diabetic complications are for cardiovascular disease as opposed to only 9% for renal disease, 6% for neurologic disease, 4% for eye disease, and 3% for other complications.[1] Cardiovascular disease is also a major cause of mortality in diabetes. For every diabetic subject diagnosed after age 20 years who dies of renal disease, nine die of coronary heart disease and two die of stroke.[2] In this chapter, we review the epidemiology of cardiovascular disease in diabetes. Several recent excellent reviews have also covered this topic.[3–9] In addition, pertinent epidemiologic data published prior to 1984 have been thoroughly compiled and discussed in a book prepared by the National Diabetes Data Group (NDDG).[9] Therefore, the objective of this chapter is to review data that have been published since the NDDG compilation and to focus attention on the outstanding questions in this area. As far as possible, studies of incidence, rather than of prevalence or mortality, are emphasized because of the well-known limitations of the latter. The epidemiology of atherosclerosis is presented separately for insulin-dependent (type I) and non-insulin-dependent (type II) diabetes mellitus. This distinction may be helpful in untangling the potentially atherosclerotic effects of hyperglycemia, present in both types of diabetes, from the effects of factors that are more characteristic of the individual types (eg, nephropathy in type I and insulin resistance and dyslipidemia in type II).

Insulin-Dependent Diabetes Mellitus

Coronary Heart Disease

Mortality

Barrett-Connor and Orchard, in their 1984 review[9] of nine clinic-based studies, concluded that heart disease is a relatively rare cause of death in the first 30 years of type I diabetes. Coronary heart disease (CHD) becomes responsible for

Portions of this chapter are adapted and reproduced with permission from a review by MP Stern and SM Haffner which appears in Diabetes Care 1991;14:1144–1159.

20% of deaths only after about 25 years' duration of this disease—that is, after more than one quarter of the patients have already died,[10] mostly from acute complications, traumatic causes, and nephropathy.[11] Clinical series indicate that CHD mortality increases dramatically after the age of 40 years.[12] Some studies,[12,13] but not others,[14] have found that the excess CHD mortality is independent of the age of onset of type I diabetes.

Unbiased mortality data for confirmed type I diabetic subjects are only now becoming available from population-based studies initiated by the Diabetes Epidemiology Research International Group.[11] Since the longest published follow-up data cover only 20 years, however, these studies are still limited in their ability to answer questions concerning CHD risk in type I diabetes. The only population-based data that are helpful with respect to this issue are those from the Wisconsin Epidemiologic Study of Diabetic Retinopathy, wherein type I diabetes was defined as diabetes diagnosed before age 30 and treated with insulin.[15] The age-standardized mortality ratios for death due to CHD (International Classification of Disease, ed 9 [ICD-9] code 410–414) were 9:1 (95% confidence interval [CI], range 6 to 13) for men and 14:1 (95% CI, range 7 to 24) for women. The excess CHD mortality associated with type I diabetes was remarkably greater than that in "older-onset diabetics" (presumably type II diabetics), which was 2.4:1 (95% CI, range 2.1 to 2.8) and 2.2:1 (95% CI, range 1.9 to 2.6) in men and women, respectively. The greater excess of CHD mortality and morbidity in women compared to men with type I diabetes and the attenuated sex differential in type II diabetes has been observed by others as well.[12–14] The Nurses' Health Study of women ages 30 to 55 has also reported a higher cardiovascular mortality ratio for type I diabetes (29:1 [95% CI, range 18 to 48]) than for type II diabetes (7:1 [95% CI, range 5 to 11]).[16]

Perhaps the most promising explanation for the excess CHD risk among type I diabetes subjects is the link between diabetic nephropathy and atherosclerosis. Two 20- to 40-year-long follow-up studies of type I diabetes patients from the Steno Memorial Hospital[13] and the Joslin Clinic[12] have demonstrated that, in patients with proteinuria, the relative mortality from CHD is 15 to 37 times higher than in the general population. For comparison, proteinuria or renal failure appears to increase the risk of fatal CHD in type II diabetes by a factor of only three to four.[17] In type II diabetic patients from Denmark, all-cause mortality adjusted for age, duration of diabetes, and serum creatinine was 1.5 to 2.3 times higher among those with albuminuria, compared to those with urine albumin concentration less than 15 μg/mL.[18] Fifty-eight percent of the deaths were caused by cardiovascular disease, whereas only 3% were caused by renal failure. Nephropathy is twice as common in type I diabetes, and renal failure is 15 times more prevalent, compared to type II diabetes.[19] Thus, nephropathy and associated CHD risk factors[20] could partially explain the excess CHD risk in type I diabetes, compared to either normal or type II diabetic subjects. However, additional CHD risk factors apparently operate in type I diabetic patients because, in those without proteinuria, CHD occurs three to four times more frequently than in the general population.[12,13] In subjects who survived at least 25 years with type I diabetes, only 37% of those with myocardial infarction, angina, stroke, or peripheral arterial disease also had overt nephropathy.[21]

Incidence

There is a paucity of data on the incidence of nonfatal CHD in type I diabetic subjects. Most studies published to date have reported data on clinic-based, rather than population-based, case series and have used nonstandardized definitions of type I diabetes. The London cohort of the World Health Organization (WHO) Multinational Study of Vascular Disease in Diabetics represents a population-based case series and has recently been reclassified into type I and type II diabetic subcohorts.[22,23] The former included subjects who had started insulin treatment within 1 year of diagnosis and who had remained on it subsequently, regardless of the age at the diagnosis; all others were regarded as having type II diabetes. In this population, initially ages 35 to 54 years, the incidence of myocardial infarction over a mean follow-up duration of 8.33 years was 17 per 1,000 person-years in the type I cohort and 19 per 1,000 person-years in the type II cohort. Among type I diabetic subjects the rates were similar in men and women, whereas among type II diabetic subjects the incidence was significantly higher in men, a pattern suggesting loss of the sex differential in CHD mortality among type I, but not type II, diabetic subjects. This pattern is at variance with other studies that report that the attenuated sex difference occurs in type II diabetes.[12–15] In the type I diabetes cohort, the risk of CHD was associated with smoking, hypertension, and duration of diabetes. Although, in this cohort, proteinuria predicted the risk of CHD only in the type II diabetic group, in patients from the Steno Hospital in Denmark it predicted CHD incidence in type I diabetics as well.[24]

Although the London study offered no comparison with a nondiabetic population, the Nurses' Health Study[16] reported the relative risk of combined fatal and nonfatal CHD in middle-aged women with diabetes compared to those without diabetes. The relative risk for type I diabetes was nearly twice that for type II and 12 times higher (95% CI, range 6 to 25) than in nondiabetic women; for type II women the risk was 7 times higher (95% CI, range 5 to 8) than in nondiabetic women. Clearly, more incidence studies are needed in the area of type I diabetes complications. Future studies should relate their findings to the patterns of CHD in the general population or, ideally, include an internal control group.

Silent Ischemia

Asymptomatic myocardial ischemia (ie, a major Q wave without a history of infarction or a positive stress test without anginal pain) is as frequent in type I diabetes subjects as clinically recognized CHD.[12] In a clinic series of 72 otherwise healthy, asymptomatic type I and 64 type II diabetic patients, ages 35 to 60 years, 24% and 36%, respectively, had ischemic changes after exercise or during 24-hour Holter monitoring or by dynamic thallium scintigraphy.[25] Significant CHD by angiography (over 50% narrowing of the arterial lumen) was found in 10% and 8%, respectively, compared to 1.3% of control subjects matched for age and sex. Much remains to be learned concerning the causes of silent myocardial ischemia in diabetics. Autonomic neuropathy is likely to play an important role in the pathophysiology, because it is associated both with a raised anginal perceptual threshold[26] and with a classic CHD risk profile (hypertension, elevated low-density lipoprotein [LDL] cholesterol, and decreased high-density lipoprotein [HDL] cholesterol[27]).

Insulin Resistance

Decreased insulin sensitivity has been proposed as a significant independent CHD risk factor in nondiabetic individuals and in those with type II diabetes.[7,28–30] The natural history of insulin resistance and its atherogenic potential has been less well studied in type I diabetes subjects. In this type of diabetes, insulin resistance appears to increase during periods of poor or average glycemic control and decrease during clinical remission[31] or intensive insulin treatment.[32] An 18-year follow-up of 51 type I diabetic patients suggested that the baseline insulin sensitivity was reproducible over the study period and significantly inversely related to the risk of cardiovascular death.[33] Thus, although the cause of insulin resistance associated with type I diabetes appears to differ from the cause of that associated with type II diabetes, its atherogenic effect may be comparable.

Ethnic Differences

There are major ethnic and international differences in the all-cause[34,35] and cause-specific[11] mortality among people with type I diabetes. It remains to be established how much of this variation is due to ethnic variability in the risk of CHD in the general populations (eg, lower CHD mortality in Japan than in Finland or the United States),[11] and how much of it results from competing causes of death or differential access to specialized health care.

Stroke

Mortality

In the three studies of insulin-treated diabetics reviewed by Jarrett,[6] mortality rates from stroke were 1.6 times higher in men and 1.4 to 2.4 times higher in women than in the general population. The Wisconsin Epidemiologic Study of Diabetic Retinopathy has found a 4.1 times higher age- and sex-standardized mortality (95% CI, range 0.8 to 11.8) for stroke in type I diabetic patients compared to a 2.0 times higher (95% CI, range 1.6 to 2.5) risk in type II diabetic patients.[15]

Incidence

The incidence of fatal and nonfatal stroke in the Nurses' Health Study cohort[16] has been reported to be ten times higher (95% CI, range 4 to 25) in women with type I diabetes and four times higher (95% CI, range 7 to 10) in women with type II diabetes than in nondiabetic women. Therefore, as in the case of CHD, the risk of cerebrovascular disease shows a greater increase in subjects with type I diabetes compared to the general population than among patients with type II diabetes.

Peripheral Vascular Disease

Prevalence

The prevalence of peripheral vascular disease (PVD) as judged by ankle–arm blood pressure ratios and/or Doppler velocimetry in a population of type I diabetic subjects with a mean duration of diabetes of 16 years has been reported to be 26% in males and 22% in females.[36] A more recent study[37] found similar rates of PVD as defined by ankle–arm blood pressure ratios at a similar point in the course of type I diabetes (ie, 34% and 26% in men and women, respectively). However, after 30 years of type I diabetes, the prevalence was significantly lower in men (11%) than in women (34%), probably reflecting increased mortality of men with PVD.

Incidence

Little is known about the incidence of PVD in type I diabetes.[38] The Wisconsin Epidemiology Study of Diabetic Retinopathy[39] has reported the incidence of lower extremity amputations in type I diabetics (diagnosis under 30 years of age and on insulin treatment) and in those with type II diabetes (diagnosis over 30 years of age). Age, history of lower extremity sores and ulcers, diastolic blood pressure, glycosylated hemoglobin, retinopathy, and smoking were significantly associated with the risk of amputation in the type I patients. In the type II patients, significant associations were found with history of lower extremity sores and ulcers, proteinuria, glycosylated hemoglobin, male gender, and duration of diabetes. The unadjusted 4-year incidence of amputations was 2.2% in both groups. However, in an earlier report from this study,[15] the prevalence of sores or ulcers on the feet or ankles after the age of 35 years was two times higher in type I patients than in type II patients, suggesting a higher incidence of clinical PVD in the former.

Non-Insulin-Dependent Diabetes Mellitus

Coronary Heart Disease

Mortality

Several studies have shown an increase in mortality in diabetic subjects. In the first National Health and Nutrition Examination Survey follow-up study (NHANES I), mortality in diabetic subjects was more than double the mortality observed in nondiabetic subjects.[40] The proportion of deaths due to cardiovascular disease in the NHANES I study was greater in diabetic than in nondiabetic subjects. The Framingham, Rancho Bernado, Evans County, Bedford, Joslin Clinic, and Israeli Heart studies have all reported a disproportionate impact of coronary heart disease in diabetic women compared with diabetic men, leading to the suggestion that diabetes eliminates or at least attenuates the well-known protection against ischemic heart disease normally enjoyed by women.[41-47] In contrast, data from the WHO showed persistent protection in diabetic women, who experienced only half as much cardiovascular mortality as diabetic men.[34] Finally, the Tecumseh study[48] and the NHANES I follow-up study[40] also found little attenutation of the sex difference in cardiovascular mortality among diabetic subjects. In the latter studies, the relative excess of cardiovascular mortality in diabetic versus nondiabetic subjects was essentially the same in both sexes.

Studies published prior to 1985 concerning CHD mortality in diabetic populations consisting exclusively or predominantly of type II diabetic patients have been reviewed elsewhere.[49] These studies show a 1.2 to 3.0-fold increase in CHD mortality in type II diabetics compared to the generally population. Table 13.1 presents mortality data from more recently published studies.[12,17,40,48,50-54] Although the definitions of both diabetes and fatal CHD varied in these studies, the data are likely to be reasonably representative of the incidence of fatal myocardial infarction among type II diabetic subjects. The excess CHD risk ratio

Table 13.1 Age-Adjusted Mortality (Per 1,000 Person-Years of Follow-Up) Due to Coronary Heart Disease (CHD) or Cardiovascular Disease (CVD) by Diabetes Status and Gender in Selected Populations

Population/Gender	Age Range (Years)	End Point	Nondiabetics	Diabetics	Risk Ratio
NHANES I[40] (NHW)[a]	40–77	Fatal CHD			
Men			10.2	28.4	2.8
Women			4.1	10.5	2.5
Tecumseh, MI[48]	40+	Fatal CHD			
Men			13.3	40.3	3.0
Women			5.9	17.8	3.0
Chicago, IL[50]	35–64	Fatal CHD			
Men			23.7	111.5	4.0
Women			3.6	30.8	5.9
Framingham[12] (NHW)	50–79	Fatal CHD			
Men			5.7	16.0	2.8
Women			2.6	11.6	4.5
Pima Indians[17]	50–79	Fatal CHD			
Men			0	10.9	—
Women			0	3.0	—
Naurans[51]	20+	Fatal CHD (crude)			
Men			2.4	7.3	3.0
Women			0.4	6.2	15.5
Paris, France[52]	43–54	Fatal CHD			
Men			1.4^b	2.9^d	2.1
			2.7^c	4.2^e	3.0
Whitehall (London)[53]	40–64	Fatal CHD			
Men			4.7^b	28.1^d	3.9
			6.7^c	$9.9–12.2^f$	1.9–2.6
Wisconsin[15]	67 ± 12 (SD)	Fatal CHD			
Men					2.4
Women					2.2
Rancho Bernardo, CA[54]	40–79	Fatal CHD			
Men					2.4
Women					3.5

[a] NHW = non-Hispanic white.
[b] Normal glucose tolerance.
[c] Impaired glucose tolerance.
[d] Newly diagnosed diabetes.
[e] Known diabetes.
[f] Known diabetes of duration between 2 and 7 years.

in diabetics compared to the general population has been consistently estimated to be between 2 and 4 in both sexes, except for the Pima Indians[17] and Naurans.[51] In these two noncaucasian populations, CHD was absent or rare among nondiabetics, which resulted in extremely high relative risks for diabetics. When standard criteria were applied, CHD mortality among diabetic Pima men and women was only 68% and 26% as high as in Framingham men and women, respectively.[17] Some studies have reported a greater increase in CHD mortality among women with type II diabetes than among men, but this phenomenon is less consistently reported in type I diabetes. The Paris Prospective Study[52] and the Whitehall Study[53] have found an increased CHD mortality in men with impaired glucose tolerance—a 1.9- and a 1.4-fold increase, respectively. The former study suggested that the risk is somewhat higher among known diabetics than among those with diabetes newly diagnosed by glucose tolerance testing, whereas the Whitehall Study showed no difference between these two groups.

Incidence

Relatively little information is available on the incidence of CHD in diabetic versus nondiabetic subjects. The incidence of all new CHD events in diabetic men and women was 1.6 and 2.1 times greater, respectively, than in nondiabetic subjects in the 18-year follow-up of the Framingham study.[55] The incidence of myocardial infarction, including both fatal and nonfatal infarctions, was 1.5 times higher in male diabetics and 2.6 times higher in female diabetics than in nondiabetic men and women, respectively. The corresponding risk ratios for angina pectoris were 1.6 and 1.9, and those for sudden death were 1.4 and 3.0. The Framingham investigators also considered the problem of "silent" myocardial infarctions. The proportion of myocardial infarctions that were clinically unrecognized, as defined by the appearance of diagnostic electrocardiographic (ECG) abnormalities at biannual examinations in subjects who had not been hospitalized for a heart attack, was found to be almost twice as high in diabetics as in nondiabetics (39% versus 22%) when both sexes were considered together.[56] The excess of "silent" myocardial infarctions in diabetic subjects is especially striking when one considers that diabetic subjects are more likely to visit a physician than nondiabetic subjects. The incidence of myocardial infarction (by ECG) was 1.5 times higher in previously diagnosed diabetic subjects and 1.4 times higher in newly diagnosed diabetic subjects than in nondiabetic subjects in the Israeli Heart Study.[46] The incidence of angina pectoris was 3.2 times higher in previously known diabetic subjects than in nondiabetic subjects.[46]

Evidence from the Joslin Clinic suggests that CHD may account for a smaller proportion of overall mortality in type I than in type II diabetes. In diabetic subjects diagnosed before the age of 20 years, the predominant cause of death was diabetic nephropathy, whereas in those in whom the onset of diabetes occurred after the age of 20 years, the predominant cause of death was cardiac.[2] However, more recent data from the Joslin Clinic indicate that, for subjects with type I disease, those with chronic renal failure have a 100-fold excess of CHD relative to a control population (Framingham), whereas those without chronic renal failure have only a two- to fourfold excess of CHD.[12]

Table 13.2 summarizes studies on the incidence of CHD among type II diabetic subjects.[16,57–62] Only the San Luis Valley Diabetes Study in Colorado[58] and the Finnish study[59] used the WHO definition for type II diabetes. These two studies found a greater excess of myocardial infarction incidence in type II diabetic men than women. Although Mexican Americans are a hybrid population with significant Native American genetic admixture, the incidence of myocardial infarction among nondiabetics was at least as high as it was among non-Hispanic whites, in contrast to the rarity of CHD in nondiabetic Pima Indians.[17] More incidence data are needed concerning CHD risk in type II diabetic subjects from noncaucasian populations, such as Hispanics, Native Americans, and African-Americans, to evaluate potentially important ethnic differences in the risk.

Table 13.2. Age-Adjusted Incidence (Per 1,000 Person-Years of Follow-Up) of Fatal and Nonfatal Coronary Events, by Diabetes Status and Gender in Selected Populations

Population/Gender	Age Range (Years)	Endpoint	Nondiabetics	Diabetics	Risk Ratio
Framingham[57] (NHW)[a]	45+	Total CHD			
Men			15	25	1.7
Women			7	18	2.6
Colorado[58] (NHW)	25–74	Total MI			
Men			14	66	4.7
Women			6	20	3.3
Colorado[58] (Hispanics)	25–74	Total MI			
Men			16	12	0.8
Women			10	13	1.3
Kuopio, Finland[59]	45–64	Total MI			
Men			6.4	39	6.1
Women			6.0	22	3.7
Gothenburg, Sweden		Total MI			
Men[60]	51–59				2.8
Women[61]	38–60				9.4
Rochester, MN[62] (NHW)	30+	Total MI			
Men					2.4
Women					4.7
US nurses[16] (NHW)	30–55	Total MI			
Women					6.7

[a] NHW = Non-Hispanic white.

Stroke

Kuller et al[63] reviewed reports published prior to 1985 concerning the risk of stroke in diabetic subjects. Table 13.3 supplements that review by summarizing more recent publications.[15,16,51,57,60,64–68] As with CHD, the risk of stroke, especially of thromboembolic stroke, is increased two- to fivefold among adults with diabetes, predominantly type II. The excess risk for females, if any, is even less impressive than in the case of CHD. The excess risk associated with diabetes appears to be similar in non-Hispanic whites, Japanese Americans,[65] and African-Americans.[66] Two European studies have suggested little difference in the risk of stroke between men with impaired glucose tolerance and men with type II diabetes.[67,68]

Peripheral Vascular Disease

The Framingham Study[69] has reported a higher age-adjusted incidence of intermittent claudication in diabetic men and women (12.6 and 8.4 per 1,000 over 20 years, respectively) compared to nondiabetic men and women (3.3 and 1.3, respectively). Using more current definitions (ie, a combination of the ankle–arm systolic blood pressure index and Doppler arterial velocity waveform analysis), the prevalence of PVD has been found to be higher in type II diabetic patients than in control subjects (22% versus 3%).[70] Over a 2-year follow-up period, the disease progressed in 87% of those with PVD at baseline and developed de novo in 14%. A study of predominantly type II patients from the

Table 13.3. Age-Adjusted Stroke Mortality or Incidence (Per 1,000 Person-Years of Follow-Up) by Diabetes Status and Gender in Selected Populations

Population/Gender	Age Range (Years)	Endpoint	Nondiabetics	Diabetics	Risk Ratio
Framingham[57] (NHW)[a]	45–74	Total ABI			
Men			1.9	4.7	2.5
Women			1.7	6.2	3.6
Rancho Bernardo, CA[64]	50–79	Total stroke			
Men			5.3	7.8	1.8
Women			4.4	8.8	2.2
Honolulu, HI[65]	45–69	Total stroke	2.7	5.2	1.9
(Japanese-Americans)		Thromboembolic stroke	1.7	3.7	2.0
Men					
Naurans[51]	20+	Total stroke (crude)			
Men			2.4	8.7	3.6
Women			1.2	1.2	1.0
NHANES I[66] (NHW)	35–74	Total stroke			
Men					2.5
Women					2.5
NHANES I[66] (blacks)	35–74	Total stroke			
Men					2.5
Women					2.4
US nurses[16] (NHW)	30–55	Total stroke			4.1
Women		Ischemic stroke			5.4
Gothenburg, Sweden[60]	51–59	Total stroke			
Men					2.7
Wisconsin[15]	67 ± 12 (SD)	Fatal stroke			
Men					1.8
Women					2.2
Paris, France[67]	43–54	Fatal stroke			2.2[a]
Men					2.5[b]
Whitehall (London)[68]	40–64	Fatal stroke			
Men					3.9[a]
					3.2[b]

Abbreviations: NHW = non-Hispanic white, ABI = atherothrombotic brain infarction.

[a] Diabetics compared to subjects with normal glucose tolerance.

[b] Subjects with impaired glucose tolerance compared to subjects with normal glucose tolerance.

Mayo Clinic[71] found a 4-year PVD incidence of 9% in diabetics compared to 1% in controls using a postexercise ankle–arm systolic blood pressure index. However, progression of the disease was similar in diabetic and nondiabetic subjects. Given the wide availability of Doppler equipment, more population-based data on the incidence of PVD in type II diabetes can be expected in the near future.

Atherosclerosis in Diabetes Mellitus

Although diabetic subjects have an excess risk of CHD relative to nondiabetic subjects even after adjustment for conventional risk factors,[41] it seems reasonable that increased atherosclerosis may be responsible for much of the excess risk in diabetic subjects. It should be noted that most epidemiologic studies of diabetes have considered only the classic risk factors, and not such risk factors as HDL, qualitative differences in lipoprotein composition, and lipoprotein (a)

(Lp[a]), which may influence the risk of CHD independently of the classic risk factors. A recent review by Schwartz et al[72] summarized the status of these nontraditional risk factors. In addition, abnormalities in cardiac muscle may partially explain the increased risk of congestive heart failure in diabetic subjects.[73-75]

Several autopsy studies have compared atherosclerosis in diabetic and nondiabetic subjects. The International Atherosclerosis Project examined 23,000 subjects in 14 countries.[76] Diabetes in older subjects was associated with an increase in fatty streaks, fibrous lesions, and complicated lesions. No analysis was made of the association between degree of atherosclerosis and type, duration, or severity of diabetes. In general, the extent of atherosclerosis in diabetic subjects tracked the extent of atherosclerosis in nondiabetic subjects from the same country. (This observation parallels the observation from the WHO study in that the prevalence of myocardial infarction in diabetic subjects followed the prevalence of myocardial infarction in nondiabetic subjects from the same country.[77]) However, even in populations at low risk for atherosclerosis, diabetic subjects had increased atherosclerosis relative to nondiabetic subjects. Kagan et al also showed an increase in atherosclerosis in diabetic subjects in an autopsy study.[78] In addition, subjects with hypertension and diabetes had increased atherosclerosis compared to diabetic subjects without hypertension.

Waller et al, in a study from the Mayo Clinic, showed that diabetic subjects had more severe narrowing of the left main coronary artery than age- and sex-matched nondiabetic subjects.[79] Among subjects with diabetes of greater than 5 years' duration, there was no association between duration of diabetes and the degree of atherosclerosis. Vigorita et al showed that diabetic subjects had greater coronary atherosclerosis, a greater number of major coronary vessels involved, and a greater diffuseness in the distribution of atherosclerotic lesions than age- and sex-matched controls.[80] In addition, neither the severity of diabetes nor its duration was related to the extent of atherosclerosis. In a small group of juvenile-onset diabetic subjects ($n = 9$), Crall and Roberts found an increase in atherosclerosis compared to nondiabetic age- and sex-matched control subjects. The diabetic subjects had more severe narrowing of the epicardial arteries than did the nondiabetic subjects.[81] Three angiography studies also have found diffuse atherosclerosis in diabetic subjects.[82-84]

In conclusion, diabetic subjects have more severe atherosclerosis than age- and sex-matched nondiabetic subjects. Although data are limited, there is little evidence that the duration of diabetes or the severity of glycemia is related to the severity of atherosclerosis in diabetic subjects.

Risk Factors for Coronary Heart Disease in Diabetics

Hyperlipidemia

The characteristic pattern of dyslipidemia in type II diabetes consists of hypertriglyceridemia and low HDL cholesterol.[85-95] Although the same pattern occurs in obesity, the greater degree of obesity typical of diabetic subjects does not fully account for their excess dyslipidemia.[88-91] Neither is it accounted for by differences between diabetic and nondiabetic subjects in various behavioral factors that influence dyslipidemia (eg, cigarette smoking, alcohol consumption, and physical activity[90,91]) Table 13.4 shows dyslipidemia prevalence data from

Table 13.4. Prevalence of Dyslipidemia (%) in Diabetic and Nondiabetic Subjects (Framingham Heart Study)

	Men		Women	
	Nondiabetic	Diabetic	Nondiabetic	Diabetic
Hypercholesterolemia				
>6.7 mmol/L in men	14	13	21	24
>7.1 mmol/L in women				
Hypertriglyceridemia				
>2.7 mmol/L in men	9	19[a]	8	17[a]
>2.3 mmol/L in women				
Low HDL cholesterol				
<0.8 mmol/L in men	12	21[a]	10	25[a]
<1.0 mmol/L in women				

(Reproduced, by permission, from Wilson PWF, Kannel WB, Anderson KM: Lipids, glucose intolerance and vascular disease: The Framingham Study. Monogr Atheroscler 1985;13:1–11.)

[a] $p < .05$.

the Framingham study that are typical.[85] In this study, the prevalence of hypercholesterolemia was similar in diabetic and nondiabetic subjects. The prevalence of hypertriglyceridemia, in contrast, was approximately doubled in the diabetic subjects, as was the prevalence of low HDL cholesterol.

The San Antonio Heart Study evaluated the number of diabetic subjects who met the National Cholesterol Education Program criteria[96] for high risk. These guidelines primarily reflect LDL cholesterol. Diabetic women, although not diabetic men, were significantly more likely to exceed these guidelines than nondiabetic subjects[97] (Table 13.5).

Walden et al[94] reported that the adverse effect of diabetes on dyslipidemia was more marked in women than men and proposed that this phenomenon might explain why diabetes eliminates or attenuates a woman's protection against ischemic heart disease. Data from the San Antonio Heart Study also demonstrate a more adverse impact of diabetes on the lipid profiles of women than of men (Table 13.5).[98] Although similar findings (ie, greater in women than in men) have been reported in other studies,[87,91] this has not been reported in all studies.[92,93]

In addition to quantitative changes, diabetic subjects may have qualitative changes in lipid and lipoprotein composition that may affect their atherogenicity. This topic has been discussed in a recent editorial.[99] For example, Biesbroeck et al[100] have shown that HDL particles from type II diabetic subjects are rich in triglyceride and poor in cholesterol, suggesting that the decrease in HDL cholesterol characteristically seen in diabetic patients is predominantly due to a reduction in the amount of cholesterol per particle rather than to a reduction in the number of particles. In addition, apolipoprotein (apo) A-I is decreased relative to apo A-II in type II diabetic subjects.[100] Because HDL_2 (the HDL subfraction thought to be more protective against CHD) has relatively more apo A-I than A-II, the decrease in total HDL may underestimate the true atherogenic potential associated with the diabetic state.[100] Taskinen et al[101] found that, although intensive insulin therapy markedly decreased the concentration of VLDL, it had only a minor effect on total HDL. However, when these investigators examined the effects of insulin therapy on the principal subfractions of HDL, they observed that HDL_2 increased by 21%, whereas HDL_3 decreased by 13%.

Table 13.5 Age-Adjusted Prevalence (%) of Dyslipidemia in Noninsulin-Dependent Diabetic and Nondiabetic Subjects (San Antonio Heart Study)

	Mexican Americans			Non-Hispanic Whites		
	Prevalence			Prevalence		
	Nondiabetic	*Diabetic*	Ratio	*Nondiabetic*	*Diabetic*	Ratio
Men						
Total cholesterol >6.2 mmol/L	21.3	21.8	1.02	21.2	25.2	1.19
Triglycerides >2.8 mmol/L	15.4	29.8	1.91[a]	14.0	25.5	1.82
HDL cholesterol <0.9 mmol/L	24.1	37.8	1.56[a]	23.1	45.9	1.99[b]
National Cholesterol Education Program criteria	48.3	53.4	1.11	46.4	54.4	1.17
Women						
Total cholesterol >6.2 mmol/L	20.2	29.3	1.45[b]	22.9	24.1	1.05
Triglycerides >2.8 mmol/L	6.5	20.6	3.17[a]	5.6	16.9	3.02[b]
HDL cholesterol <0.9 mmol/L	8.0	21.6	2.70[a]	4.6	17.5	3.80[b]
National Cholesterol Education Program criteria	24.9	45.6	1.83[a]	26.0	43.7	1.68[c]

(Adapted from Stern MP, Haffner SM: Dyslipidemia in type II diabetes. Implication for therapeutic intervention. Diabetes Care 1991;14:1144–1159.)

[a] $p < .001$, diabetic versus nondiabetic.

[b] $p < .01$, diabetic versus nondiabetic.

[c] $p < .05$, diabetic versus nondiabetic.

Thus, the benefits of insulin therapy may be underestimated if only its effect on total HDL is monitored.

LDL composition may also be altered in type II diabetes. Polydispersion of LDL particle size has been reported in association with hypertriglyceridemia in both diabetic and nondiabetic subjects.[102,103] In nondiabetic hypertriglyceridemic subjects, polydispersion is associated with increased numbers of small, dense LDL particles, which are thought to be more atherogenic than normal LDL particles.[104] Increased glycosylation of LDL is also characteristic of the diabetic state, although this modification of LDL has not been shown to increase coronary risk, either in diabetic or in nondiabetic subjects.[105] Oxidized LDL, by comparison, may increase the risk of CHD because it is believed to be more atherogenic than native LDL.[106] Increased peroxidation of LDL, which may reflect increased oxidation, has been described in diabetic subjects.[107] Although it is apparent why glycosylated LDL would be elevated in diabetic subjects, it is less clear why oxidized LDL would also be elevated. A possible mechanism is suggested by the data of Steinbrecher and Witztum,[108] which indicated that glycosylation of LDL may slow its removal via the LDL–apo B-100 receptor pathway. Such slowing could allow more time for oxidization to take place. Thus far, however, no study has examined whether concentrations of glycosylated and oxidized LDL are correlated in diabetic subjects or whether glycosylation of LDL predisposes it to oxidation.

Elevations in the free cholesterol–lecithin ratio have also been described in diabetic subjects, a change that in nondiabetic subjects has been shown to be a strong predictor of CHD, comparable in effect to LDL cholesterol.[109] Fielding et al[110] and Bagdade et al[111] have shown that, in diabetic subjects, VLDL is enriched with free cholesterol and also that the free cholesterol–lecithin ratio is increased in subjects whose triglyceride concentrations are elevated. These changes are not reversed by improved metabolic control achieved by intensive insulin therapy.[111] Recently, Lane et al[112] described a compositional change in normolipidemic diabetic subjects, specifically, an increase in the free cholesterol–lecithin ratio of the HDL_2 subfraction. The mechanisms whereby changes in the composition of surface and core lipids could enhance atherosclerotic risk are obscure but may relate to the ability of HDL to exchange cholesteryl ester with other lipoproteins and to transport free cholesterol from cell membranes to circulating lipoproteins.[113]

Recent data have suggested that in nondiabetic subjects Lp(a) is a strong independent risk factor for CHD.[114] However, few data are available on Lp(a) concentrations in patients with type II diabetes. Schernthaner et al[115] found no difference in mean or median Lp(a) concentrations between diabetic and non-diabetic subjects. However, 14% of diabetic subjects had Lp(a) concentrations greater than 20 mg/dL, compared with only 5% of control subjects. No distinction was made between type I and type II diabetes in this study. Arauz et al[116] found in type I subjects that the concentration of Lp(a) correlated with glycosylated hemoglobin level, but a corresponding correlation was not seen in type II diabetic subjects. This pattern is concordant with the results of several studies that have reported declines in Lp(a) concentration after improved glycemic control in type I diabetic patients[117–119] but not in type II diabetic patients.[120,121] However, in one study of improved glucose control in type II diabetic subjects using both oral agents and insulin, lower Lp(a) concentrations were seen in the intensively controlled group.[122] Lp(a) levels were not elevated in type II diabetics compared to normoglycemic controls in two studies.[121,123] Lp(a) is increased in type I diabetic subjects with microalbuminuria[124] or with chronic renal failure.[125] Few data are available on whether Lp(a) is related to CHD in diabetic subjects, but in one small study of types I and II diabetic subjects, Lp(a) levels were not higher in subjects who died of CHD than in those who remained alive 4 years later.[126] The mechanism whereby Lp(a) might increase the risk of CHD is unknown, but because apo (a) shares homology with plasminogen,[127] Lp(a) could provide a link between the lipoprotein and clotting pathways. Further studies are needed to establish whether Lp(a) is a risk factor for coronary heart disease in diabetic subjects.

The risk of macrovascular complications in diabetics is related to classic cardiovascular risk factors, including lipids and lipoproteins. For example, major Q waves were associated with cholesterol and triglyceride concentrations and also with systolic blood pressure in diabetic subjects examined in the WHO Multinational Study[128] (Table 13.6). These data are cross-sectional, but prospective data from the Framingham Study confirm that the same risk factors that influence cardiovascular disease in nondiabetic subjects (ie, cholesterol, triglyceride, systolic blood pressure, etc) also operate in diabetic subjects.[129] Additional prospective data on 5,245 diabetic subjects who participated in

Table 13.6 Risk Factors for Ischemic Heart Disease
in Diabetic Subjects (WHO Multinational Study)

Risk Factor	Percentage with Major Q Wave Abnormalities (%)
Plasma glucose (mmol/L)	
<8.3	5.3
8.3–13.8	4.7
>13.8	5.2
p value	NS
Duration (yr)	
<7	4.8
7–14	5.2
>15	5.1
p value	NS
Cholesterol (mmol/L)	
<5.2	4.6
5.2–7.2	4.8
>7.2	8.0
p value	<.05
Triglyceride (mmol/L)	
<1.1	4.5
1.1–2.8	5.6
>2.8	10.2
p value	<.01
Systolic blood pressure (mm Hg)	
<120	3.0
120–149	4.6
>150	7.1
p value	<.001

(Adapted from West KM, Ahuja MMS, Bennett PH, et al: The role of circulating glucose and triglyceride concentrations and their interactions with other "risk factors" as determinants of arterial disease in nine diabetic population samples from the WHO Multinational Study. Diabetes Care 1983;6:361–369.)

screening for the Multiple Risk Factor Intervention Trial further confirm that serum cholesterol, blood pressure, and cigarette smoking are independent risk factors for coronary and cardiovascular mortality among diabetic subjects.[130] At any given level of these risk factors, the risk in diabetic subjects was markedly higher than in nondiabetic subjects, indicating that diabetes itself confers additional risk. However, among diabetic subjects the traditional risk factors operated in essentially the same way as they did in the nondiabetic population.

Although the role of triglyceride concentrations as a cardiovascular risk factor has been challenged by Hulley et al,[131] considerable data suggest that they may be a risk factor in diabetic subjects. This is of importance in the present context, because hypertriglyceridemia is the characteristic lipid abnormality of diabetic subjects (Tables 13.4 and 13.5). The fundamental criticism made by Hulley et al was that, whereas triglyceride can be shown to be a univariate predictor of coronary disease, in most cases its predictive effect is no longer statistically significant once other cardiovascular risk factors are taken into account with multivariate analyses. It is fair to ask whether this limitation extends to diabetic subjects. Although the analyses presented in Table 13.6 are univariate,[128] multivariate analyses were also carried out in the WHO Multinational Study. In these analyses, serum triglyceride concentration remained significantly associated with major Q wave abnormalities even after controlling for other risk factors.[128] In contrast, cholesterol ceased to be statistically significant in multivariate analyses in diabetics.[128] Thus, the results suggested that, for diabetic subjects, triglyceride could be a more important cardiovascular risk factor than cholesterol. The WHO Multinational Study, however, was cross-sectional. Recent prospective data from the Paris Prospective Study tend further to rehabilitate triglyceride as an independent cardiovascular risk factor among diabetic subjects.[52] In this study, 943 middle-aged men with either impaired glucose tolerance or diabetes were followed for 11 years. Cholesterol, triglyceride, and fasting and 2-hour insulin levels were all significant univariate predictors of CHD mortality, but only triglyceride was a significant predictor in multivariate analyses. Thus, triglyceride again emerged as a stronger predictor of coronary mortality than cholesterol in these diabetic subjects. The authors expressed the view that this powerful effect of triglyceride may be relatively unique to glucose-intolerant subjects because, in their overall population (ie, nondiabetic subjects included), triglyceride ceased to be significantly predictive in multivariate analyses, just as in other studies of the general population. It is unfortunate that HDL data were not reported from the Paris Prospective Study, because it would be of interest to know whether triglyceride remains independently predictive once the effect of HDL is taken into account.

Glycemia and Diabetes Duration

There is a large body of literature suggesting that degree and duration of hyperglycemia are the principal risk factors for the microvascular complications of diabetes.[77,132–135] These, however, are not the principal risk factors for macrovascular complications. In the WHO Multinational Study,[128] no relationship was found between either plasma glucose concentration or diabetes duration and major Q wave abnormalities (Table 13.6). Similarly, in a population-based study of type I and type II diabetic subjects in Denmark, Nielsen and Ditzel[136] found no association between glycosylated hemoglobin levels and the prevalence of macrovascular complications, although they did confirm that diabetic control was correlated with diabetic retinopathy. The two studies just cited are cross-sectional, but prospective studies have also failed to uncover an association between the duration of clinical diabetes (ie, the duration of hyperglycemia) and macrovascular complications.[46,137] Also, in the London cohort of the WHO Multinational Study, which was followed prospectively, no effect of diabetes duration on cardiovascular mortality was observed among type II diabetic subjects.[14]

Hypertension

An excellent review of diabetes and hypertension has recently appeared.[138] Christieb et al, in a study from the Joslin Clinic, reported that blood pressure was higher in diabetic subjects than in normal subjects from the Framingham Study.[139] In this study, the onset of hypertension occurred in the same decade of life as the development of renal disease, suggesting that the hypertension could have been a consequence of the renal failure.

Several studies have shown an increase in hypertension in type II diabetic subjects.[75,140-144] The relationship of duration of diabetes to hypertension is disputed, with some studies showing a positive association[75] and other studies no association.[144] Impaired glucose tolerance also appears to be associated with an increased prevalence of hypertension.[47,143,145]

Few prospective data are available on the relationship of blood pressure to the incidence of cardiovascular disease in diabetic subjects. However, hypertension is related to cardiovascular mortality in both type I[146] and type II[57,130] subjects.

Hyperinsulinemia and Insulin Resistance

Several prospective studies have shown that insulin concentrations predict the incidence of cardiovascular disease in the general population.[28-30] Laakso et al[147] have recently shown that insulin resistance (as measured by the euglycemia clamp technique) is related to carotid and femoral atherosclerosis. The available data in diabetic subjects are less convincing. In cross-sectional studies, insulinemia has been associated with ECG abnormalities.[75,148-151] In addition, Standl and Janka have shown a relationship between fasting C-peptide levels and peripheral vascular disease.[152]

Hyperinsulinemia and/or insulin resistance could be associated with CHD either by a direct effect on the arterial wall or through its effect on other risk factors such as lipids or blood pressure. Stout has recently reviewed the area of insulin and atherosclerosis.[7] Stout et al[153] and Pfeifle and Ditschuneit[154] have shown that insulin may have a direct effect on the arterial wall. Many investigators have shown cross-sectional relationships between hyperinsulinemia and several cardiovascular risk factors, including lipids and lipoproteins[155-157] and blood pressure.[143,157,158] It is not certain whether hyperinsulinemia or insulin resistance is more important, although, in a few studies, insulin resistance was more closely related to lipid and lipoprotein abnormalities than were insulin concentrations.[159-161] Reaven has used the term "syndrome X" to refer to the cluster of insulin resistance, cardiovascular risk factors, and coronary artery disease.[162] Although there is considerable evidence to support such a cluster (see also the section on prediabetics, below), recent data have suggested weaker relationships. For instance, Saad et al have described an association between blood pressure and insulin sensitivity in caucasians, but not in blacks or Pima Indians.[163]

Cardiovascular Risk Factors in Prediabetic Subjects

A possible explanation for the lack of association between severity and duration of hyperglycemia and risk of macrovascular complications is that the latter are influenced by the metabolic derangements that precede diabetes—that is, those that are present during the prediabetic phase. Prospective data from a number of epidemiologic studies,[164,165] including the San Antonio Heart Study,[166] have established that a prolonged period (perhaps decades) of hyperinsulinemia precedes the onset of clinical diabetes. This hyperinsulinemia is presumed to be a compensatory response to insulin resistance, which is also characteristic of the prediabetic phase. Moreover, prospective studies in both whites[167] and Pima Indians[168] have shown that insulin resistance can predict the later occurrence of type II diabetes.

As already noted above, there is a considerable body of evidence suggesting that hyperinsulinemia is a cardiovascular risk factor, both by virtue of its contributions to other established cardiovascular factors, specifically dyslipidemia and hypertension, and because of a possible direct atherogenic effect on the arterial wall.[7] Moreover, there is direct empirical evidence suggesting that serum insulin concentration is an independent risk factor for future cardiovascular disease.[28-30] These findings, combined with the fact that the prediabetic phase is characterized by hyperinsulinemia, suggest that prediabetic subjects should have an atherogenic pattern of risk factors. Indeed, this has been directly demonstrated in prediabetics identified retrospectively in prospective epidemiologic studies.[169-172] Because many prediabetic subjects have impaired glucose tolerance, and because impaired glucose tolerance is a condition that is known to be associated with an adverse pattern of cardiovascular risk factors, one could postulate that the excess of such risk factors observed in prediabetic subjects is entirely due to impaired glucose tolerance. However, in the San Antonio Heart Study, even after eliminating prediabetic subjects with impaired glucose tolerance, the remaining prediabetic subjects whose glucose tolerance was entirely normal had, in addition to hyperinsulinemia, an excess of other cardiovascular risk factors[172] (Table 13.7). Note that this excess was observed even though these normal glucose-tolerant prediabetic subjects were not overweight relative to individuals who maintained normal glucose tolerance throughout the follow-up period. We have summarized the above concepts using the "ticking clock" metaphor: in the case of microvascular complications, for which the principal risk factors are degree and duration of hyperglycemia, "the clock starts ticking" at the onset of clinical diabetes (ie, at the onset of hyperglycemia). In contrast, for macrovascular complications, in which insulin resistance with its concomitant metabolic derangements, including compensatory hyperinsulinemia, are important risk factors, "the clock starts ticking" years or even decades earlier in the prediabetic phase.

The above data suggest that the insulin resistance syndrome (syndrome X) may be important in the pathogenesis of CHD in type II diabetic subjects. Interestingly, we have recently shown that pre-*hypertensive* subjects also have

Table 13.7 Cardiovascular Risk Factors in Prediabetic Subjects With Normal Glucose Tolerance at Baseline (San Antonio Heart Study)

Risk Factor	Confirmed Prediabetic Subjects ($n = 18$)	Normal Subjects ($n = 490$)	p value
Total cholesterol (mmol/L)	5.79	5.48	$<.001$
HDL cholesterol (mmol/L)	1.14	1.29	.045
Triglyceride (mmol/L)	1.83	1.28	.006
Blood pressure (mm Hg)	117/76	109/72	$<.050$
Body mass index (kg/m^2)	28	27	.462
Subscapula-to-triceps skinfold ratio	1.38	1.16	.078
Fasting glucose (mmol/L)	5.28	5.00	.032
Two-hour glucose (mmol/L)	6.44	5.78	.011
Fasting insulin (pmol/L)	158	79	.006

(Reproduced, by permission, from Haffner SM, Stern MP, Hazuda HP, et al: Cardiovascular risk factors in confirmed prediabetics: Does the clock for coronary heart disease start ticking before the onset of clinical diabetes? JAMA 1990;263:2893–2898.)

decreased HDL cholesterol, increased triglyceride concentrations, and hyper-insulinemia prior to the onset of clinical hypertension.[173] The magnitude of hyperinsulinemia in prehypertensive subjects,[173] however, is much less than in prediabetic subjects,[172] perhaps because fasting insulin predicts the incidence of hypertension in lean individuals only. We have also shown that fasting insulin concentrations predict the incidence of multiple metabolic disorders, including low HDL cholesterol and elevated triglyceride levels.[174]

Conclusions

CHD is increased in both types I and II diabetic subjects. In type I diabetic subjects, the rate of CHD is particularly increased in subjects who have developed renal disease. In type II diabetic subjects, the increase in CHD is related neither to the duration of clinical diabetes nor to the extent of glycemia, suggesting that the increased risk may be due to the hyperinsulinemia and/or insulin resistance of the prediabetic state. Coronary risk in diabetic subjects appears to be related to the conventional risk factors for CHD (ie, lipids, lipoproteins, blood pressure, and cigarette smoking), and triglyceride levels are more closely related to CHD in diabetic than in nondiabetic subjects.

References

1. Center for Economic Studies in Medicine: *Direct and Indirect Cost of Diabetes in the United States in 1987*. Alexandria, VA, American Diabetes Association, 1988.
2. Marks HH, Krall LP: Onset, course, prognosis, and mortality in diabetes mellitus, in Marble A, White P, Bradley RF (eds): *Joslin's Diabetes Mellitus* ed 11. Philadelphia, Lea & Febiger, 1971, pp 227–228.
3. Pyörälä K, Laakso M, Uusitupa M: Diabetes and atherosclerosis: An epidemiologic view. *Diabetes* 1987;3:463–524.
4. Dunn FL: Hyperlipidemia in diabetes mellitus. *Diabetes* 1990;6:47–61.
5. Stern MP, Haffner SM: Dyslipidemia in type II diabetes: Implications for therapeutic intervention. *Diabetes Care* 1991;14:1144–1159.
6. Jarrett RJ: Cardiovascular disease and hypertension in diabetes mellitus. *Diabetes Metab Rev* 1989;5:547–558.
7. Stout RW: Insulin and atheroma: 20-yr perspective. *Diabetes Care* 1990;13:631–654.
8. Merrin PK, Feher MD, Elkeles RS: Diabetic macrovascular disease and serum lipids: Is there a connection? *Diabetes Med* 1992;9:914.
9. Barrett-Connor E, Orchard T: Diabetes and heart disease, in Harris MI, Hamman RF (eds): *Diabetes in America*, NIH publication No 85-1468. Bethesda, MD, National Institutes of Health, 1985, vol XVI, pp 1–41.
10. Dorman JS, LaPorte RE, Kuller LH, et al: The Pittsburgh insulin-dependent diabetes mellitus (IDDM) morbidity and mortality study. Mortality results. *Diabetes* 1984;33:271–276.
11. DERI Mortality Study Group: International evaluation of cause-specific mortality and IDDM. *Diabetes Care* 1991;14:55–60.
12. Królewski AS, Kosinski EJ, Warram JH, et al: Magnitude and determinants of coronary artery disease in juvenile-onset insulin-dependent diabetes mellitus. *Am J Cardiol* 1987;59:750–755.
13. Borch-Johnsen K, Kreiner S: Proteinuria: Value as predictor of cardiovascular mortality in insulin dependent diabetes mellitus. *BMJ* 1987;294:1651–1654.

14. Morrish NJ, Stevens LK, Head J, et al: A prospective study of mortality among middle-aged diabetic patients (the London cohort of the WHO Multinational Study of Vascular Disease in Diabetics) II: Associated risk factors. *Diabetologia* 1990;33:542–548.
15. Moss SE, Klein R, Klein BEK: Cause-specific mortality in a population-based study of diabetes. *Am J Public Health* 1991;81:1158–1162.
16. Manson JE, Colditz GA, Stampfer MJ, et al: A prospective study of maturity-onset diabetes mellitus and risk of coronary heart disease and stroke in women. *Arch Intern Med* 1991;151:1141–1147.
17. Nelson RG, Sievers ML, Knowler WC, et al: Low incidence of fatal coronary heart disease in Pima Indians despite high prevalence of non-insulin-dependent diabetes. *Circulation* 1990;81:987–995.
18. Schmitz A, Vaeth M: Microalbuminuria: A major risk factor in non-insulin-dependent diabetes. A 10-year follow-up study of 503 patients. *Diabetic Med* 1988;5:126–134.
19. Herman WH, Teutsch SM: Kidney diseases associated with diabetes, in Harris MI, Hamman RF (eds): *Diabetes in America*, NIH Publication no. 85-1468. Bethesda, MD, National Institute of Health, 1985, vol XIV, pp 1–31.
20. Jones SL, Close CF, Mattock MB, et al: Plasma lipid and coagulation factor concentrations in insulin dependent diabetics with microalbuminuria. *BMJ* 1989;298:487–490.
21. Orchard TJ, Dorman JS, Maser RE, et al: Factors associated with avoidance of severe complications after 25 yr of IDDM: Pittsburgh Epidemiology of Diabetes Complications Study I. *Diabetes Care* 1990;13:741–747.
22. Morrish NJ, Stevens LK, Fuller JH, et al: Incidence of macrovascular disease in diabetes mellitus: The London cohort of the WHO Multinational Study of Vascular Disease in Diabetics. *Diabetologia* 1991;34:584–589.
23. Morrish NJ, Stevens LK, Fuller JH, et al: Risk factors for macrovascular disease in diabetes mellitus: The London cohort of the WHO Multinational Study of Vascular Disease in Diabetics. *Diabetologia* 1991;34:590–594.
24. Jensen T, Borch-Johnsen K, Kofoed-Enevoldsen A, et al: Coronary heart disease in young type I (insulin-dependent) diabetic patients with and without diabetic neuropathy: Incidence and risk factors. *Diabetologia* 1987;30:144–148.
25. Koistinen MJ: Prevalence of asymptomatic myocardial ischemia in diabetic subjects. *BMJ* 1990;301:92–95.
26. Ambepityia G, Kopelman PG, Ingram D, et al: Exertional myocardial ischemia in diabetes: A quantitative analysis of anginal perceptual threshold and the influence of autonomic function. *J Am Coll Cardiol* 1990;15:72–77.
27. Maser RE, Pfeifer MA, Dorman JS, et al: Diabetic autonomic neuropathy and cardiovascular risk. Pittsburgh Epidemiology of Diabetes Complications Study III. *Arch Intern Med* 1990;150:1218–1222.
28. Welborn TA, Wearne K: Coronary heart disease incidence and cardiovascular mortality in Busselton with reference to glucose and insulin concentrations. *Diabetes Care* 1979;2:154–160.
29. Pyörälä K, Savolainen E, Kaukola S, et al: Plasma insulin as coronary heart disease risk factor: Relationship to other risk factors and predictive value during 9½ year follow-up of the Helsinki Policemen Study population. *Acta Med Scand Suppl* 1985;701:38–52.
30. Fontbonne A, Charles MA, Thibult N, et al: Hyperinsulinemia as a predictor of coronary heart disease mortality in a healthy population: The Paris Prospective Study, 15-year follow-up. *Diabetologia* 1991;34:356–361.
31. Yki-Järvinen H, Koivisto VA: Natural course of insulin resistance in type I diabetes. *N Engl J Med* 1986;315:224–230.
32. Revers RR, Kolterman OG, Scarlett JA, et al: Lack of in vivo insulin resistance in controlled insulin-dependent type I diabetic patients. *J Clin Endocrinol Metab* 1984;58:353–358.

33. Martin FIR, Hopper JL: The relationship of acute insulin sensitivity to the progression of vascular disease in long-term type I (insulin-dependent) diabetes mellitus. *Diabetologia* 1987;30:149–153.

34. Head J, Fuller JH: International variation in mortality among diabetic patients: The WHO Multinational Study of Vascular Disease in Diabetics. *Diabetologia* 1990;33: 477–481.

35. DERI Mortality Study Group: Major cross-country difference in risk of dying for people with IDDM. *Diabetes Care* 1991;14:49–54.

36. Beach KW, Brunzell JD, Conquest LL, et al: The correlation of arteriosclerosis obliterans with lipoproteins in insulin-dependent and non-insulin-dependent diabetes. *Diabetes* 1979;28:836–840.

37. Orchard TJ, Dorman JS, Maser RE, et al: Prevalence of complications in IDDM by sex and duration. Pittsburgh Epidemiology of Diabetes Complications Study II. *Diabetes* 1990;39:1116–1124.

38. Palumbo PJ, Melton LJ: Peripheral vascular disease and diabetes, in Harris MI, Hamman RF (eds): *Diabetes in America*, NIH Publication no. 85-1468. Bethesda, MD, National Institutes of Health, 1985, vol XV, p 11.

39. Moss S, Klein R, Klein BEK: Incidence of lower extremity amputations in a diabetic population [abstract]. *Am J Epidemiol* 1991;134:741.

40. Kleinman JC, Donahue RP, Harris MI, et al: Mortality among diabetics in a national sample. *Am J Epidemiol* 1988;128:389–401.

41. Kannel WB, McGee DL: Diabetes and glucose tolerance as risk factors for cardiovascular disease: The Framingham Study. *Diabetes Care* 1979;2:120–126.

42. Barrett-Connor E, Wingard DL: Sex differential in ischemic heart disease mortality in diabetics: A prospective population-based study. *Am J Epidemiol* 1983;118:489–496.

43. Hayden S, Heiss G, Bartel AG, et al: Sex differences in coronary heart disease among diabetics in Evans County, Georgia. *J Chronic Dis* 1980;33:265–273.

44. Entmacher PS, Root HF, Marks HH: Longevity of diabetic patients in recent years. *Diabetes* 1964;13:373–377.

45. Westlund K: Mortality of diabetics. Life Insurance Companies Institute for Medical Statistics at the Oslo City Hospital, report no. 13, Universitetsforlaget, 1969.

46. Herman JB, Medalie JH, Goldbourt U: Differences in cardiovascular morbidity and mortality between previously known and newly diagnosed adult diabetics. *Diabetologia* 1977;13:229–234.

47. Jarrett RJ, McCartney P, Keen H: The Bedford study: Ten year mortality rates in newly diagnosed diabetics, borderline diabetics and normoglycemic controls and risk indices for coronary heart disease in borderline diabetics. *Diabetologia* 1982; 22:79–84.

48. Butler WJ, Ostrander LD, Carman WJ, et al: Mortality from coronary heart disease in the Tecumseh Study: Long term effect of diabetes mellitus, glucose tolerance and other risk factors. *Am J Epidemiol* 1985;121:541–547.

49. Panzram G: Mortality and survival in type 2 (non-insulin-dependent) diabetes mellitus. *Diabetologia* 1987;30:123–131.

50. Pan W-H, Cedres LB, Liu K, et al: Relationship of clinical diabetes and asymptomatic hyperglycemia to risk of coronary heart disease mortality in men and women. *Am J Epidemiol* 1986;123:504–516.

51. Zimmet PZ, Finch CF, Schooneveldt MG, et al: Mortality from diabetes in Nauru. Results of 4-yr follow-up. *Diabetes Care* 1988;11:305–310.

52. Fontbonne A, Eschwege E, Cambien F, et al: Hypertriglyceridemia as a risk factor for coronary heart disease in subjects with impaired glucose tolerance or diabetes: Results from the 11-year follow-up of the Paris Prospective Study. *Diabetologia* 1989; 32:300–304.

53. Jarrett RJ, Shipley MJ: Type 2 (non-insulin-dependent) diabetes mellitus and car-

diovascular disease—putative association via common antecedents; further evidence from the Whitehall Study. *Diabetologia* 1988;31:737–740.

54. Barrett-Connor E, Wingard DL: Sex differential in ischemic heart disease mortality in diabetics: A prospective population-based study. *Am J Epidemiol* 1983;118:489–496.

55. Kannell WB, Hjortland M, Castelli WP: Role of diabetes in cardiac disease: Conclusions from population studies. The Framingham Study. *Am J Cardiol* 1974;34:29–34.

56. Margolis JR, Kannel WB, Feinleib M, et al: Clinical features of unrecognized myocardial infarction—silent and symptomatic. Eighteen year follow-up: The Framingham Study. *Am J Cardiol* 1973;32:1–7.

57. Kannel WB, McGee DL: Diabetes and cardiovascular disease. The Framingham Study. *JAMA* 1979;241:2035–2038.

58. Rewers M, Shetterly SM, Baxter J, et al: Insulin and cardiovascular disease in Hispanics and non-Hispanic whites (NHW): The San Luis Valley Diabetes Study [abstract]. *Circulation* 1992;85:4.

59. Uusitupa MIJ, Niskanen LK, Siitonen O, et al: 5-year incidence of atherosclerotic vascular disease in relation to general risk factors, insulin level, and abnormalities in lipoprotein composition in non-insulin-dependent diabetic and non-diabetic subjects. *Circulation* 1990;82:27–36.

60. Rosengren A, Welin L, Tsipogianni A, et al: Impact of cardiovascular risk factors on coronary heart disease and mortality among middle aged diabetic men: A general population study. *BMJ* 1989;299:1127–1131.

61. Lapidus L, Bengtsson C, Blohme G, et al: Blood glucose, glucose tolerance and manifest diabetes in relation to cardiovascular disease and death in women. *Acta Med Scand* 1985;218:455–462.

62. Palumbo PJ, Elveback LR, Connolly DC: Coronary heart disease in the diabetic: Epidemiological aspects. The Rochester Diabetes Project, in Scott RC (ed): *Clinical Cardiology and Diabetes*. Mount Kisco, NY, Futura Publishing Company, Inc, 1987, vol 1, pp 13–27.

63. Kuller LH, Dorman JS, Wolf PA: Cerebrovascular disease and diabetes, in Harris MI, Hamman RF (eds): *Diabetes in America*, NIH Publication no. 85-1468. Bethesda, MD, National Institutes of Health, 1985, vol XVIII, p 2.

64. Barrett-Connor E, Khaw KT: Diabetes mellitus: An independent risk factor for stroke? *Am J Epidemiol* 1988;128:116–123.

65. Abbott RD, Donahue RP, MacMahon SW, et al: Diabetes and the risk of stroke. The Honolulu Heart Program. *JAMA* 1987;257:949–952.

66. Kittner SJ, White LR, Losonczy KG, et al: Black-white difference in stroke incidence in a national sample. The contribution of hypertension and diabetes mellitus. *JAMA* 1990;264:1267–1270.

67. Balkau B, Eschwege E, Ducimetiere P, et al: The high risk of death by alcohol related diseases in subjects diagnosed as diabetic and impaired glucose tolerant: The Paris Prospective Study after 15 years of follow-up. *J Clin Epidemiol* 1991;41:465–474.

68. Fuller JH, Shipley MJ, Rose G, et al: Mortality from coronary heart disease and stroke in relation to degree of glycaemia: The Whitehall Study. *BMJ* 1983;287:867–870.

69. Widmer LK, Greensher A, Kannel WB: Occlusion of peripheral arteries: A study of 6,400 working subjects. *Circulation* 1964;30:836–852.

70. Beach KW, Bedford GR, Bergelin RO, et al: Progression of lower-extremity arterial occlusive disease in type II diabetes mellitus. *Diabetes Care* 1988;11:464–472.

71. Osmundson PJ, O'Fallon WM, Zimmerman BR, et al: Course of peripheral occlusive arterial disease in diabetes. Vascular laboratory assessment. *Diabetes Care* 1988; 11:143–152.

72. Schwartz CJ, Valente AJ, Sprague EA, et al: Pathogenesis of the atherosclerotic lesion: Implications for diabetes mellitus. *Diabetes Care* 1992;15:1156–1157.

73. Fein FS, Sonnenblick EH: Diabetic cardiomyopathy. *Prog Cardiovasc Dis* 1985;27: 255–270.

74. Kannel WB, Hjörtland M, Castelli WP: Role of diabetes in congestive heart failure: The Framingham Study. *Am J Cardiol* 1974;34:29–34.

75. Uusitupa M, Siitonen O, Aro A, et al: Prevalence of coronary heart disease, left ventricular failure and hypertension in middle-aged, newly diagnosed type 2 (non-insulin-dependent) diabetic subjects. *Diabetologia* 1985;28:22–27.

76. Robertson WB, Strong JP: Atherosclerosis in persons with hypertension and diabetes mellitus. *Lab Invest* 1968;18:538–551.

77. Diabetes Drafting Group: Prevalance of small vessel and large vessel disease in diabetic patients from 14 centres: The World Health Organization Multinational Study of Vascular Disease in Diabetics. *Diabetologia* 1985;28:615–640.

78. Kagan AR, Uemura K, Sternby NH, et al: Atherosclerosis of the aorta and coronary arteries in five towns. *Bull WHO* 1976;53:485–638.

79. Waller BF, Palumbo PJ, Lie JT, et al: Status of the coronary arteries at necropsy in diabetes mellitus with onset after age 30 years. Analysis of 229 diabetic patients with and without clinical evidence of coronary heart disease and comparison to 183 control subjects. *Am J Med* 1980;69:498–506.

80. Vigorita VJ, Morre GW, Hutchens GM: Absence of correlation between coronary arterial atherosclerosis and severity or duration of diabetes mellitus of adult onset. *Am J Cardiol* 1980;46:535–542.

81. Crall FV, Roberts WC: The extramural and intramural coronary arteries in juvenile diabetes mellitus before age 15 years. *Am J Med* 1978;64:221–230.

82. Verska JJ, Walker WJ: Aortacoronary bypass in the diabetic patient. *Am J Cardiol* 1975;35:774–777.

83. Hamby RI, Sherman L, Mehta J, et al: Reappraisal of the role of the diabetic state in coronary artery disease. *Chest* 1976;70:251–257.

84. Dortimer AC, Shenoy PN, Shiroff RA, et al: Diffuse coronary artery disease in diabetic patients: Fact or fiction? *Circulation* 1978;57:133–136.

85. Wilson PWF, Kannel WB, Anderson KM: Lipids, glucose intolerance and vascular disease: The Framingham Study. *Monogr Atheroscler* 1985;13:1–11.

86. Hanefeld M, Schulze J, Fischer S, et al: The Diabetes Intervention Study (DIS): A cooperative multi-intervention trial with newly manifested type II diabetics: Preliminary results. *Monogr Atheroscler* 1985;13:98–103.

87. Assmann G, Schulte H: The Prospective Cardiovascular Munster (PROCAM) Study: Prevalence of hyperlipidemia in persons with hypertension and/or diabetes mellitus and their relationship to coronary heart disease. *Am Heart J* 1988;116:1713–1724.

88. Haffner SM, Stern MP, Hazuda HP, et al: Do upper-body and centralized adiposity measure different aspects of regional body fat distribution? Relationship to non-insulin dependent diabetes mellitus, lipids and lipoproteins. *Diabetes* 1987;36:13–51.

89. Barrett-Connor E, Grundy SM, Holdbrook MI: Plasma lipids and diabetes mellitus in an adult community. *Am J Epidemiol* 1982;115:657–663.

90. Barrett-Connor E, Witztum JL, Holdbrook M: A community study of high density lipoproteins in adult non-insulin dependent diabetics. *Am J Epidemiol* 1983;117: 186–192.

91. Laakso M, Barrett-Connor E: Asymptomatic hyperglycemia is associated with lipid and lipoprotein changes favoring atherosclerosis. *Arteriosclerosis* 1989;9:665–672.

92. Falko JM, Parr JH, Simpson RN, et al: Lipoprotein analyses in varying degrees of glucose tolerance: Comparison between non-insulin-dependent diabetic, impaired glucose tolerant and control populations. *Am J Med* 1987;83:641–647.

93. Briones ER, Mao SJT, Palumbo PJ, et al: Analyses of plasma lipids and apolipoproteins in insulin-dependent and non-insulin-dependent diabetics. *Metabolism* 1984; 33:42–49.

94. Walden CE, Knopp RH, Wahl PW, et al: Sex differences in the effect of diabetes mellitus on lipoprotein triglyceride and cholesterol concentrations. *N Engl J Med* 1984;311:953–959.

95. Lopes-Virella MFL, Stone PG, Colwell JA: Serum high density lipoprotein cholesterol in diabetic patients. *Diabetologia* 1977;13:285–291.

96. The Expert Panel: Report of the National Cholesterol Education Program expert panel on detection, evaluation and treatment of blood cholesterol in adults. *Arch Intern Med* 1988;148:36–69.

97. Stern MP, Patterson JK, Haffner SM, et al: Lack of awareness and treatment of hyperlipidemia in type II diabetes in a community survey. *JAMA* 1989;262:360–364.

98. Stern MP, Mitchell BD, Haffner SM, et al: Does glycemic control of type II diabetes suffice to control diabetic dyslipidemia? A community perspective. *Diabetes Care* 1992;15:638–644.

99. Haffner SM: Compositional changes in lipoproteins of subjects with non-insulin dependent diabetes mellitus. *J Lab Clin Med* 1991;118:111–112.

100. Biesbroeck B, Albers JJ, Wahl PW, et al: Abnormal composition of high density lipoproteins in non-insulin dependent diabetics. *Diabetes* 1982;31:126–131.

101. Taskinen MR, Huasi T, Helve E, et al: Insulin therapy induces antiatherogenic changes of serum lipoproteins in non-insulin dependent diabetes. *Arteriosclerosis* 1988;8:168–177.

102. Fisher WR: Heterogeneity of plasma low density lipoproteins: Manifestations of the physiologic phenomenon in man. *Metabolism* 1983;32:283–291.

103. Vega GL, Grundy SM: Kinetic heterogeneity of low density lipoproteins in primary hypertriglyceridemia. *Arteriosclerosis* 1986;6:395–406.

104. Austin MA, Breslow JA, Hennekens CH, et al: Low density lipoprotein subclass pattern and risk of myocardial infarction. *JAMA* 1988;260:1917–1921.

105. Lyons TJ: Oxidized low density lipoproteins: A role in the pathogenesis of atherosclerosis in diabetes? *Diabetic Med* 1991;8:411–419.

106. Steinberg D, Parthasarathy S, Carew TE, et al: Beyond cholesterol: Modifications of low density lipoprotein that increase its atherogenicity. *N Engl J Med* 1989;320:913–924.

107. Nishigaki I, Hagihara M, Tsunekawa H, et al: Lipid peroxide levels of serum lipoprotein fractions of diabetic patients. *Biochem Med* 1981;25:373–378.

108. Steinbrecher UP, Witztum JL: Glucosylation of low density lipoproteins to an extent comparable to that seen in diabetes slows their catabolism. *Diabetes* 1984;33:130–134.

109. Kuksis A, Myher JJ, Geher K, et al: Decreased plasma phosphotidyl-choline (free cholesterol) ratio as an indicator of risk for ischemic vascular disease. *Arteriosclerosis* 1982;2:296–302.

110. Fielding CJ, Reaven GM, Fielding P: Human non-insulin-dependent diabetes mellitus: Identification of a defect in plasma cholesterol transport normalized in vivo by insulin and in vitro by selective immunoabsorption of apolipoprotein. *Proc Natl Acad Sci USA* 1982;79:6365–6369.

111. Bagdade JD, Buchanan WE, Kuasi T, et al: Persistent abnormalities in lipoprotein composition in non-insulin dependent diabetes following intensive insulin therapy. *Arteriosclerosis* 1990;10:232–239.

112. Lane JGT, Subbiah PU, Otto ME, et al: Lipoprotein composition and HDL particle distributions in women with non-insulin dependent diabetes mellitus and the effect of probucol treatment. *J Lab Clin Med* 1991;118:552–560.

113. Morton RE: Interaction of lipid transfer protein with plasma lipoproteins and cell membranes. *Experentia* 1990;46:552–560.

114. Saad M, Hoppichler F, Reaveley D, et al: Relationship of serum lipoprotein (a) concentration to coronary heart disease in patients with familial hypercholesterolemia. *N Engl J Med* 1990;322:1494–1499.

115. Schernthaner G, Kostner GM, Dieplinger H, et al: Apolipoproteins (A-I, A-II, B), Lp(a) lipoprotein and lecithin cholesterol acyltransferase activity in diabetes mellitus. *Atherosclerosis* 1983;49:277–293.

116. Arauz C, Lackner C, Ramirez LC: Lipoprotein (a) level in diabetic patients and its correlation with the metabolic control [abstract]. *Diabetes* 1990;39(suppl 1):64A.

117. Bruckert E, Davidoff P, Grimaldi A, et al: Increased serum lipids and lipoprotein (a) in diabetes mellitus and their reduction with glycemic control [letter]. *JAMA* 1990; 263:35–36.

118. Haffner SM, Tuttle KR, Rainwater DL: Decrease of Lp(a) with improved glycemic control in subjects with insulin dependent diabetes mellitus. *Diabetes Care* 1991; 14:302–307.

119. Levitsky LL, Scanu AM, Gould SH: Lipoprotein (a) levels in black and white children and adolescents with IDDM. *Diabetes Care* 1991;14:283–286.

120. Haffner SM, Tuttle KR, Rainwater DL: Preliminary report: Lack of change of Lp(a) concentration with improved metabolic control in subjects with type II diabetes. *Metabolism* 1992:41:194–197.

121. Taskinen MR, Enholm C, Juahianen M, et al: The concentration of Lp(a) is not influenced by the degree of glycemic control in type II diabetes. Presented at the 9th International Symposium on Atherosclerosis, Rosemont, IL, Oct 6–11, 1991.

122. Garber AJ, Jones PH, Ghanem KK, et al: Response of plasma lipoprotein (a) levels to diabetes control therapy. Presented at the 9th International Symposium on Atherosclerosis, Rosemont, IL, Oct 6–11, 1991.

123. Haffner SM, Morales PA, Stern MP, et al: Lp(a) concentrations in non-insulin dependent diabetes mellitus. *Diabetes*, to be published.

124. Jenkins AJ, Steele JS, Janus ED, et al: Increased plasma apolipoprotein (a) levels in IDDM patients with microalbuminuria. *Diabetes* 1991;40:787–790.

125. Haffner SM, Gruber K, Aldrete G, et al: Increased Lp(a) concentrations in chronic renal failure. *J Am Soc Nephrol*, to be published.

126. Haffner SM, Klein BEK, Moss SE, et al: Lack of association between Lp(a) concentrations and coronary heart disease mortality in diabetics: The Wisconsin Epidemiologic Survey of Diabetic Retinopathy. *Metabolism* 1992;41:194–197.

127. McLean JW, Tomlinson JE, Kuang WJ, et al: cDNA sequence of human apolipoprotein (a) is homologous to plasminogen. *Nature* 1987;330:132–137.

128. West KM, Ahuja MMS, Bennett PH, et al: The role of circulating glucose and triglyceride concentrations and their interactions with other "risk factors" as determinants of arterial disease in nine diabetic population samples from the WHO Multinational Study. *Diabetes Care* 1983;6:361–369.

129. Kannel WB, McGee DL: Diabetes and cardiovascular risk factors: The Framingham Study. *Circulation* 1979;59:8–13.

130. Stamler J, Wentworth D, Neaton J, et al: Diabetes and risk of coronary, cardiovascular, and all causes mortality: Findings for 356,000 men screened by the Multiple Risk Factor Intervention Trial (MRFIT). *Circulation* 1984;70(suppl 2):161.

131. Hulley SB, Rosenman RH, Bawol BD, et al: Epidemiology as a guide to clinical decisions: The association between triglyceride and coronary heart disease. *N Engl J Med* 1980;302:1383–1418.

132. Ballard DJ, Melton LJ, Dwyer MS, et al: Risk factors for diabetic retinopathy: A population-based study in Rochester, Minnesota. *Diabetes Care* 1986;9:334–342.

133. Klein R, Klein BEK, Moss SE, et al: Glycosylated hemoglobin predicts the incidence and progression of diabetic retinopathy. *JAMA* 1988;260:2864–2871.

134. Humphrey LL, Ballard DJ, Frohnert PP, et al: Chronic renal failure in non-insulin dependent diabetes mellitus: A population-based study. Rochester, Minnesota. *Ann Intern Med* 1989;111:788–796.

135. Pugh JA: The epidemiology of diabetic nephropathy. *Diabetes Metab Rev* 1989;5: 531–545.

136. Nielsen NV, Ditzel J: Prevalence of macro- and microvascular disease as related to glycosylated hemoglobin in type I and type II diabetic subjects: An epidemiologic study in Denmark. *Horm Metab Res Suppl* 1985;15:19–23.

137. Fuller JH, Shipley MJ, Rose G, et al: Coronary heart disease risk and impaired glucose tolerance: The Whitehall Study. *Lancet* 1980;1:1373–1376.

138. Epstein M, Sowers JR: Diabetes and hypertension. *Hypertension* 1992;19:403–418.

139. Christlieb AR, Warram JH, Krolewski AS, et al: Hypertension: The major risk factor in juvenile-onset insulin-dependent diabetics. *Diabetes* 1981;30(suppl 2):90–96.

140. Garcia MJ, McNamara PM, Gordon T, et al: Morbidity and mortality in diabetics in the Framingham population. Sixteen year follow-up study. *Diabetes* 1974;23:105–111.

141. Ostrander LD, Francis T, Hayner NS, et al: The relationship of cardiovascular disease to hyperglycemia. *Ann Intern Med* 1965;62:1188–1198.

142. Barrett-Connor E, Criqui MH, Klauber MR, et al: Diabetes and hypertension in a community of older adults. *Am J Epidemiol* 1981;13:276–284.

143. Modan M, Halkin H, Almog S, et al: Hyperinsulinemia. A link between hypertension, obesity and glucose intolerance. *J Clin Invest* 1985;75:809–817.

144. Jarrett RJ, Keen H, McCartney M, et al: Glucose tolerance and blood pressure in two population samples: Their relation to diabetes mellitus and hypertension. *Int J Epidemiol* 1978;63:54–64.

145. Cederholm J, Wibell L: Glucose intolerance in middle-aged subjects—a cause of hypertension. *Acta Med Scand* 1985;217:363–371.

146. Goodkin G: Mortality factors in diabetes. *J Occup Med* 1975;17:716–721.

147. Laakso M, Sarlund H, Salonen R, et al: Asymptomatic atherosclerosis and insulin resistance. *Arterioscler Thromb* 1991;11:1068–1076.

148. Santen RJ, Willis PW, Fajans SS: Atherosclerosis in diabetes mellitus. Correlations with serum lipid levels, adiposity and serum insulin level. *Arch Intern Med* 1972;130:833–843.

149. Hillson RM, Hockaday TDR, Mann JI, et al: Hyperinsulinemia is associated with development of electrocardiographic abnormalities in diabetics. *Diabetes Res* 1984;1:143–149.

150. Kashyap ML, Magill F, Rojas L, et al: Insulin and non-esterified fatty acid metabolism in asymptomatic diabetics and atherosclerotic subjects. *Can Med Assoc J* 1970;102:1165–1169.

151. Rönnemaa T, Laakso M, Pyörälä K, et al: High fasting plasma insulin is an indicator of coronary heart disease in non-insulin dependent diabetic and nondiabetic subjects. *Arterioscler Thromb* 1991;11:80–90.

152. Standl E, Janka HU: High serum insulin concentrations in relation to other cardiovascular risk factors in macrovascular disease of type II diabetes. *Horm Metab Res Suppl* 1985;15:46–51.

153. Stout RW, Bierman EL, Ross R: Effect of insulin on the proliferation of cultured primate arterial smooth muscle cells. *Circ Res* 1975;36:319–327.

154. Pfeifle B, Ditschuneit H: Effect of insulin in growth of human arterial smooth muscle cells. *Diabetologia* 1981;20:155–118.

155. Zavaroni I, Bonora E, Pagliara M, et al: Risk factors for coronary heart disease in healthy persons with hyperinsulinemia and normal glucose tolerance. *N Engl J Med* 1989;320:702–706.

156. Orchard TJ, Becker DJ, Bates M, et al: Plasma insulin and lipoprotein concentrations: An atherogenic association? *Am J Epidemiol* 1983;118:326–337.

157. Haffner SM, Fong D, Hazuda HP, et al: Hyperinsulinemia, upper body adiposity and cardiovascular risk factors in non-diabetic subjects. *Metabolism* 1988;37:338–345.

158. Ferrannini E, Buzzigoli G, Bonadonna R, et al: Insulin resistance in essential hypertension. *N Engl J Med* 1987;317:350–357.

159. Abbott WGH, Lillioja S, Young AA, et al: Relationship between plasma lipoprotein

concentrations and insulin action in an obese hyperinsulinemic population. *Diabetes* 1987;36:897–904.

160. Garg A, Helderman JH, Koffler M, et al: Relationship between lipoprotein levels and in vivo insulin action in normal white men. *Metabolism* 1988;37:982–987.

161. Laakso M, Sarlund H, Mykkanen L: Insulin resistance is associated with lipid and lipoprotein abnormalities in subjects with varying degrees of glucose tolerance. *Arteriosclerosis* 1990;10:223–231.

162. Reaven GM: Role of insulin resistance in human disease. Banting Lecture. *Diabetes* 1988;37:1595–1607.

163. Saad MF, Lillioja S, Nyomba BL, et al: Racial differences in the relation between blood pressure and insulin resistance. *N Engl J Med* 1991;324:733–739.

164. Saad MF, Knowler WC, Pettit DJ, et al: The natural history of impaired glucose tolerance in Pima Indians. *N Engl J Med* 1988;319:1500–1506.

165. Sicree RA, Zimmet PZ, King HOM, et al: Plasma insulin response among Nauruans: Prediction of deterioration of glucose tolerance over six years. *Diabetes* 1987;36:179–186.

166. Haffner SM, Stern MP, Mitchell BD, et al: Incidence of type II diabetes in Mexican Americans predicted by fasting insulin and glucose levels, obesity, and body fat distribution. *Diabetes* 1990;39:283–288.

167. Warram JH, Martin BC, Krolewski AS, et al: Slow glucose removal rate and hyperinsulinemia precede the development of type II diabetes in the offspring of diabetic parents. *Ann Intern Med* 1990;113:909–915.

168. Bogardus C, Lillioja S, Foley J, et al: Insulin resistance predicts the development of non-insulin dependent diabetes mellitus in Pima Indians [abstract]. *Diabetes* 1987;36(suppl 1):47A.

169. Medalie JH, Papier CM, Goldbourt U, et al: Major factors in the development of NIDDM in 10,000 men. *Arch Intern Med* 1975;135:811–817.

170. Pell S, d'Alonzo CA: Some aspects of hypertension in diabetes mellitus. *JAMA* 1967;202:104–110.

171. McPhillips JB, Barrett-Connor E, Wingard DL: Cardiovascular disease risk factors prior to the diagnosis of impaired glucose tolerance and non-insulin dependent diabetes mellitus in a community of older adults. *Am J Epidemiol* 1990;131:443–453.

172. Haffner SM, Stern MP, Hazuda HP, et al: Cardiovascular risk factors in confirmed prediabetics: Does the clock for coronary heart disease start ticking before the onset of clinical diabetes? *JAMA* 1990;263:2893–2898.

173. Haffner SM, Ferrannini E, Hazuda HP, et al: Clustering of cardiovascular risk factors in confirmed prehypertensive individuals. *Hypertension* 1992;20:38–45.

174. Haffner SM, Valdez RA, Hazuda HP, et al: Prospective analysis of the insulin resistance syndrome (syndrome X). *Diabetes* 1992;41:715–722.

Chapter 14

Heart Disease in Patients With Diabetes Mellitus

Allan Sniderman, MD, Caroline Michel, MD, and Normand Racine, MD

With therapy to regulate the concentration of glucose in their blood, diabetics survive and, for long periods of time, are apparently well. Notwithstanding their seeming good health, their systemic arteries and ventricles are often under insidious, sustained, and severe attack by processes still only dimly understood. Too frequently, the end result is that two or three decades later, often without prior warning, the clinical complications of vascular disease explode in close succession throughout their arterial tree. The sequence is most dramatic in juvenile diabetes but may be just as real and malignant in the adult form, and so we consider both together.

The hallmarks of diabetic vascular disease are the range and number of vessels involved. Macrovascular and microvascular disease occur in varying proportions in different anatomic beds, with one or another or both occupying center stage at different times. In the kidney, for example, macrovascular disease is common, but it is the microvascular involvement that is classic and so often ruinous to function. In the heart, the balance is reversed. Microvascular disease can occur and on occasion may be clinically significant. Nevertheless, by far the greatest proportion of problems are due to narrowing or obstruction of the major epicardial vessels.

Coronary artery disease by any measure is more common in diabetics than nondiabetics, leaving the diabetics from two to four times as likely to die from myocardial infarction or heart failure as the nondiabetic.[1-10] An increased frequency of severe epicardial coronary disease in diabetics has been repeatedly confirmed in angiographic studies,[11-15] and a series of epidemiologic studies have delineated just how adverse an impact on long-term survival diabetes produces.[16-19] The remarkable propensity of the premenopausal diabetic female to all the complications of coronary heart disease is a particularly striking clinical feature,[16,17,20,21] as is the extraordinary vigor with which coronary disease advances in diabetics with proteinuria.[22,23] In the end, about half of diabetics will die a cardiac death[8,9,24] and vascular disease in one vital organ or another will play an important clinical role in almost all. Inexplicably, the extent of coronary artery disease cannot be linked directly to the severity and duration of the diabetic state.[5,14,25]

There can be no doubt, however, that the risk of premature coronary disease is elevated substantially in diabetics. Two excellent recent reviews detail this body of evidence, and there seems little reason to repeat it here,[24,26] particularly because we show later that important differences in clinical outcome have now been achieved. Accordingly, we place our emphasis elsewhere and try to integrate the pathology of diabetes with some of its most distinctive clinical features. The two most interesting of these are the frequency of clinical heart failure and the phenomena of silent ischemia and infarction. In both, we are convinced that dysfunction of the cardiac sympathetics plays a more important role than often is appreciated, and the syndromes that result are different from much of what is usually designated as cardiac autonomic neuropathy.

Frequency of Coronary Artery Disease in Diabetes

Diabetes destroys and distorts the walls of both large and small arteries. The intima becomes thickened and encroaches on the vessel lumen. A sudden fracture through the endothelial surface often causes an acute thrombosis that abruptly markedly diminishes or completely obliterates the lumen of the vessel. The sequelae of such an anatomic catastrophe are well known and include unstable angina, myocardial infarction, and sudden death. Although disease of major coronary vessels so often dominates the clinical picture in diabetics, curiously, there is nothing about the gross pathologic appearance of the lesion that seems distinctive except the rate and degree to which it so often occurs.

Although not all agree, the small and medium vessels that penetrate the ventricular wall seem altered to a greater extent in diabetics than would be expected by chance alone. Endothelial proliferation, excessive deposits of glycoproteins, and occlusion of the lumen by platelet aggregates or atheromatous debris are the characteristic features of these lesions, not deposition of lipid.[27] Could these lesions be responsible for the sometimes widespread fibrosis seen in the absence of large vessel coronary disease? They may, although clear proof is lacking. At a more distal level yet, the microcirculation itself may be involved in diabetics: the endothelium may be damaged and the basement membrane thickened at sites at which microthrombi of platelets and sometimes clumps of red cells also may be found.[28] Excess glycoproteins may be present in the walls of these vessels,[29] and microaneurysms have been demonstrated in the coronary circulation, although not in intimate association with areas of myocardial damage.[30] Unfortunately, however, the functional significance of these findings remains unclear.

Ventricular Dysfunction in Diabetes

The left ventricle often suffers severely under the multipronged assault of diabetes. Widespread areas of infarction and fibrosis are common and, when sufficiently extensive, are followed by heart failure. Sometimes heart failure appears in the absence of large vessel disease, and from such reports has emerged the concept of a diabetic cardiomyopathy. The pathologic features consist of diffuse subendocardial fibrosis plus extensive interstitial deposition of glycoproteins.[31] The latter might be metabolic in origin, the former perhaps the consequence of microvascular disease, but other elements come into play. Hypertension is common in diabetics and its impact on the ventricle is real. Factor and his colleagues[32] found severe systolic dysfunction in diabetics without coronary disease only in the presence of hypertension. Moreover, they believe that hypertension may play a more important role in the genesis of vasospastic microvascular disease than has been appreciated to date.[32] Diabetes now accounts for the largest proportion of patients entering dialysis programs, and the impact of end-stage renal disease also must be taken into account. Anemia and the arteriovenous fistula necessary for hemodialysis cause cardiac output to rise, and both the right and left ventricles hypertrophy to meet this challenge.[33,34] However produced, left ventricular hypertrophy adversely affects long-term outcome,[35–41] and detecting and attempting to reverse hypertrophy would now appear to be prudent clinical practice.

Not only is the pathogenesis of diabetic cardiomyopathy still obscure, but even its clinical sequence and characteristics are far from clear. The first reports emphasized severe heart failure with marked systolic dysfunction. At autopsy, coronary disease was absent and marked ventricular dilation with scarring was present.[31] Patients with profound systolic dysfunction and heart failure without anatomic coronary disease have also been documented by cardiac catheterization. In such patients left ventricular end-diastolic volumes and pressures are elevated and ejection fraction reduced.[42] In contrast, so-called diastolic dysfunction of the left ventricle has also been observed; in these patients, ventricular end-diastolic volume is normal, end-diastolic pressure elevated, and ejection fraction normal.[31] The pathophysiologic basis for this syndrome is unclear, but one possible explanation is reduction in left ventricular diastolic compliance as a result of interstitial deposition of glycoproteins or subendocardial fibrosis. A second is destruction of the cardiac sympathetic efferents, a hypothesis we consider later.

Although both patterns of heart failure have been reported in the absence of coronary disease, their frequency in unreferred clinical practice is difficult to judge. In our experience, systolic or diastolic ventricular dysfunction sufficiently severe to produce evidence of heart failure at rest but without significant coronary disease is unusual. Whether lesser but still important degrees of abnormality are present more often remains to be determined. It should be appreciated that the capacity of such patients to exercise normally might be substantially reduced but the examination at rest remains normal.

Involvement of the Cardiac Autonomic Nervous System in Diabetes

One of the hallmarks of diabetes is its propensity to destroy components of the autonomic nervous system, and those that supply the heart and peripheral vascular system are no exceptions to this rule. The three classic cardiovascular manifestations of autonomic neuropathy are resting tachycardia, postural hypotension, and silent ischemia or infarction. The first is due to altered parasympathetic function,[43,44] the second is due to abnormal peripheral circulatory sympathetic innervation,[45] and the third takes us closer to home—destruction of the cardiac sympathetic fibers themselves.[46] These last are likely the most common, and certainly the least appreciated, of the group.

Cardiac Parasympathetic Nerve Dysfunction

The parasympathetic cardiac nerves play a major role in the regulation of heart rate. Damage elevates resting rate, although the change is usually not extreme, with values being more often between 90 and 100 than above.[47,48] Occasionally, however, rates of even 120 and greater are seen at rest. The conclusion that parasympathetic control is impaired in some diabetics is based on pharmacologic studies that have shown that heart rate rises little in such patients after atropine but responds normally to propranolol.[47] Adequacy of parasympathetic control can be assessed at the bedside.[47] Among the most popular tests are (1) effect of the Valsalva maneuver on heart rate, (2) heart rate variation during deep breathing, and (3) heart rate change on standing. These test the integrity of parasympathetic function, and abnormalities here are much more common and appear much earlier in the course of the disease than is the case for the next group, which depend on impaired sympathetic interaction with the peripheral vascular system.

Peripheral Circulatory Sympathetic Nerve Dysfunction

The peripheral circulatory autonomic axis consists of vasoconstrictor fibers in muscles, skin, and the splanchnic bed, and dysfunction of this system is typically a late manifestation of sympathetic nerve dysfunction, often associated with more diffuse neuropathy.[48] The two maneuvers that have been used most often clinically to test the integrity of this axis are the blood pressure response to standing (a fall of 30 mm Hg or more in systolic pressure is abnormal) and the rise in diastolic blood pressure with isometric exercise (diastolic blood pressure should rise more than 15 mm Hg with sustained handgrip maintained at 30% of maximum, and an increase of 10 mm Hg or less is considered abnormal).

Abnormal circulatory reflexes account for the enhanced sensitivity of some diabetic patients to vasoactive medications. Undue drop in blood pressure is a well-known, although not that common, scenario after nitroglycerin administration. Such patients may or may not have clinical evidence of peripheral sympathetic nerve dysfunction.[49] A test dose of nitroglycerin while seated is always reasonable, and even more so for diabetics, but the fragile balance of their circulation can also be unmasked by anticalcium agents (nifedipine is foremost here) and occasionally can be seen as well with angiotensin-converting enzyme (ACE) inhibitors.[50]

Cardiac Sympathetic Nerve Dysfunction

The clinical effects just discussed are largely due to interference with peripheral circulatory efferent pathways. However, we believe there is a more common and even more significant interruption in sympathetic nerve activity involving the afferents from, and efferents to, the heart itself. Destruction of the afferents is almost certainly the key event responsible for silent ischemia, a phenomenon that is classic in diabetics but by no means restricted to them, whereas destruction of the efferents likely contributes importantly to the extraordinary frequency of heart failure in diabetics.

The sympathetic nerves destined for the heart leave the spinal column, synapse in the cervical ganglia, and then reach the heart. Once there, these postganglionic efferent fibers run beside the coronary arteries, branching as they do, and covering a greater and greater area of the heart. If a sympathetic nerve were to be injured proximally in its course (i.e., close to the origin of a coronary artery), everything downstream would degenerate. If it were injured more distally, the denervated area would be smaller. Based on the results of Zipes,[51] it appears that efferent sympathetics run in the subepicardium; those destined for that particular area then dive more deeply into the ventricle itself, whereas those heading for more remote regions remain superficial. Afferent fibers begin within the ventricle, join this superficial pathway, and then return toward the brain.

That the phenomenon of cardiac sympathetic injury should be more common in diabetics than nondiabetics should not be surprising. They are at greater risk for many reasons, not least because their coronary disease is often more extensive and severe. Also, diabetic sympathetic autonomic fibers are exposed to metabolic insults that those in the nondiabetic do not face. What will be the consequences of such injuries? With interruption of the afferent pathways, the heart can no longer signal its distress, and so lack of pain with ischemia or infarction should be an expected, not surprising, presentation. In reality, however, many so-called silent infarcts are not asymptomatic: nausea, vomiting, weakness, dyspnea, and death—everything but pain itself—mark their occurrence.

However, there is another, perhaps even more important, consequence if the sympathetic efferents are destroyed. The ventricle needs little or no inotropic support from the sympathetics to function at rest. With exercise, the normal heart can call two principal adaptive mechanisms into play. With one, the Frank-Starling mechanism, output increases with longer diastolic fiber length. This mechanism is well known but quantitatively less important than the second—increase in sympathetic efferent tone. Sympathetic stimulation of the sinoatrial and atrioventricular nodes causes heart rate to increase, although withdrawal of parasympathetic tone also contributes to the jump in heart rate with exercise. More importantly, however, release of norepinephrine from the sympathetic axons distributed throughout the ventricle causes cardiac myocytes to shorten more rapidly and to a greater extent than before, with the result that more blood is ejected more rapidly from both ventricles into the circulations they serve.

However, systole and diastole are intertwined far more closely than usually is appreciated. Normally, most ventricular filling occurs in the first third of diastole, and notwithstanding that its volume is rapidly increasing, pressure in the ventricle continues to fall or, at the least, not rise during this brief but vital period of time. The ventricle behaves, therefore, like a spring that has been compressed during systole by shortening of the myofilaments and deformation of the elastic elements of the interstitial tissue. At the end of systole, as the calcium rapidly and synchronously leaves the active sites of the myofilaments, the potential energy generated during systole is suddenly released and the ventricle recoils open. It is the extreme efficiency of this recoil phase that permits the normal ventricle to fill so rapidly during early diastole without any rise in pressure.

Stimulation of sympathetic efferents will not only increase systolic performance but will increase diastolic recoil as well.[52,53] With exercise, diastole shortens more than systole as heart rate rises, but the rate of diastolic filling increases even further because of sympathetic stimulation, and this allows the normal ventricle to fill more effectively than at rest. If the cardiac sympathetic nerves are damaged, there is, of course, a backup system in place: the adrenal medulla can release catecholamines into the circulation, which then reach the heart. Such release requires time, however, and even then the exercise response is not normal. This has been neatly demonstrated in studies in heart transplant patients, whose ventricles are almost always completely denervated. Such patients increase their cardiac output with exercise, but do so at the cost of elevated ventricular diastolic pressures.[54–56] Loss of sympathetic efferent function in the diabetic heart, therefore, will diminish the systolic effectiveness of whatever viable muscle persists and will also tend to produce diastolic dysfunction. As a consequence of these effects, destruction of the cardiac sympathetics may play a critical role in increasing the frequency of heart failures in diabetics, magnifying the impact of ventricular dysfunction produced by macrovascular or microvascular disease.

The sympathetics also influence repolarization of the cardiac myocytes,[51,57] and sympathetic injury may explain the prolonged Q-T interval that can be seen in diabetics.[58] The risk of disastrous arrhythmia appears to be influenced by the duration of repolarization in the ventricle, and prolonged repolarization is reflected in a prolonged Q-T interval in the surface electrocardiogram.[59,60] These relations may underlie the increased chance of sudden death documented in diabetics with sympathetic denervation.[47]

Clinical Aspects of Coronary Artery Disease in Diabetics

Silent Ischemia and Infarction

A very substantial proportion of diabetics with coronary disease, very likely the majority in fact, at least some of the time have either symptoms of typical angina or a recognizable anginal equivalent, such as dyspnea on exertion. Nevertheless, in some of these patients ischemia is truly silent. Although silent ischemia is frequent in coronary disease in general, the weight of evidence indicates that, whether assessed by treadmill exercise testing, ambulatory Holter monitoring, or exercise radionuclide studies, silent ischemia is even more common in diabetics than nondiabetics.[61–65] Similarly, there is little doubt that myocardial infarction without severe pain occurs more often in diabetics than nondiabetics.[66,67] This matters clinically because the frequency of adverse events following silent infarction or with silent ischemia after infarction is just as high as that following infarcts that were symptomatic.[68,69]

Many investigators have examined the correlation in diabetics between silent ischemia and the presence of either parasympathetic cardiac or peripheral sympathetic autonomic neuropathy. The conclusions from the various studies are much the same, and these, based on the discussion above, should not be surprising. Silent coronary disease is more common in, but by no means restricted to, diabetics with "classic" autonomic neuropathy.[70–74] Because different regions of the autonomic nervous system may be involved at different times in diabetes, there is no reason the correlation should be exact between damage to the sympathetics to the heart and damage to autonomic nerves elsewhere.

Noninvasive Testing

Given the frequency of silent ischemia in diabetics, when appropriate, the physician must search actively for significant coronary disease in diabetics. A wide variety of noninvasive tests are now available for this purpose, but before briefly reviewing these, one important principle must be stressed: none tests directly for the presence or absence of large vessel coronary disease. Rather, all search for consequences of abnormal coronary flow to areas of the heart. Not all coronary lesions significantly limit flow reserve, and because the majority of energy loss occurs in the arterioles, the relation between flow limitation in an epicardial vessel and the severity of a coronary stenosis within it is asymmetric. Until the lesion in the epicardial coronary artery is fairly severe, no clinically significant effect on flow will be evident.[75]

Noninvasive tests are often sought of as being positive or negative for coronary disease, whereas, in fact, they either demonstrate, or do not, changes consistent with myocardial ischemia. The extreme example of this point would be an area of myocardium well supplied by collateral vessels, which might not become ischemic on exercise even though the native vessel supplying that area is completely occluded. The point is not academic. Small lesions that will escape detection also can be fatal if they suddenly fracture and thrombose. It is only that the chance of such a catastrophe is low compared to the risk with larger lesions. One should not conclude, therefore, that patients with negative noninvasive tests are free from coronary disease, but only that flow to most of the myocardium at rest and at exercise is within the normal range at that moment. Tests of Coronary Flow Reserve.

Stress Electrocardiography. With treadmill testing, the physician can determine not only whether the myocardial ischemia occurs with exercise but the threshold at which this occurs. The lower the heart rate–blood pressure product at which clinical or electrocardiographic evidence of myocardial ischemia appears, generally, the more severe the stenosis. An inadequate rise in pulse pressure, disproportionate dyspnea and tachypnea, evidence of heart failure following exercise—all of these can be invaluable clues not just to the diagnosis but as to how quickly and aggressively the patient should be investigated and treated. Twenty-four–hour ST segment recording is an extension of this approach. If the system used allows accurate ST segment recordings, it can yield important information as to the frequency and severity of ischemic episodes.

Stress Radionuclide Imaging. Notwithstanding its strengths, stress electrocardiography has important limitations. The electrocardiogram sees some areas of the heart much better than others. For example, the posterior and high lateral walls of the left ventricle are remote from the electrodes, and ischemia in these regions can be missed. Changes in ST segments that were abnormal at rest cannot be interpreted with confidence, and more than ischemia can change an ST segment, digitalis being a notorious confounder of clinical interpretation in everyday clinical life. Appropriate radionuclide tracers avoid these problems and generally allow more accurate anatomic localization of the problem area.[76]

These tests are based on the existence of a direct relationship between myocardial flow and myocardial uptake of radioisotopes such as thallium 201 and technetium 99–labeled methoxyisobutyl isonitrile.[76,77] A "hole" on the scan taken at rest usually identifies an area in which myocytes have been destroyed and replaced. By far the most common reason for this is ischemic damage, but many other pathologies are possible, including tumor and a variety of infectious agents. A hole that appears with exercise points to an area of myocardium supplied by vessels with limited capacity to increase flow on demand.

This capacity to increase flow on demand can be examined either by performing the stress radionuclide examination at peak exercise on a treadmill or by inducing maximal coronary dilation pharmacologically with dipyridamole.[65,78-80] The principle here is that arterioles dilate to maintain flow in territories supplied by diseased vessels. In consequence, there is less vasodilator reserve in such areas compared to the normal ones and, as a result, flow to the normal zones can increase more than flow to the abnormal ones.

Stress Echocardiography. In the last few years, there has been a growing experience with, and enthusiasm for, this approach. Regional ventricular contraction is monitored with two-dimensional echocardiography at rest and following stress. Echocardiograms have been done before and after treadmill stress and administration of dobutamine or dipyridamole. All three types of stress have induced reduced efficiency of ventricular contraction in areas supplied by stenosed vessels.[81-83]

Tests of Ventricular Function. The clinician also has a variety of tests to examine ventricular function objectively. The most common response of the ventricle to injury is dilation, and chest radiography allows at least a rough assessment of heart size. Newer technologies such as rapid computed tomography and magnetic resonance imaging provide exciting and informative images of the contracting heart. However, they are not essential to clinical practice because the tools that already exist, such as gated ventricular radionuclide scanning and two-dimensional echocardiography, are enormously powerful.[84-86] This applies particularly to echocardiography, which allows repeated and detailed examination of global and regional ventricular function.

Tests of Cardiac Sympathetic Function. The cardiac sympathetics can be visualized following injection of the appropriately iodinated radiotracer, monoiodobenzylguanidine (MIBG).[87] Injury to the sympathetic nerves may be regional or global and may or may not be associated with areas of ventricular damage.[88] Thus, following a myocardial infarction, the MIBG hole is usually larger than the thallium hole.[89] However, other clinical patterns exist. For example, we have described a clinical syndrome—the phantom infarct syndrome[90]—in which patients present with the typical pain of a myocardial infarction and over 2 to 3 days the T waves in a local area of the heart become symmetrically and deeply negative. Characteristically, no ST segment or QRS complex abnormalities are present or evolve. Moreover, other objective tests of myocyte injury remain normal. That is, serum enzyme levels do not increase and there is no evidence of regional wall dysfunction on either echocardiographic or radionuclide examination. MIBG scanning, however, demonstrates a defect that corresponds to the area of the negative T waves, although thallium scanning documents normal perfusion and myocyte uptake in this region. We believe the vascular supply to the sympathetic nerve to the region has been occluded and the nerve infarcted, but the muscle not affected. Such patients almost always have severe proximal coronary lesions in the appropriate area and are at high risk for death versus the case of true infarction. Finally, there may be complete loss of MIBG uptake in the heart in diabetics corresponding to diffuse cardiac sympathetic injury.[91] Such patients often, but not always, have evidence of the other elements of autonomic vascular neuropathy.

Invasive Assessment of Coronary and Cardiac Function

The coronary angiogram remains by far the most informative technique to examine the integrity of the coronary tree and, at the same time, allows ventricular and valvular function to be assessed in detail. The most important limitation here is risk.[92] Renal failure following cardiac catheterization is an important complication, particularly in the diabetic patient.[93] D'Elia and colleagues prospectively studied the clinical relevance of pre-existing chronic renal insufficiency in 378 hospitalized patients undergoing angiography. They demonstrated a 25-fold increase in the incidence of acute renal dysfunction (ie, creatinine rise of 1.0 mg/dL or more) induced by angiographic contrast material in patients with pre-existing azotemia compared to those with normal renal function (17.4% versus 0.7%, respectively). Furthermore, the combination of pre-existing azotemia and diabetes mellitus increased the risk still further.[94] Of importance, Byrd and Sherman as well as others have argued that it is not diabetes itself but its related nephropathy that places these patients at high risk for subsequent acute renal dysfunction.[95,96]

The use of nonionic radiographic contrast agents has not diminished the incidence of renal toxicity after cardiac catheterization significantly.[97,98] Because of this, left heart and coronary studies must be used judiciously, principally to determine whether surgery or angioplasty is necessary at that moment. By contrast, right heart study, which allows hydrostatic pressure in the cardiac chambers to be assessed, is probably underused. Diastolic dysfunction can be very difficult to recognize clinically, and echocardiography remains an imperfect tool in this regard as well. Right heart study carries little risk, and recognition of abnormal diastolic function may change the clinical management dramatically.

Myocardial Infarction

The Classic Outlook

Not only do they face a higher risk of myocardial infarction but, in the event one occurred, diabetics have done substantially worse than nondiabetics.[67,99–101] A typical report is that from Kouvaras et al[102] in a study of 548 patients with a first myocardial infarction. Even though the diabetics were on average 14 years younger (50 versus 64; $p < .05$), their in-hospital mortality was double that of the nondiabetics (30% versus 16%; $p < .001$). In addition, heart failure was more common in diabetics, as was death due to heart failure.

Not only is the immediate outcome after myocardial infarction more unfavorable in diabetics but the long-term outlook is also much grimmer.[20,67,103] The report of Herlitz and his colleagues is representative.[104] They examined the 5-year outcome in 78 diabetics and 709 nondiabetics who had been enrolled in the Goteborg Metroprolol Trial. Mortality was substantially higher in the diabetics (55% versus 30%; $p < .001$). Reinfarction was also significantly higher (42% versus 25%; $p < .001$), and these differences remained significant even after correction for other known prognostic factors.

Of considerable interest, heart failure in diabetics with myocardial infarction has been shown to be more common and more severe than would be predicted from the size of the infarct alone. Jaffe and his colleagues were among the first to document this fascinating phenomenon.[105] Their study compared the outcome in 100 consecutive diabetic patients with myocardial infarction to 426 nondiabetics with infarction. Based on estimates derived from measurements of creatine kinase (CK) release, the diabetics had smaller infarcts (16.2 versus 19.2 CK g-Eq/m^2; $p < .02$) but more frequent heart failure (31.2% versus 15.7%;$p < .02$). The results of the MILIS Study Group are also important in this regard.[106] Serial studies of left ventricular function were done in 85 diabetics and 415 nondiabetics. During the hospital phase, postinfarction angina, infarct extension, heart failure, and death were all more common in the diabetics than the non-diabetics, notwithstanding that the former had smaller estimated infarct sizes than the latter and that left ventricular function differed little between the two groups. More detailed analyses of ventricular function have revealed additional findings of interest. For example, early after infarction, increased contractility has often been observed in noninfarcted areas of the ventricle, and this com-pensatory response appears to be blunted in diabetics.

Why, then, is heart failure so common in diabetics following myocardial infarction, particularly when infarct size does not appear to be the answer? No conclusion is certain, but we believe that impaired efferent cardiac sympathetic nerve function might well be the basis for the clinical observations. Destruction of the sympathetic nerves would reduce the inotropic reserve of the viable muscle within the infarct zone. If sympathetic efferents were affected in non-infarcted regions as well, the lack of compensatory response of these zones also would be explained. Finally, loss of sympathetic augmentation of early relaxation would be expected to result in diastolic dysfunction.

Unlike in the general population, myocardial infarction affects diabetic women as frequently as men. Also, diabetic women seem to face higher in-hospital mortality rates during acute myocardial infarction than do diabetic men (46.6% versus 39.1%, respectively).[67] In addition, Weaver and colleagues showed that women with newly diagnosed adult-onset diabetes have a higher prevalence of ischemic heart disease than men, although no reason for this was evident.[107]

Marked hyperglycemia on admission has on several occasions been asso-ciated with a worse clinical outcome.[4,67] However, the degree of metabolic dis-array may simply reflect the severity of the infarct. In contrast, outcome has been reported to be improved with aggressive control of blood sugar during infarction, although not all agree.[108,109] In our view, as discussed below, although good metabolic control is obviously a reasonable and achievable objective, em-phasis must fall on modern cardiologic management of the event and its complications.

The Modern Outlook

Therapy of myocardial infarction has evolved remarkably over the past few decades, and the pace of change continues to accelerate with the widespread use of agents such as aspirin and β-blockers and the introduction of thrombolysis and early surgical or medical revascularization for postinfarction ischemia. Taken together, these new therapies, particularly when initiated early after the onset of acute myocardial infarction (ie, within 6 hours), have improved the in-hospital and 1-year prognoses remarkably. In the present context, it is critical to note that diabetics have also benefited. Both in-hospital as well as discharge-to–1-year mortality rates appear to have dropped dramatically. This improve-

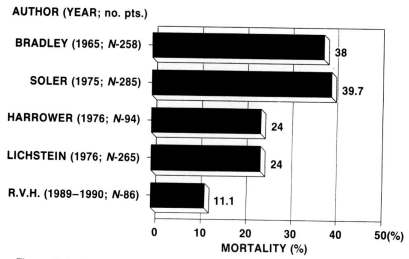

Figure 14.1. Acute myocardial infarction in-hospital mortality rate in diabetics.

ment in clinical outcome is illustrated in Figure 14.1 (in-hospital mortality rates) and Figure 14.2 (discharge-to-1-year mortality rates).

In 1965, Partamian and Bradley[20] reported an in-hospital mortality rate of 38% in 258 diabetic patients who had suffered an acute myocardial infarction. A very similar result was reported by Soler et al in 1975,[67] with an in-hospital mortality rate of 39.7% in 285 diabetic acute infarct patients. By this time, however, others had noted drops in the death rate, with Harrower and Clarke[108] and Lichstein et al[109] recording mortality rates of 24% in their series. Because few recent data are available, we reviewed our own experience: in 86 consecutive diabetic patients admitted with acute infarctions in 1989–1990, our in-hospital mortality rate was only 11.8% compared to 7.8% for the 179 consecutive non-diabetics, a value much lower than previously reported.[67,108–111]

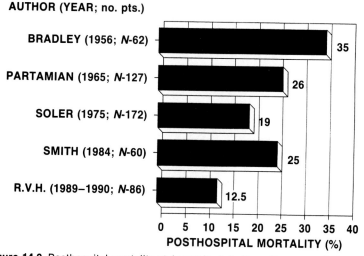

Figure 14.2 Posthospital mortality at 1 year in diabetics with myocardial infarction.

To date, no study has directly evaluated the potential benefit of thrombolysis in diabetics with acute infarctions. However, we have extracted data from the published TIMI study that appear to be of interest. In this study, 425 diabetic patients and 2,836 nondiabetic patients were randomized within 4 hours of acute myocardial infarction to thrombolytic therapy. The 6-week mortality rates were 8.5% and 3.6%, respectively.[111] Although the mortality rate of the diabetics remained higher than that of the nondiabetics, taken together with our recent experience, there seems reason to believe that the short-term outcome in diabetics following acute myocardial infarction has improved substantially.

Happily, a similar trend has also been documented in the follow-up period from hospital discharge to 1-year after infarction, as illustrated in Figure 14.2. In 1956, just over one in three postinfarct diabetic patients died in the first year after discharge[110]; by 1989–1990, the death rate had fallen to one in 10. These results argue for treating diabetics with infarction with the same aggressive approach as is now applied to other infarct patients. As noted above, the main-stays of modern management of myocardial infarction are thrombolysis[112] followed by either oral anticoagulants or aspirin and β-blocker therapy if contraindications are not present.[113,114] Also, ischemic threshold during the hospital period is assessed, usually with a treadmill exercise test.[115–117] Coronary angiography should follow promptly if either spontaneous ischemia or low-threshold ischemia is documented, and in such cases, if coronary anatomy warrants, revascularization should proceed either with coronary angioplasty or coronary bypass surgery.[118–120] The same approach should apply to diabetics. For reasons discussed above, the physician must always keep in mind that ventricular diastolic function may be worse than appears to be the case clinically, and that silent ischemia is closer to the rule than the exception. These considerations, along with a reasonable likelihood of multivessel disease even at the time of first infarction, may lower somewhat the usual clinical threshold for invasive assessment.

Today, mechanical revascularization can be achieved either with coronary bypass surgery or angioplasty, and the short-term benefits of these procedures in restoring adequate flow in the coronary tree are indisputable.[121–123] Surgery in patients with diffuse vascular disease is undoubtedly more complicated and hazardous than in those with disease limited to the coronary tree. However, the most important determinants of outcome will be those that apply to all patients—the adequacy of the distal vessels and the rate at which disease progresses in the long term. The short-term results with surgery and angioplasty have both been very acceptable, although with the latter there may be a somewhat higher re-stenosis rate in diabetics than nondiabetics.[124,125]

Long-Term Strategies

Such therapies, although often life-saving in the short term, do not alter the basic disease process, and changing this should become a principal clinical objective. There is now convincing angiographic evidence that the progression of coronary disease can be halted in many patients and, indeed, that regression not infrequently occurs with therapies that markedly lower the plasma levels of low-density lipoproteins (LDLs) and increase those of high-density lipoproteins.[126–129] The trials to date have excluded diabetics, perhaps based on the view that lipoproteins do not play as critical role in the pathogenesis of vascular disease in diabetics as they do in nondiabetics. However, vascular disease may not be inevitable in the diabetic. In populations in which the incidence of coronary disease is low, diabetics largely escape as well.[130] This has been documented in several countries, including Japan,[131] Africa,[132] and Central America.[133] Within the United States, the relatively low incidence of vascular disease in the Navajo, a group in whom diabetes is common, further testifies to the validity of this concept.[134,135]

How can this be explained? Until recently, almost all emphasis in the study of atherogenesis fell on events with the arterial lumen. The two most popular targets for study and therapeutic intervention were the hydrostatic pressure within vessels and the concentration of the plasma lipoproteins. By contrast, events within the wall itself received much less attention, perhaps not unreasonably since only recently has the technology to study such sequences emerged. However, we now know that entry of atherogenic lipoproteins, in particular LDLs, into the vessel appear to be a necessary but not sufficient cause for arteriosclerosis. What matters most is what happens next.

Three outcomes are possible for any LDL particle that has entered a vessel wall. First, the LDL particle may promptly leave the vessel, or, second, it may be degraded by a cell possessing an LDL receptor. These outcomes are both harmless. The third outcome is oxidation, and that is anything but harmless because, once an LDL particle has been oxidized, it becomes fully competent to initiate the atherogenic process. The adverse consequences that follow oxidation of LDL within the vessel wall range from converting macrophages to foam cells, to altering endothelial function so as to increase the risk of thrombosis and spasm, to inducing death of a series of cells within the vessel wall.[136]

Most cases of premature coronary disease result from increased numbers of LDLs entering the vessel wall because their numbers in plasma are increased.[137–139] Nevertheless, although dyslipoproteinemias in diabetics occur, they often do not seem striking enough, or common enough, to explain the remarkable frequency and severity of the clinical problem. However, were the arterial wall to be affected such that it became "stickier" than normal—that is, if LDL bound to the ground substance of the arterial wall with increased avidity— atherogenesis would be accelerated even if LDL particle number in plasma was not strikingly elevated. Equally, if the LDL of diabetics were more likely to oxidize than normal LDL, atherogenesis would be more aggressive than predicted from the serum levels of LDL alone. In addition, glycation of LDL or the glycosaminoglycans, or both, might well increase the likelihood of oxidation and therefore of atherogenesis.

At the moment, notwithstanding impressive evidence in animals,[140,141] no clinical trials in humans of agents that reduce the likelihood of LDL oxidizing within arterial walls have been conducted. However, because the entry rate of LDL particles into arterial walls is a function of their number in plasma, the option that is at hand is to aggressively reduce that number with diet and pharmacologic therapy. The success of the angiographic trials to inhibit the progression of coronary disease plus the epidemiologic evidence of varying incidence of vascular disease in different diabetic populations suggests to us that this option may turn out to be reasonable in diabetics as well.

References

1. Root HF, Bland EF, Gordon WH, et al: Coronary atherosclerosis in diabetes mellitus: A post-mortem study. *JAMA* 1939;113:27.
2. Stearns S, Schlesinger MJ, Rudy A: Incidence and clinical significance of coronary artery disease in diabetes mellitus. *Arch Intern Med* 1947;80:463.
3. Liebow IM, Hellerstein HK, Miller M: Arteriosclerotic heart disease in diabetes mellitus. A clinical study of 383 patients. *Am J Med* 1955;18:438–447.
4. Bryfogle JW, Bradley RF: The vascular complications of diabetes mellitus. A clinical study. *Diabetes* 1957;6:159–167.
5. Waller BF, Palumbo PJ, Lie JT, et al: Status of the coronary arteries of necropsy in diabetes mellitus with onset after age 30 years. Analysis of 229 diabetic patients with and without clinical evidence of coronary heart disease and comparison to 183 control subjects. *Am J Med* 1980;69:498–506.
6. Bell ET: A postmortem study of vascular disease in diabetics. *Arch Pathol* 1952;53: 444.
7. Robertson WB, Strong JP: Atherosclerosis in persons with hypertension and diabetes mellitus, in HC McGill Jr (ed): *Geographical Pathology of Atherosclerosis.* Baltimore, Williams & Wilkins, 1968.
8. Kessler II: Mortality experience of diabetic patients. A twenty-six year follow-up study. *Am J Med* 1971;51:715–724.
9. Krolewski AS, Czyzyk A, Janeczko D, et al: Mortality from cardiovascular diseases among diabetics. *Diabetologia* 1977;13:345–350.
10. Hayward RE, Lucena BC: An investigation into the mortality of diabetics. *J Inst Actuaries* 1979;91:8.
11. Hamby RI, Sherman L, Mehta J, et al: Reappraisal of the role of the diabetic state in coronary artery disease. *Chest* 1976;70:251–257.
12. Dortimer AC, Shenoy PN, Shiroff RA, et al: Diffuse coronary artery disease in diabetic patients. Fact or fiction? *Circulation* 1978;57:133–136.
13. Wilson CS, Gau GT, Fulton RE, et al: Coronary artery disease in diabetic and non-diabetic patients: A clinical and angiographic comparison. *Clin Cardiol* 1983;6:440–446.
14. Lemp GF, Vander Zwaag R, Hughes JP, et al: Association between the severity of diabetes mellitus and coronary arterial atherosclerosis. *Am J Cardiol* 1987;60:1015–1019.
15. Freedman DS, Gruchow HW, Bamrah VS, et al: Diabetes mellitus and arteriographically-documented coronary artery disease. *J Clin Epidemiol* 1988;41:659–668.
16. Ostrander LD Jr, Francis T Jr, Hayner NS, et al: The relationship of cardiovascular disease to hyperglycemia. *Ann Intern Med* 1965;62:1188–1198.
17. Kannel WB, McGee DL: Diabetics and cardiovascular risk factors: The Framingham study. *Circulation* 1979;59:8–13.
18. Lapidus L, Bengtsson C, Blohme G, et al: Blood glucose, glucose intolerance and manifest diabetes in relation to cardiovascular disease and death in woman. A 12-year follow-up of participant in the population study of women in Gothenburg, Sweden. *Acta Med Scand* 1985;218:455–462.
19. Eschwege E, Richard JL, Thibult N, et al: Coronary heart disease mortality in relation with diabetes, blood glucose and plasma insulin levels. The Paris Prospective Study ten years later. *Horm Metab Res Suppl* 1985;15:41–46.
20. Partamian JO, Bradley RF: Acute myocardial infarction in 258 cases of diabetes. Immediate mortality and five-year survival. *N Engl J Med* 1965;273:455–461.
21. Kleinman JC, Donahue RP, Harris MI, et al. Mortality among diabetics in a national health sample. *Am J Epidemiol* 1988;128:389–401.
22. Jensen T, Borch-Johnsen K, Kofoed-Enevoldsen A, et al: Coronary heart disease in

young type 1 (insulin-dependent) diabetic patients with and without diabetic nephropathy: Incidence and risk factors. *Diabetologia* 1987;30:144–148.

23. Earle K, Walker J, Hill C, et al: Familial clustering of cardiovascular disease in patients with insulin-dependent diabetes and nephropathy. *N Engl J Med* 1900;326: 673–677.

24. Leland OS, Maki PC: Heart disease and diabetes mellitus, in Marble A (ed): *Joslin's Diabetes Mellitus.* Philadelphia, Lea & Febiger, 1985, pp 553–582.

25. Vigorita VJ, Moore GW, Hutchins GM: Absence of correlation between coronary arterial atherosclerosis and severity or duration of diabetes mellitus of adult onset. *Am J Cardiol* 1980;46:535–542.

26. Fein FS, Scheuer J: Heart disease in diabetes, in Rifkin H, Forte D (eds): *Diabetes Mellitus: Theory and Practice.* New York, Elsevier Publishing Co, 1990, pp 812–823.

27. Blumenthal HT, Morris A, Goldenberg S: A study of lesions of the intramural coronary artery branches in diabetes mellitus. *Arch Pathol* 1960;70:13–28.

28. Colwell JA: Pathogenesis of diabetic vascular disease: New concepts, in Podolsky S (ed): *Clinical Diabetes: Modern Management.* New York, Appleton-Century-Crofts, 1980, pp 363–372.

29. Williamson JR, Kilo C: Basement-membrane thickening and diabetic microangiopathy. *Diabetes* 1976;25(suppl 2):925–927.

30. Factor SM, Okun EM, Minase T: Capillary microaneurysms in the human diabetic heart. *N Engl J Med* 1980;302:384–388.

31. Regan TJ, Lyons MM, Ahmed SS, et al: Evidence for cardiomyopathy in familial diabetes mellitus. *J Clin Invest* 1977;60:885–899.

32. Factor SM, Minase T, Sonnenblick EH: Clinical and morphological features of human hypertensinve-diabetic cardiomyopathy. *Am Heart J* 1980;99:446–458.

33. Anderson CB, Codd JR, Graff RA, et al: Cardiac failure in upper extremity arteriovenous dialysis fistulae. *Arch Intern Med* 1976;136:292–297.

34. Silberberg JS, Rahal DR, Patton DR, et al: Role of anemia in the pathogenesis of left ventricular hypertrophy in end-stage renal failure. *Am J Cardiol* 1989;64:222–224.

35. London GM, Fabiani F, Marchais SJ, et al: Uremic cardiomyopathy: An inadequate left ventricular hypertrophy. *Kidney Int* 1987;31:973–980.

36. Gordon T, Kannel WB: Premature mortality from coronary heart disease. The Framingham Study. *JAMA* 1971;215:1617–1625.

37. Messerli FH, Ventura HO, Elizardi DJ, et al: Hypertension and sudden death: Increased ventricular ectopic activity in left ventricular hypertrophy. *Am J Med* 1984; 77:18–22.

38. Anderson KP: Sudden death, hypertension and hypertrophy. *J Cardiovasc Pharmacol* 1984;6(suppl 3):S498–S503.

39. Silberberg JS, Barre P, Prichard S, et al: The impact of left ventricular hypertrophy on survival in end-stage renal failure. *Am J Cardiol* 1989;64:222–224.

40. Levy D, Garrison RJ, Savagh DD, et al: Left ventricular mass predicts coronary disease events independent of the standard risk factors. *Circulation* 1987;76(suppl IV): IV-435.

41. Casale P, Devereux R, Milner M, et al: Value of echocardiographic measurement of left ventricular mass in predicting cardiovascular morbid events in hypertensive men. *Ann Intern Med* 1986;105:173–178.

42. Hamby RI, Zoneraich S, Sherman L: Diabetic cardiomyopathy. *JAMA* 1974;229:1749–1754.

43. Wheeler T, Watkins PJ: Cardiac denervation in diabetes. *BMJ* 1973;4:584–586.

44. Lloyd-Mostyn RH, Watkins PJ: Defective innervation of heart in diabetic autonomic neuropathy. *BMJ* 1975;3:15–17.

45. Roy TM, Peterson HR, Snider HL, et al: Autonomic influence on cardiovascular performance in diabetic subjects. *Am J Med* 1989;87:382–388.

46. Faerman I, Faccio E, Milei J, et al: Autonomic neuropathy and painless myocardial

infarction in diabetic patients: Histologic evidence of their relationship. *Diabetes* 1977;26:1147–1158.

47. Ewing DJ, Campbell IW, Clarke BF: Assessment of cardiovascular effects in diabetic autonomic neuropathy and prognostic implications. *Ann Intern Med* 1980;92:308–311.

48. Ewing DJ: Cardiovascular reflexes and autonomic neuropathy. *Clin Sci Mol Med* 1978; 55:321–327.

49. Vaisrub S: Diabetes and the heart: The autonomic connection, in Zoneraich S (ed): *Diabetes and the Heart.* Springfield, IL, Charles C Thomas, 1978, pp 161–174.

50. Packer M, Lee WH, Medina N, et al: Influence of diabetes mellitus on changes in left ventricular performance and renal function produced by converting enzyme inhibition in patients with severe chronic heart failure. *Am J Med* 1987;82:1119–1126.

51. Zipes DP: Influence of myocardial ischemia and infarction on autonomic innervation of the heart. *Circulation* 1990;82:1095–1105.

52. Grossman W, McLaurin LP: Diastolic properties of the left ventricle. *Ann Intern Med* 1976;84:316–326.

53. Katz AM: Influence of altered inotropy and lusitropy on ventricular pressure-volume loops. *J Am Coll Cardiol* 1988;11:438–445.

54. Kavanagh T, Yacoub MH, Mertens DJ, et al: Cardiorespiratory responses to exercise training after orthotopic cardiac-transplantation. *Circulation* 1988;77:162–171.

55. Banner NR, Lloyd MH, Hamilton RD, et al: Cardiopulmonary response to dynamic exercise after heart and combined heart-lung transplantation. *Br Heart J* 1989;61:215–223.

56. Von Scheidt W, Newdert J, Erdmann E, et al: Contractility of the transplanted denervated human heart. *Am Heart J* 1991;121:1480–1488.

57. Kammerling JM, Green FJ, Watanabe AM, et al: Denervation supersensitivity of refractoriness in noninfarcted areas apical to transmural infarction. *Circulation* 1987; 76:383–393.

58. Kahn JK, Sisson JC, Vinik AI: QT interval prolongation and sudden cardiac death in diabetic autonomic neuropathy. *J Clin Endocrinol Metab* 1987;64:751–754.

59. Inoue H, Zipes DP: Results of sympathetic denervation in the canine heart: Supersensitivity that may be arrhythmogenic. *Circulation* 1987;75:877–887.

60. Zipes DP: Plenary lecture. Cardiac electrophysiology: Promises and contributions. *J Am Coll Cardiol* 1989;13:1329–1352.

61. Chipkin SR, Frid D, Alpert JS, et al: Frequency of painless myocardial ischemia during exercise tolerance testing in patients with and without diabetes mellitus. *Am J Cardiol* 1987;59:61–65.

62. Valderova J, Valek J, Vondra K, et al: The significance of glycosylated hemoglobin in patients with ischemic heart disease and disorders of saccharide tolerance. *Am Heart J* 1985;110:529–534.

63. Marin Huerta E, Rayo I, Lara JI, et al: Silent myocardial ischemia during Holter monitoring in patients with diabetes mellitus. *Rev Esp Cardiol* 1989;42:519–529.

64. Nesto RW, Phillips RT: Asymptomatic myocardial ischemia in diabetic patients. *Am J Med* 1986;80(4C):40–47.

65. Nesto RW, Phillips RT, Kett KG, et al: Angina and exertional myocardial ischemia in diabetic and nondiabetic patients: Assessment by exercise thallium scintigraphy. *Ann Intern Med* 1988;108:170–175.

66. Bradley RF, Schonfeld A: Diminished pain in diabetic patients with acute myocardial infarction. *Geriatrics* 1962;17:322–326.

67. Soler NG, Bennett MA, Pentecost BL, et al: Myocardial infarction in diabetes. *Q J Med* 1975;44:125–132.

68. Kannel WB, Abbott RD: Incidence and prognosis of unrecognized myocardial infarction. An update on the Framingham Study. *N Engl J Med* 1984;311:1144–1147.

69. Tzivoni D, Gavish A, Zin D, et al: Prognostic significance of ischemic episodes in patients with previous myocardial infarction. *Am J Cardiol* 1988;62:661–664.
70. Langer A, Freeman MR, Josse RG, et al: Detection of silent myocardial ischemia in diabetes mellitus. *Am J Cardiol* 1991;67:1073–1078.
71. Murray DP, O'Brien T, Mulrooney R, et al: Autonomic dysfunction and silent myocardial ischaemia on exercise testing in diabetes mellitus. *Diabetic Med* 1990;7:580–584.
72. Hume L, Oakley GD, Boulton AJ, et al: Asymptomatic myocardial ischemia in diabetes and its relationship to diabetic neuropathy: An exercise electrocardiography study in middle-aged diabetic men. *Diabetes Care* 1986;9:384–388.
73. Theron HD, Steyn AF, du Raan HE, et al: Autonomic neuropathy and atypical myocardial infarction in a diabetic clinic population. *S Afr Med* 1987;72:253–254.
74. Niakan E, Harati Y, Rolak LA, et al: Silent myocardial infarction and diabetic cardiovascular autonomic neuropathy. *Arch Intern Med* 1986;146:2229–2230.
75. Gould KL, Lipscomb K: Effects of coronary stenoses on coronary flow reserve and resistance. *Am J Cardiol* 1974;34:48–55.
76. Seldin DW, Johnson LL, Blood D, et al: Myocardial perfusion imaging with technetium-99m SQ30217: Comparison with thallium-201 and coronary anatomy. *J Nucl Med* 1989;30:312–319.
77. Wackers FJT, Berman DS, Maddahi J, et al: Technetium-99m-hexakis 2 methoxyisobutyl isonitrile: Human biodistribution, dosimetry, safety and preliminary comparison to thallium-201 for myocardial perfusion imaging. *J Nucl Med* 1989;30:301–311.
78. Kaul S: A look at 15 years of planar thallium-201 imaging. *Am Heart J* 1989;118:581–601.
79. Gould KL: Noninvasive assessment of coronary stenoses by myocardial perfusing imaging during pharmacologic coronary vasodilatation. 1. Physiologic basis and experimental validation. *Am J Cardiol* 1978;41:267–278.
80. Zhu YY, Chung WS, Botvinick EH, et al: Dipyridamole perfusion scintigraphy: The experience with its application in one hundred seventy patients with known or suspected unstable angina. *Am Heart J* 1991;121:33–43.
81. Armstrong WF, O'Donnell J, Ryan T, et al: Effect of prior myocardial infarction and extent and location of coronary disease on accuracy of exercise echocardiography. *J Am Coll Cardiol* 1987;10:531–538.
82. Berthe C, Pierard LA, Hiernaux M, et al: Predicting the extent and location of coronary artery disease in acute myocardial infarction by echocardiography during dobutamine infusion. *Am J Cardiol* 1986;58:1167–1172.
83. Picano E, Severi S, Michelassi C, et al: Prognostic importance of dipyridamole-echocardiography test in coronary artery disease. *Circulation* 1989;80:450–457.
84. Abraham RD, Harris PG, Roubin GS, et al: Usefulness of ejection fraction response to exercise one month after acute myocardial infarction in predicting coronary anatomy and prognosis. *Am J Cardiol* 1987;60:225–230.
85. Ahnve S, Gilpin E, Henning H, et al: Limitations and advantages of the ejection fraction for defining high risk after myocardial infarction. *Am J Cardiol* 1986;58:872–878.
86. Shiina A, Tajik AJ, Smith HC, et al: Prognostic significance of regional wall motion abnormality in patients with prior myocardial infarction: A prospective correlative study of two-dimensional echocardiography and angiography. *Mayo Clin Proc* 1986;61:254–262.
87. Sisson JC, Lynch JJ, Johnson J, et al: Scintigraphic detection of regional disruption of adrenergic neurons in the heart. *Am Heart J* 1988;116:67–76.
88. McGhie AI, Corbett JR, Akers MS, et al: Regional cardiac adrenergic function using I-123-metaiodobenzylguanidine tomographic imaging after acute myocardial infarction. *Am J Cardiol* 1991;67:236–242.

89. Stanton MS, Tuli MM, Radtke NL, et al: Regional sympathetic denervation after myocardial infarction in humans detected noninvasively using I-123-metaiodobenzylguanidine. *J Am Coll Cardiol* 1989;14:1519–1526.

90. Ferguson J, Lisbona R, Rahal D, et al: Correlative electrocardiographic studies in myocardial infarction. *Cardiol Clin* 1984;2(1):47–62.

91. Sisson JC, Wieland DM, Sherman RL, et al: Metaiodobenzylguanidine as an index of the adrenergic nervous system integrity and function. *J Nucl Med* 1987;28:1620–1624.

92. Wyman RM, Safian RD, Portway V, et al: Current complications of diagnostic and therapeutic cardiac catheterization. *J Am Coll Cardiol* 1988;12:1400–1406.

93. Wish JB, Moritz CE: Preventing radiocontrast-induced acute renal failure. How to identify patients at highest risk for a common problem. *J Critical Illness* 1990;5:16–31.

94. D'Elia JA, Gleason RE, Alday M, et al: Nephrotoxicity from angiographic contrast material: A prospective study. *Am J Med* 1982;72:719–725.

95. Byrd L, Sherman RL: Radiocontrast-induced acute renal failure. A clinical and pathophysiologic review. *Medicine* 1979;58:270–279.

96. Parfrey PS, Griffiths SM, Barrett BJ, et al: Contrast material-induced renal failure in patients with diabetes mellitus, renal insufficiency or both: A prospective controlled trial. *N Engl J Med* 1989;320:143–149.

97. Schwab SJ, Hlatky MA, Pieper KS, et al: Contrast nephrotoxicity: A randomized controlled trial of nonionic and an ionic radiographic contrast agent. *N Engl J Med* 1989;320:149–153.

98. Davidson CJ, Hlatky MA, Morris KG, et al: Cardiovascular and renal toxicity of a nonionic radiographic contrast agent after cardiac catheterization. A prospective trial. *Ann Intern Med* 1989;110:119–124.

99. Czyzyk A, Krolewski AS, Szabowska A, et al: Clinical course of myocardial infarction among diabetic patients. *Diabetes Care* 1980;3:526.

100. Weitzman S, Wagner GS, Heiss G, et al: Myocardial infarction site and mortality in diabetes. *Diabetes Care* 1982;5:31–35.

101. Smith JW, Marcus FI, Serokman R, et al: Prognosis of patients with diabetes mellitus after acute myocardial infarction. *Am J Cardiol* 1984;54:718–721.

102. Kouvaras G, Cokkinos D, Spyropoulou M: Increased mortality of diabetics after acute myocardial infarction attributed to diffusely impaired left ventricular performance as assessed by echocardiography. *Jpn Heart J* 1988;29:1–9.

103. Tansey MJB, Opie LH, Kennelly BM: High mortality in obese women diabetics with acute myocardial infarction. *BMJ* 1977;1:1624–1626.

104. Herlitz J, Malmberg K, Karlson BW, et al: Mortality and morbidity during a five-year follow-up of diabetics with myocardial infarction. *Acta Med Scand* 1988;224:31–38.

105. Jaffe AS, Spadaro JJ, Schechtman K, et al: Increased congestive heart failure after myocardial infarction of modest extent in patients with diabetes mellitus. *Am Heart J* 1984;108:31–37.

106. Stone PH, Muller JE, Harwell T, et al: The effect of diabetes mellitus on prognosis and serial left ventricular function after acute myocardial infarction: Contribution of both coronary disease and diastolic left ventricular dysfunction to the adverse prognosis. The MILIS Study Group. *J Am Coll Cardiol* 1989;14:49–57.

107. Weaver JA, Bhatia SK, Boyle D, et al: Cardiovascular state of newly discovered diabetic women. *BMJ* 1970;1:783–786.

108. Harrower AD, Clarke BF: Experience of coronary care in diabetes. *BMJ* 1976;1:126–128.

109. Lichstein E, Kuhn LA, Goldberg E, et al: Diabetic treatment and primary ventricular fibrillation in acute myocardial infarction. *Am J Cardiol* 1976;38:100–102.

110. Bradley RF, Bryfogle JW: Survival of diabetic patients after myocardial infarction. *Am J Med* 1956;20:207–216.

111. Hillis LD, Forman S, Braunwald E, et al: Risk stratification before thrombolytic therapy in patients with acute myocardial infarction. *J Am Coll Cardiol* 1990;16:313–315.

112. Verstaete M: Thrombolytic treatment in acute myocardial infarction. *Circulation* 1990;82(suppl II):II-96–II-109.

113. Yusuf S, Peto R, Lewis J, et al: Beta blockade during and after myocardial infarction: An overview of the randomized trials. *Prog Cardiovasc Dis* 1985;27:335–371.

114. Gunderson T, Kjekshus J: Timolol treatment after myocardial infarction in diabetic patients. *Diabetes Care* 1983;6:285–290.

115. DeBusk RF: Specialized testing after recent acute myocardial infarction. *Ann Intern Med* 1989;110:470–481.

116. ACC/AHA Task Force on Early Management of Acute Myocardial Infarction: Guidelines for the early management of patients with acute myocardial infarction. Strategies for predischarge or early postdischarge exercise evaluation. *J Am Coll Cardiol* 1990;16:249–292.

117. Krone RJ: The role of risk stratification in the early management of a myocardial infarction. *Ann Intern Med* 1992;116:223–237.

118. The TIMI Study Group: Comparison of invasive and conservative strategies after treatment with intravenous tissue plasminogen activator in acute myocardial infarction. Results of the thrombolysis in myocardial infarction (TIMI) Phase II Trial. *N Engl J Med* 1989;320:618–627.

119. Phillips SJ, Zeff RH, Skinner JR, et al: Reperfusion protocol and results in 738 patients with evolving myocardial infarction. *Ann Thorac Surg* 1986;41:119–125.

120. DeWood MA, Notske RN, Berg R, et al: Medical and surgical management of early Q wave myocardial infarction. I. Effects of surgical reperfusion on survival, recurrent myocardial infarction, sudden death and functional class at 10 or more years of follow-up. *J Am Coll Cardiol* 1989;14:65–78.

121. Devineni R, McKenzi FN: Surgery for coronary artery disease in patients with diabetes mellitus. *Can J Surg* 1985;28:367–370.

122. Lawrie GM, Morris GC Jr, Glaeser DH: Influence of diabetes mellitus on the results of coronary bypass surgery: Follow-up of 212 diabetic patients ten to fifteen years after surgery. *JAMA* 1986;256:2967–2971.

123. Johnson WD, Pedraza PM, Kayser KL: Coronary artery surgery in diabetics: 261 consecutive patients followed four to seven years. *Am Heart J* 1982;104(4, Pt 1):823–827.

124. Holmes DR, Vlietstra RE, Smith HC, et al: Restenosis after percutaneous transluminal coronary angioplasty (PTCA): A report from the PTCA Registry of the National Heart, Lung and Blood Institute. *Am J Cardiol* 1984;53:77c–81c.

125. Lambert M, Bonan R, Coté G, et al: Multiple coronary angioplasty. A model to discriminate systemic and procedural factors related to restenosis. *J Am Coll Cardiol* 1988;12:310–314.

126. Blakenhorn DH, Nessim SA, Johnson RL, et al: Beneficial effects of combined colestipol niacin therapy on coronary atherosclerosis and coronary venous bypass grafts. *JAMA* 1987;257:3233.

127. Brown BG, Albers JJ, Fisher LD, et al: Regression of coronary artery disease as a result of intensive lipid-lowering therapy in men with high levels of apolipoprotein B. *N Engl J Med* 1990;323:1289–1298.

128. Ornish D, Brown SE, Scherwitz LW, et al: Can lifestyle changes reverse coronary heart disease? *Lancet* 1990;1:129.

129. Buchwald H, Varco RL, Tats PJ, et al: Effect of partial ileal bypass surgery on mortality and morbidity from coronary heart disease in patients with hypercholesterolemia: Report of the Program on the Surgical Control of Hyperlipidemia (POSCH). *N Engl J Med* 1990;323:946.

130. Gordon T, Garcia-Palmieri MR, Kagan A, et al: Differences in coronary heart disease in Framingham, Honolulu and Puerto Rico. *J Chronic Dis* 1974;27:329–344.

131. Goto Y, Fukuhara N: Cause of death in 933 diabetic autopsy cases. *J Jpn Diabetic Soc* 1968;11:197.

132. Greenwood BM, Taylor JR: The complications of diabetes in Nigerians. *Trop Geogr Med* 1968;20:1.

133. West KM, Kalbfleisch JM: Diabetes in Central America. *Diabetes* 1970;19:656–663.

134. West KM: Diabetes in American Indians and other native populations of the New World. *Diabetes* 1974;23:841–855.

135. Prosnitz LR, Mandell GL: Diabetes mellitus among Navajo and Hopi Indians: The lack of vascular complications. *Am J Med Sci* 1967;253:700.

136. Witztum J, Steinberg D: Role of oxidized low density lipoprotein in atherogenesis. *J Clin Invest* 1991;88:1785–1792.

137. Leary T: The genesis of atherosclerosis. *Arch Pathol* 1941;32:507.

138. Parthasarathy S, Quinn MT, Schwenke DC, et al: Oxidative modification of beta-very low density lipoprotein. Potential role in monocyte recruitment and foam cell formation. *Atherosclerosis* 1989;1:293.

139. Vackson RL, Gotto AM Jr: Hypothesis concerning membrane structure, cholesterol, and atherosclerosis, in Paoletti R, Gotto AM Jr (eds): *Atherosclerosis Reviews.* New York, Raven Press, 1976, vol 1, p 1.

140. Carew T, Schwenke DC, Steinberg D: Antiatherogenic effect of probucol unrelated to its hypocholesterolemic effect: Evidence that the antioxidants in vivo can selectively inhibit low density lipoprotein degradation in macrophage-rich fatty streaks and slow the progression of atherosclerosis in the Watanabe heritable hyperlipidemic (WHHL) rabbit. *Proc Natl Acad Sci USA* 1987;84:7725–7729.

141. Kita T, Nagano Y, Yokode M, et al: Probucol prevents the progression of atherosclerosis in Watanabe heritable hyperlipidemic rabbit, an animal model for familial hypercholesterolemia. *Proc Natl Acad Sci USA* 1987;84:5928–5931.

Diabetes and Hypertension

Chapter 15

Mechanisms of Hypertension in Diabetes Mellitus

Luciano Rossetti, MD, and Simona Frontoni, MD

Diabetes and hypertension are common diseases that frequently coexist and dramatically affect the patient's clinical outcome. Hypertension is approximately twice as common in diabetic subjects as in the general population. Essential hypertension and diabetic nephropathy account for the great majority of cases of hypertension in diabetic individuals. However, the prevalence of essential hypertension in diabetic subjects remains a controversial issue. In fact, the independent effects of obesity and diabetic nephropathy were not taken in account in some of the early epidemiologic studies.[1,2] Recent studies have firmly established an increased prevalence of hypertension in diabetic individuals independent of age, obesity, and renal disease.[3-6] In individuals with non-insulin-dependent diabetes mellitus (NIDDM), there is a significant prevalence of hypertension at the time of diagnosis that appears to be related to the obesity common in these patients.[7-9] However, even when this factor (obesity) is taken into account, a significant increase in the prevalence of hypertension is still observed.[4] In individuals with insulin-dependent diabetes mellitus (IDDM), hypertension typically begins several years after the onset of hyperglycemia. Blood pressure increases slightly but significantly during the microalbuminuric stage and progressively rises with the development of clinically overt nephropathy.[10-13]

Many of the epidemiologic data concerning individuals with IDDM are based on a definition of diastolic hypertension greater than 95 mm Hg, which may be inappropriate for this young patient population. Using this diastolic pressure criterion, the prevalence of hypertension becomes higher than in the general population only in the second decade after diagnosis, mostly in association with the onset of proteinuria and incipient diabetic nephropathy.[14,15] However, recent reports have suggested an increased prevalence of mild hypertension in IDDM subjects before the onset of renal disease[10,16,17] Some evidence suggests that, in IDDM subjects, mild hypertension may precede the onset of nephropathy and may represent a major risk factor for its development. In this regard, it is of interest that parents of individuals with IDDM who have diabetic nephropathy manifest an increased incidence of essential hypertension.[18,19]

In summary, epidemiologic data suggest that hypertension is more frequent in the diabetic population as a whole compared to the general population. These observations suggest one of two primary possibilities: (1) that a genetic predisposition that contributes along with environmental factors, to the development of hypertension exists with an increased prevalence in diabetic individuals; or (2) that some peculiar pathogenetic mechanism(s) of hypertension are present in diabetic compared to nondiabetic subjects. This review focuses on the mechanism(s) of hypertension that have been suggested to be characteristic of the diabetic state.

Pathogenesis of Hypertension in Diabetes

The pathogenesis of the association between diabetes and hypertension is still poorly understood. However, several theories have been advanced that may explain the increased prevalence of hypertension in diabetes. The great majority of hypertension in diabetic individuals is essential hypertension and/or obesity-related hypertension. Two major hypotheses can be postulated to explain the prevalence and pathogenesis of hypertension in diabetes: (1) diabetes itself, through metabolic and hormonal abnormalities, may result both in renal damage and hypertension; and (2) the two diseases are genetically linked and environmental factors may contribute to the development of both diabetes and hypertension. In the presence of a genetic predisposition for the development of hypertension, some metabolic and/or hemodynamic alterations that accompany the diabetic state may determine an increased penetrance of the phenotype in diabetic individuals.

Relation of Metabolic and/or Hemodynamic Abnormalities of Diabetes to Hypertension

Role of Sodium

Several studies have independently demonstrated that both normotensive and hypertensive diabetic subjects have approximately a 10% increase in the exchangeable body sodium pool compared to nondiabetic subjects.[20-22] Although a further increase in exchangeable sodium has been shown in diabetic subjects with microalbuminuria or nephropathy,[23] this alteration has been clearly demonstrated in patients with diabetes mellitus even when normotensive, in good metabolic control, and free of complications.[24-26] Although the mechanism(s) of sodium retention are not clear, some hypotheses have been formulated. It is known that both glucose and ketone bodies are actively resorbed at the level of the proximal renal tubulus as Na^+ salt.[27,28] As a consequence, the moderate increases in blood concentrations of glucose and ketone bodies that can be observed in patients with diabetes mellitus determine an enhanced resorption of Na^+ salt, resulting in sodium retention. Consistent with this view, Brenner's group recently reported that the hyperglycemia-induced chronic volume expansion results in increased sodium resorption in streptozotocin-diabetic rats.[29] Additionally, the achievement of a significant improvement in metabolic control in NIDDM patients is associated with a decrease in blood pressure.[30,31]

In contrast, both insulin-treated IDDM and NIDDM patients usually present peripheral hyperinsulinemia, and the acute "in vivo" administration of insulin is followed by a significant antinatriuretic effect.[22,32,33] This effect may be responsible for the increased tubular sodium absorption and consequent volume expansion.

Finally, a blunted secretory response of atrial natriuretic peptide (ANP) to isotonic volume expansion has been shown in IDDM patients,[22,34] and this alteration has been reproduced in normal subjects by insulin administration.[22] In contrast, increased plasma levels of ANP have been demonstrated in overnight-fasted IDDM subjects, despite normal rates of Na$^+$ excretion, thus suggesting the presence of resistance to the hormonal action of ANP.[22] Thus, both impaired ANP secretion and action may contribute to the increased sodium retention and extracellular volume expansion in IDDM.

In summary, diabetic patients tend to have an increased changeable pool of sodium and a larger extracellular liquid compartment. Hyperglycemia, hyperosmolarity, hyperinsulinemia, and impaired ANP secretion and action may all contribute to this phenomenon. Increased extracellular volume is a hemodynamic condition that is usually associated with increased cardiac output and ultimately contributes to the onset of hypertension in the context of a feedback mechanism aimed to counterbalance the expansion of the plasma compartment. However, it is important to point out that the increased pool of exchangeable sodium and extracellular liquid compartment is common to hypertensive and normotensive diabetic individuals. Thus, this factor alone cannot explain the pathogenesis of hypertension in diabetes. Rather, it is conceivable that the impaired natriuresis that accompanies the diabetic state contributes to the onset of hypertension in a subgroup of diabetic individuals with enhanced susceptibility to hypertension.

Renin-Angiotensin System in Diabetes

The renin-angiotensin system in diabetic hypertensive subjects has received considerable attention.[35,36] In patients with metabolically stable diabetes, plasma active renin, angiotensin II, and aldosterone concentrations are usually normal or reduced.[20,35,37] The prevalence of low plasma renin and aldosterone levels increases with the progression of impaired kidney function.[36,38,39] It has therefore been commonly assumed that hyperreninism and hyperaldosteronism play no direct role in the impaired natriuresis, hypertension, and nephropathy of diabetes mellitus. However, it may be argued that plasma renin activity, and the plasma levels of aldosterone and angiotensin II, are minimally and therefore "inappropriately" suppressed by volume expansion (sodium excess) in diabetic subjects. In accordance with the latter speculation, improved glycemic control decreases plasma angiotensin II concentrations in individuals with NIDDM,[40] and the inhibition of the angiotensin-converting enzyme effectively decreases blood pressure in diabetic hypertensive patients.[41–45] Thus, although a direct role of high circulating levels of aldosterone and angiotensin II in the pathogenesis of hypertension in diabetes appears to be improbable, a permissive role in the form of insufficient suppression has been suggested.

The biologic vasopressor response to angiotensin II has also been an object of investigation.[46–50] Several studies have shown an increased vascular sensitivity to angiotensin II in both diabetic patients and animals.[24,51,52] The dose of angiotensin II required to increase diastolic blood pressure by 20 mm Hg was significantly less in nonazotemic diabetic subjects compared to nondiabetic controls[24] (Figure 15.1). This hypersensitivity was clearly demonstrated in nor-

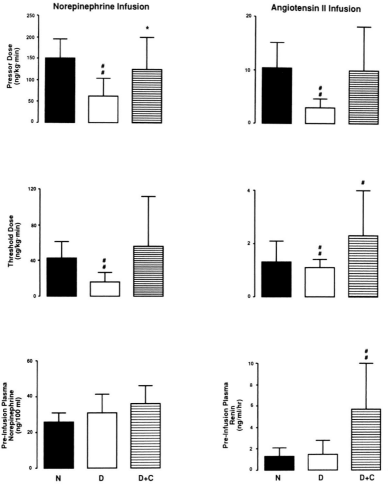

Figure 15.1 Norepinephrine and angiotensin II pressor and threshold doses, and preinfusion plasma norepinephrine and renin levels in age-matched untreated nondiabetic control group (N; solid bars) and in hypertensive diabetic (D) patients on placebo (open bars) and after chlorthalidone (C) treatment (D+C; hatched bars). $^* = p < .02$ versus untreated diabetic patients; $\# = p < .01$ versus untreated diabetic patients; $\#\# = p < .001$ versus normal subjects and untreated diabetic patients. *(Reprinted, by permission, from Weidmann P, Beretta-Piccoli C, Keusch G, et al: Sodium volume factor, cardiovascular reactivity and hypotensive mechanisms of diuretic therapy in mild hypertension associated with diabetes mellitus. Am J Med 1979;67:779–784.)*

motensive diabetic patients in the absence of complications,[53] and may play a role in the development of diabetes-associated hypertension.

Several factors may contribute to the increased vascular response to angiotensin II. The leading candidate is sodium retention, which is known to increase vascular reactivity to vasopressor stimuli. However, short-term sodium restriction lowers the blood pressure response to angiotensin II in nondiabetic subjects but is ineffective in hypertensive individuals with NIDDM.[54] The observation that the pressor effect of angiotensin II was blunted by calcium channel blockade[55] suggests that the diabetes-associated cardiovascular hyperreactivity could be at least in part mediated by an increase in cytosolic calcium.

Role of the Sympathetic Nervous System

Plasma and urinary catecholamine concentrations are usually normal or low in patients with metabolically stable diabetes.[20,23,56–58] Because norepinephrine clearance has been reported to be unaffected in diabetic subjects,[59] it is conceivable that the circulating norepinephrine level would be proportional to the overall spillover from neuronal synapses.

In contrast, it is well documented that acute insulin infusions, determining plasma hormone levels within the physiologic range, increase sympathetic outflow[60–63] even in the absence of concomitant hypoglycemia. Anderson et al have demonstrated increased sympathetic nerve activity by direct electrophysiologic recording of nerve activity during euglycemic insulin clamp studies in healthy volunteers[64] (Figure 15.2).

Thus, a role for chronically increased activation of the sympathetic nervous system in the pathogenesis of hypertension in diabetes cannot be ruled out. In this regard, the importance of the nutritional state in the evaluation of sympathetic nervous system activity in hypertensive diabetic patients should be emphasized.

Increased cardiovascular reactivity has also been documented in mild hypertension associated with diabetes mellitus[24] (Figure 15.1). The dose of infused norepinephrine that increases blood pressure by 20 mm Hg was significantly decreased in diabetic compared to nondiabetic subjects.[24,51] A recent report demonstrating increased cardiovascular reactivity to norepinephrine following exogenous insulin infusion in healthy humans[65] appears to suggest that peripheral hyperinsulinemia plays a role in this enhanced sensitivity.

Alterations in Intracellular Electrolytes

Hyperinsulinemia and insulin resistance may have a major impact on the activity of several pump systems that regulate the transmembrane transport of electrolytes. Insulin-induced stimulation of Na^+/K^+ adenosine triphosphatase (ATPase) tends to produce a decline in intracellular sodium,[66–67] whereas insulin's activation of the Ca^{2+}-Na^+ antiporter, Na^+-H^+ antiporter, and Na^+ aminoacid cotransporter will all tend to elevate the intracellular sodium concentration.[68–73] In contrast, insulin tends to increase the intracellular calcium level through the inhibition of Ca^{2+}/Mg^{2+}-ATPase.[74–76] Increased intracellular Ca^{2+} has been reported in circulating platelets and erythrocytes and in isolated adipose cells from essential hypertensive[77,78] and diabetic hypertensive[79] patients. Furthermore, the insulin-stimulated Mg^{2+} uptake is decreased in red blood cells of NIDDM patients.[80] Thus, the available evidence suggests that, in diabetic subjects, there is an increased concentration of intracellular calcium and a concomitant decrease in intracellular magnesium levels.[81]

Intracellular Ca^{2+} is critical to cardiac and smooth muscle contraction.[82,83] Thus, calcium plays a fundamental role in both cardiac output and vascular resistance. It is therefore not surprising that several investigators have focused their attention on cellular Ca^{2+} handling in hypertension and diabetes. A strong correlation has been demonstrated between the level of blood pressure and the intraplatelet[77] (Figure 15.3) or the erythrocyte[78] cytosolic free Ca^{2+} content in

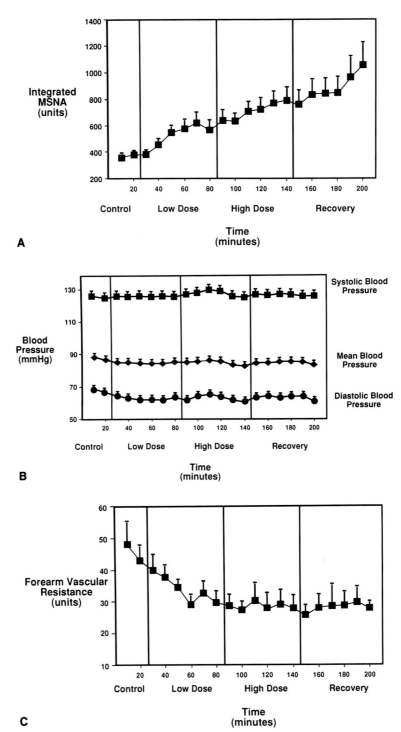

Figure 15.2 (A) Muscle sympathetic nerve activity (MSNA), expressed as integrated activity (ie, burst frequency × mean burst amplitude), rose after 20 minutes of low-dose (38 mU/m^2/min) insulin and continued to rise during both high-dose (76 mU/m^2/min) insulin and the 1-hour recovery period. (B) Systolic, diastolic, and mean blood pressures during control, low-dose, and high-dose insulin infusion, and recovery. Systolic blood pressure did not change significantly during the study. In contrast, diastolic and mean pressures declined significantly

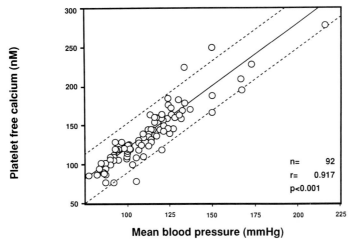

Figure 15.3 Correlation between mean blood pressure and intracellular free calcium concentrations in platelets of 38 normotensive subjects, 9 patients with borderline hypertension, and 45 patients with essential hypertension. Broken lines indicate 95 percent confidence limits. *(Reprinted, by permission of The New England Journal of Medicine, from Erne P, Bolli P, Burgisser E, et al: Correlation of platelet calcium with blood pressure: Effect of antihypertensive therapy. N Engl J Med 1984;310:1084–1088.)*

hypertensive subjects. In contrast, an inverse correlation has also been demonstrated between the blood pressure level and the Mg^{2+} concentration in red blood cells of hypertensive humans[81] and spontaneously hypertensive rats.[84] Furthermore, recent studies in both nondiabetic[85] and diabetic[86] individuals have demonstrated a strong direct correlation of blood pressure levels with fasting plasma insulin and cytosolic Ca^{2+} levels in erythrocytes and an inverse correlation with intracellular Mg^{2+} and pH. Interestingly, the increased cytosolic Ca^{2+} and the decreased Mg^{2+} concentrations were also common to diabetic normotensive patients, whereas the decrease in intracellular pH was characteristic of hypertensive diabetic patients. Thus, it has been proposed that a peculiar alteration in the intracellular ion metabolism may represent the link between alterations in carbohydrate metabolism and blood pressure regulation.[87]

Genetic Predisposition

Essential hypertension is a complex polygenic disease with a strong environmental component. One of the most common alterations in membrane ion transport in essential hypertension is the elevation in erythrocyte Na^+-Li^+ ex-

at 10 minutes of low-dose insulin and remained below control levels during both high-dose insulin and recovery. (C) Forearm vascular resistance declined during the 1-hour low-dose insulin infusion and remained stable during the high-dose insulin infusion and during the 1-hour recovery period. *(Reprinted, by permission of the American Society for Clinical Investigation, from Anderson EA, Hoffman RP, Thomas WB, et al: Hyperinsulinemia produces both sympathetic neural activation and vasodilation in normal humans. J Clin Invest 1991;87:2246–2252.)*

change.[88-90] Interestingly, the average Na^+-Li^+ countertransport activity has also been reported to be elevated in normotensive first-degree relatives of patients with essential hypertension compared to first-degree relatives of normotensive individuals.[88] Although there is a strong degree of overlap of Na^+-Li^+ countertransport activity between groups, these results suggest that a subgroup of essential hypertensive patients may have inherited an overactivity of this ion exchange system. Enhanced Na^+-Li^+ countertransport activity has also been reported in diabetic patients with microalbuminuria,[17] glomerular hyperfiltration,[91] and proteinuria,[92] leading to the hypothesis that elevated Na^+-Li^+ countertransport activity is an early marker of diabetic nephropathy. In this regard, it is of interest that the subgroup of patients with essential hypertension who manifest Na^+-Li^+ countertransport overactivity has been associated with a positive family history of cardiovascular and kidney diseases.[93-95] Thus, it has been hypothesized that a subgroup of IDDM patients inherited a predisposition to hypertension and to diabetic nephropathy that is associated with an increased Na^+-Li^+ countertransport activity in red blood cells.[96]

In NIDDM subjects there is increasing evidence that insulin resistance is at least partially inherited.[97-101] Recent studies have also shown the presence of severe insulin resistance in a subset of nondiabetic patients with essential hypertension.[102,103] To compensate for the defect in insulin action, the pancreatic beta cells tend to secrete more insulin. The consequent hyperinsulinemia has been suggested to play a role in the pathophysiology of essential hypertension.[104] It is therefore conceivable to hypothesize that a "genetic" form of insulin resistance may represent a link between NIDDM, obesity, and hypertension.

Conclusion

Hypertension is more common in the diabetic than in the nondiabetic population. The mechanism(s) behind this association are still obscure; however, several provocative hypothesis have been advanced. Increased exchangeable sodium and enhanced cardiovascular reactivity are common in both IDDM and NIDDM patients. Similarly, increased intracellular Ca^{2+} and decreased Mg^{2+} have been reported in diabetic and in hypertensive patients. The majority of the proposed mechanisms for the development of hypertension in diabetic states are shared by normotensive and hypertensive diabetic individuals. This observation suggests that these factors, if combined with a susceptible genetic background, may determine the onset of hypertension. In this regard, two genetic markers have attracted the attention of several investigators: the Na^+-Li^+ countertransport in a subset of IDDM subjects and the inherited form of insulin resistance in NIDDM subjects.

References

1. Hamilton M, Pickering GW, Robert JAF, et al: The aetiology of essential hypertension: I. The arterial pressure in the general population. *Clin Sci* 1954;13:11–35.
2. Pell S, D'Alonzo CA: Some aspects of hypertension in diabetes mellitus. *JAMA* 1966; 202:104–110.

3. Christlieb AR, Warram JH, Krolewski AS, et al: Hypertension, the major risk in juvenile-onset insulin-dependent diabetics. *Diabetes* 1981;30(suppl 2):90–96.
4. Barrett-Connor E, Criqui MH, Klauber MR, et al: Diabetes and hypertension in a community of older adults. *Am J Epidemiol* 1981;113:276–284.
5. Keen H, Chloverakis C, Fuller JH, et al: The concomitants of raised blood sugar: Studies in the newly detected hyperglycaemics. II. Urinary albumin excretion, blood pressure and their relation to blood sugar levels. *Guy's Hosp Rep* 1969;118:247–254.
6. Modan M, Halkin H, Almog S, et al: Hyperinsulinemia. A link between hypertension, obesity and glucose intolerance. *J Clin Invest* 1985;75:809–817.
7. Heyden S: The working man's diet. II: Effect of weight reduction in obese patients with hypertension, diabetes, hyperuricaemia and hyperlipidaemia. *Nutr Metab* 1978; 22:141–159.
8. Tuck ML, Sowers J, Dornfeld L, et al: The effect of weight reduction on blood pressure, plasma renin activity and plasma aldosterone levels in obese patients. *N Engl J Med* 1981;304:930–933.
9. Salans LB, Knittle JL, Hirsch J: Obesity, glucose intolerance and diabetes mellitus, in Ellenberg M, Rifkin H (eds): *Diabetes Mellitus, Theory and Practice.* New Hyde Park, NY, Medical Examination 1983, pp 469–479.
10. Wiseman M, Viberti GC, Mackintosh D, et al: Glycaemia, arterial blood pressure and microalbuminuria in type 2 (insulin-dependent) diabetes mellitus. *Diabetologia* 1984;26:401–405.
11. Feldt-Rasmussen B, Borch-Johnsen K, Mathiesen ER: Hypertension in diabetes as related to nephropathy: Early blood pressure changes. *Hypertension* 1985;7(6, suppl 2):18–20.
12. Berglund J, Lins P-E, Adamson U, et al: Microalbuminuria in long-term insulin-dependent diabetes mellitus. *Acta Med Scand* 1987;222:333–338.
13. Gall M, Skott P, Damsbo P, et al: The prevalence of micro- and macroalbuminuria, retinopathy, arterial hypertension and large vessel disease in non-insulin dependent diabetes mellitus [abstract]. *Diabetologia* 1988;31:492A.
14. Krolewski AS, Warram JH, Cupples A, et al: Hypertension, orthostatic hypotension, and the microvascular complications of diabetes. *J Chrinic Dis* 1985;38:432.
15. A multicenter study: United Kingdom Prospective Diabetes Study III. Prevalence of hypertension and hypotensive therapy in patients with newly diagnosed diabetes. *Hypertension* 1985;7(6, suppl 2):8–13.
16. Mathiesen ER, Oxenboll D, Johansen K, et al: Incipient nephropathy in type I insulin-dependent diabetes. *Diabetologia* 1984;26:406–410.
17. Mogensen CE, Christensen CK: Predicting diabetic nephropathy in insulin-dependent patients. *N Engl J Med* 1984;311:89–93.
18. Viberti GC, Keen H, Wiseman MJ: Raised arterial pressure in parents of proteinuric insulin-dependent diabetics. *BMJ* 1987;295:515–517.
19. Krolewski AS, Canessa M, Warram JH, et al: Predisposition to hypertension and susceptibility to renal disease in insulin-dependent diabetes mellitus. *N Engl J Med* 1988;318:140–145.
20. De Chatel R, Weidmann P, Flammer J, et al: Sodium, renin, aldosterone, catecholamines and blood pressure in diabetes mellitus. *Kidney Int* 1977;12:412–421.
21. O'Hare JA, Anderson JV, Millar ND, et al: The relationship of the renin-angiotensin-aldosterone system to atrial natriuretic peptide and the natriuresis of volume expansion in diabetics with and without proteinuria. *Postgrad Med J* 1988;64:35–38.
22. Trevisan R, Fioretto P, Semplicini A, et al: Role of insulin and atrial natriuretic peptide in sodium retention in insulin-treated IDDM patients during isotonic volume expansion. *Diabetics* 1990;39:289–298.
23. Feldt-Rasmussen B, Mathiesen ER, Deckert T, et al: Central role for sodium in the pathogenesis of blood pressure changes independent of angiotensin II, aldosterone and catecholamines in type I diabetes mellitus. *Diabetologia* 1987;30:610–617.

24. Weidmann P, Beretta-Piccoli C, Keusch G, et al: Sodium-volume factor, cardiovascular reactivity and hypotensive mechanism of diuretic therapy in mild hypertension associated with diabetes mellitus. *Am J Med* 1979;67:779–784.

25. Weidmann P, Beretta-Piccoli C, Trost BN: Pressor factors and responsiveness in hypertension accompanying diabetes mellitus. *Hypertension* 1985;7(6, suppl 2):33–42.

26. O'Hare JA, Ferriss JB, Brady D, et al: Exchangeable sodium and renin in hypertensive diabetic patients with and without nephropathy. *Hypertension* 1985;7(6, suppl 2):43–48.

27. Ditzel J, Brochner-Mortesen J: Tubular reabsorption rates as related to elevated glomerular filtration in diabetic children. *Diabetes* 1983;32(suppl 2):28–33.

28. Sapir DG, Owen OE: Renal conservation of ketone bodies during starvation. *Metabolism* 1975;24:23–33.

29. Ortola FV, Ballermann BJ, Anderson S, et al: Glomerular hyperfiltration in diabetic rats is associated with high circulating atrial natriuretic peptide (ANP) levels and reversed by specific ANP antiserum insulin [abstract]. Program of the 2nd World Congress on Biologically Active Atrial Peptides, New York, 1987, p 196.

30. DeFronzo RA, Sherwin RS, Hendler R, et al: Insulin binding to monocytes and insulin action in human obesity, starvation and refeeding. *J Clin Invest* 1978;62:204–213.

31. DeFronzo RA: Insulin secretion, insulin resistance and obesity. *Int J Obes* 1982;6(suppl 1):72–82.

32. DeFronzo RA: The effect of insulin on renal sodium metabolism: A review with clinical implications. *Diabetologia* 1981;21:165–171.

33. Baum M: Insulin stimulates volume absorption in the rabbit proximal convolute tubule. *J Clin Invest* 1987;79:1104–1109.

34. De Chatel R, Toth M, Barra I: Exchangeable body sodium: Its relationship with blood pressure and atrial natriuretic factor in patients with diabetes mellitus. *J Hypertens* 1986;4:S256–S258.

35. Christlieb AR, Kaldany A, D'Elia JA: Plasma renin activity and hypertension in diabetes mellitus. *Diabetes* 1976;25:969–974.

36. Christlieb AR: Nephropathy, the renin system and hypertensive vascular disease in diabetes mellitus. *Cardiovasc Med* 1978;2:417–431.

37. Weidmann P, Beretta-Piccoli C, Ziegler WH, et al: Age versus urinary sodium for judging renin, aldosterone and catecholamine levels: Studies in normal subjects and patients with essential hypertension. *Kidney Int* 1978;14:619–628.

38. Christlieb AR, Kaldany A, D'Elia JA, et al: Aldosterone responsiveness in patients with diabetes mellitus. *Diabetes* 1978;27:732–736.

39. Campbell IW, Ewing DJ, Anderton JL, et al: Plasma renin activity in diabetic autonomic neuropathy. *Eur J Clin Invest* 1976;6:381–385.

40. Sullivan PA, Gonggrijp H, Crowley MJ, et al: Plasma angiotensin II and the control of diabetes mellitus. *Clin Endocrinol (Oxf)* 1980;13:387–392.

41. Prince M, Stuart C, Padia M, et al: Metabolic effects of hydrochlorthiazide and enalapril during treatment of the hypertensive diabetic patient. *Arch Intern Med* 1988;148:2363–2368.

42. Elving L, DeNobel E, Van Lier J, et al: A comparison of the hypotensive effects of captopril and athenolol in the treatment of hypertension in diabetic patients. *J Clin Pharmacol* 1989;29:316–320.

43. Corcoran J, Perkins J, Hoffbrand B, et al: Treating hypertension in non-insulin dependent diabetes: A comparison of athenolol, nifedipine and captopril combined with bendrofluazide. *Diabetic Med* 1987;4:164–168.

44. Gall M, Rossing P, Hommel E, et al: Metabolic and hemodynamic effects of captopril, metoprolol, and hydrochlorthiazide in hypertensive non-insulin dependent diabetic (NIDDM) patients [abstract]. *Diabetes* 1990;39(suppl 1):124A.

45. Sullivan P, Kelleher M, Twomey M, et al: Effects of converting enzyme inhibition on

blood pressure, plasma renin activity (PRA) and plasma aldosterone in hypertensive diabetics compared to patients with essential hypertension. *J Hypertens* 1985;3:359–363.

46. Phillip T, Distler A, Cordes U: Sympathetic nervous system and blood-pressure control in essential hypertension. *Lancet* 1978;2:959.

47. Weidmann P, Keusch G, Flammer J: Increased ratio between changes in blood pressure and plasma norepinephrine in essential hypertension. *J Clin Endocrinol Metab* 1979;48:727.

48. Kaplan N, Silah JG: The effect of angiotensin II on the blood pressure in humans with hypertensive disease. *J Clin Invest* 1964;43:659.

49. Weidmann P, Endres P, Siegenthaler W: Plasma renin and angiotensin pressor dose in hypertension. Correlation and diagnostic implications. *BMJ* 1968;3:154.

50. Distler A, Barth C, Liebau H: The effect of tyramine, noradrenaline and angiotensin on blood pressure in hypertensive patients with aldosteronism and low plasma renin. *Eur J Clin Invest* 1970;1:196.

51. Beretta-Piccoli C, Weidmann P: Exaggerated pressor responsiveness to norepinephrine in non-azotemic diabetes mellitus. *Am J Med* 1981;71:829–835.

52. Christlieb AR: Vascular reactivity to angiotensin II and to norepinephrine in diabetic subjects. *Diabetes* 1976;25:268–274.

53. Drury PL, Smith GM, Ferriss JB: Increased vasopressor responsiveness to angiotensin II in uncomplicated type I (insulin-dependent) diabetes. *Diabetologia* 1984;27:174–179.

54. Tuck M, Corry D, Trujillo A: Salt-sensitive blood pressure and exaggerated vascular reactivity in the hypertension of diabetes mellitus. *Am J Med* 1990;68:210–216.

55. Trost BN, Weidmann P: Hypertension accompanying diabetes mellitus: Antihypertensive and metabolic effects of calcium antagonism [abstract]. Proceedings of the IXth International Congress of Nephrology, Los Angeles, CA, June 11–16, 1984, p 228A.

56. Christensen NJ: Plasma catecholamines in long-term diabetics with and without neuropathy and in hypophysectomized subjects. *J Clin Invest* 1972;51:779–787.

57. Beretta-Piccoli C, Weidmann P, De Chatel R, et al: Plasma catecholamines and renin in diabetes mellitus: Relationship with age, posture, sodium and blood pressure. *Klin Wochenschr* 1979;57:681–691.

58. Christensen NJ: Catecholamines and diabetes mellitus. *Diabetologia* 1979;16:211–224.

59. Beretta-Piccoli C, Weidmann P: Total plasma clearance of infused norepinephrine in non azotemic diabetes mellitus. *Klin Wochenschr* 1982;60:555–560.

60. Christensen NJ, Gundersen HJG, Hegedus L, et al: Acute effects of insulin on plasma noradrenaline and the cardiovascular system. *Metabolism* 1980;29:1138–1145.

61. Rowe JW, Young JB, Minaker KL, et al: Effect of insulin and glucose infusions on sympathetic nervous system activity in normal man. *Diabetes* 1981;30:219–225.

62. Landsberg L, Young JB: Insulin-mediated glucose metabolism in the relationship between dietary intake and sympathetic nervous system activity. *Int J Obes* 1985;9:63–68.

63. Berne C, Fagius J: Sympathetic response to oral carbohydrate administration: Evidence from microelectrode nerve recordings. *J Clin Invest* 1989;84:1403–1409.

64. Anderson EA, Hoffman RP, Thomas WB, et al: Hyperinsulinemia produces both sympathetic neural activation and vasodilation in normal humans. *J Clin Invest* 1991;87:2246–2252.

65. Gans ROB, Bilo HJB, van Maarschalkerweerd WWA, et al: Exogenous insulin augments in healthy volunteers the cardiovascular reactivity to noradrenaline but not to angiotensin II. *J Clin Invest* 1991;88:512–518.

66. Gavryck WA, Moore RD, Thompson RC: Effect of insulin upon membrane-bound ($Na^+ + K^+$)-ATPase extracted from frog skeletal muscle. *J Physiol (Lond)* 1975;252:43–58.

67. Moore RD, Munford JW, Popolizio M: Effect of streptozotocin-induced diabetes upon intracellular sodium in rat skeletal muscle. *FEBS Lett* 1979;106:375–378.

68. Moore RD, Fidelman ML, Seeholzer SH: Correlation between insulin action upon glycolysis and change in intracellular pH. *Biochem Biophys Res Commun* 1979;91:905–910.

69. Fidelman ML, Seeholzer SH, Walsh KB, et al: Intracellular pH mediates action of insulin on glycolysis in frog skeletal muscle. *Am J Physiol* 1982;242:C87–C93.

70. Mullins LJ: Steady-state calcium fluxes: Membrane versus mitochondrial control of ionized calcium in axoplasm. *Fed Proc* 1976;35:2583–2588.

71. Mullins LJ: A mechanism for Na/Ca transport. *J Gen Physiol* 1977;70:681–695.

72. Eddy AA: The amino acid pumps of living cells. *Sci Prog* 1981;67:245–270.

73. Christensen HN: Linked ion and amino acid transport, in Bittar EE (ed): *Membranes and Ion Transport.* London, Wiley-Interscience, 1970, vol 1, pp 365–395.

74. Pershadsingh HA, McDonald JM: Direct addition of insulin inhibits a high affinity Ca^{2+}-ATPase in isolated adipocyte plasma membranes. *Nature* 1979;281:495–497.

75. Pershadsingh HA, McDonald JM: $(Ca^{2+} + Mg^{2+})$-ATPase in adipocyte plasmalemma: Inhibition by insulin and concanavalin A in the intact cell. *Biochem Int* 1981;2:243–248.

76. Elbrink J, Bihler I: Membrane transport: Its relation to cellular metabolic rates. *Science* 1975;188:1177–1184.

77. Erne P, Bolli P, Burgisser E, et al: Correlation of platelet calcium with blood pressure: Effect of antihypertensive therapy. *N Engl J Med* 1984;310:1084–1088.

78. Zemel MB, Kraniak J, Standley PR, et al: Erythrocyte metabolism in salt-sensitive blacks as affected by dietary sodium and calcium. *Am J Hypertens* 1988;1:386–392.

79. Zemel MB, Bedford BA, Zemel PC, et al: Altered cation transport in non-insulin-dependent diabetic hypertension: Effect of dietary calcium. *J Hypertens* 1988;6(suppl 4):288–230.

80. Paolisso G, Sgambato S, Giugliano D, et al: Impaired insulin-induced erythrocyte magnesium accumulation is correlated to impaired insulin-mediated glucose disposal in type 2 (non-insulin-dependent) diabetic patients. *Diabetologia* 1988;31:910–915.

81. Resnick LM, Gupta RK, Laragh JH: Intracellular free magnesium in erythrocytes of essential hypertension: Relation to blood pressure and serum divalent cations. *Proc Natl Acad Sci USA* 1984;81:6511–6515.

82. Ringer S: A third contribution regarding the infusion of the inorganic constituents of the blood on the ventricular contraction. *J Physiol (Lond)* 1883;4:222–225.

83. Kuriyama H, Uyshi I, Sueuk H, et al: Factors modifying contract-relation cycle in vascular smooth muscles. *Am J Physiol* 1982;243:H641–H662.

84. Matsuura T, Kohno M, Kanayama Y, et al: Decreased intracellular free magnesium in erythrocytes of spontaneously hypertensive rats. *Biochem Biophys Res Commun* 1987;143:1012–1017.

85. Resnick LM, Gupta RK, Laragh JH: RBC cytosolic free calcium levels in hypertension: Relation to blood pressure and other cations [abstract]. *Am J Hypertens* 1990;3:59A.

86. Resnick LM, Gupta RK, Bhargava BK, et al: Cellular ions in hypertenstion, diabetes and obesity: An NMR spectroscopic study. *Hypertension* 1991;17:951–957.

87. Resnick LM: Calcium metabolism in hypertension and allied metabolic disorders. *Diabetes Care* 1991;14:505–520.

88. Canessa M, Adragna N, Solomon H, et al: Increased sodium-lithium countertransport in red cells of patients with essential hypertension. *N Engl J Med* 1980;302:772–776.

89. Smith JB, Ash KO, Hunt SC: Three red cell sodium transport system in hypertensive and normotensive Utah adults. *Hypertension* 1984;6:159–166.

90. Livne A, Balffe JW, Veitch R, et al: Increased platelet Na^+/H^+ exchange rates in essential hypertension: Application of a novel test. *Lancet* 1987;1:533–536.

91. Carr S, Mbanya JC, Thomas T, et al: Increase in glomerular filtration rate in patients

with insulin-dependent diabetes and elevated erythrocyte sodium-lithium counter-transport. *N Engl J Med* 1990;322:500–505.

92. Mangili R, Bending JJ, Scott G, et al: Increased sodium-lithium countertransport activity in red cells of patients with insulin-dependent diabetes and nephropathy. *N Engl J Med* 1988;318:146–150.

93. Carr SJ, Thomas TH, Wilkinson R: Erythrocyte sodium-lithium countertransport in primary and renal hypertension: Relation to family history. *Eur J Clin Invest* 1989; 19:101–106.

94. Turner ST, Weidman WH, Michels VV, et al: Distribution of sodium-lithium countertransport and blood pressure in caucasians five to eighty-nine years of age. *Hypertension* 1989;13:378–391.

95. Morgan DB, Stewart AD, Davidson C: Relationship between erythrocyte lithium efflux, blood pressure and family history of hypertension and cardiovascular disease: Studies in a factory work force and hypertension clinic. *J Hypertens* 1986;4:609–615.

96. Nosadini R, Fioretto P, Trevisan R, et al: Insulin-dependent diabetes mellitus and hypertension. *Diabetes Care* 1991;14:210–219.

97. Barnett AH, Eff C, Leslie RD, et al: Diabetes in identical twins: A study of 200 pairs. *Diabetologia* 1981;20:87–93.

98. Leslie RDF, Pyke DA: Genetics of diabetes, in Alberti KGMM, Krall LP (eds): *Diabetes Annual/3*. Amsterdam, Elsevier, 1987, pp 39–54.

99. Newman B, Selby JV, King MC, et al: Concordance for type 2 (non-insulin-dependent) diabetes mellitus in male twins. *Diabetologia* 1987;30:763–768.

100. Kobberling J, Tillil H: Empirical risk figures for first-degree relatives of non-insulin-dependent diabetics, in Kobberling J, Tattersal R (eds): *The Genetics of Diabetes Mellitus*. London, Academic, 1982, pp 201–210.

101. Eriksson J, Franssila-Kallunki A, Edstrand A, et al: Early metabolic defects in persons at increased risk for non-insulin-dependent diabetes mellitus. *N Engl J Med* 1989; 321:337–343.

102. Ferrannini E, Buzzigoli G, Bonadonna R, et al: Insulin resistance in essential hypertension. *N Engl J Med* 1987;317:350–357.

103. Pollare T, Lithell H, Berne C: Insulin resistance is a characteristic feature of primary hypertension independent of obesity. *Metabolism* 1990;39:167–174.

104. DeFronzo RA, Ferrannini E: Insulin resistance. A multifaced syndrome responsible for NIDDM, obesity, hypertension, dyslipidemia and atherosclerotic cardiovascular disease. *Diabetes Care* 1991;14:173–194.

Chapter 16

Hypertension, Insulin Function, and Calcium

Jeffrey L. Ram, PhD, Paul R. Standley, PhD, and James R. Sowers, MD

Hypertension is common in industrialized societies, and its frequency is increasing as our society ages. Currently, the basic mechanisms that initiate and sustain hypertension are poorly understood. Frequent associations between hypertension and abnormalities in calcium (Ca^{2+}) function, as reviewed in this chapter, indicate that studies of Ca^{2+} function and the factors that regulate it may be critical in understanding the mechanisms underlying hypertension. Furthermore, these abnormalities are frequently associated with hormonal imbalances, including those that occur in diabetes and obesity. A variety of mechanisms undoubtedly play a role in the development and maintenance of high blood pressure, and these must be taken into account in its treatment. However, the perspective taken in this review is that abnormal insulin function is particularly important and may be a nexus between hypertension and calcium function in many forms of hypertension. This perspective is supported not only by clinical associations between diabetes and hypertension, but also by experimental studies of interactions between insulin and calcium function both in animal models and in in vitro tissue and cell systems.

Human Studies

Increases in Cell Ca^{2+} in Essential Hypertension

A number of abnormalities of Ca^{2+} metabolism have been reported in patients with essential hypertension. Utilizing fluorescent dye indicator techniques, a number of investigators have observed an elevation of cytosolic intracellular Ca^{2+} ($[Ca^{2+}]_i$) levels in hypertensive individuals. Measurement of $[Ca^{2+}]_i$ in humans has been done on circulating blood cells because levels have not been determined in intact vascular smooth muscle from hypertensive and normal human subjects. At least 14 investigative teams have reported elevated basal platelet $[Ca^{2+}]_i$ in patients with essential hypertension.

A positive relationship between platelet $[Ca^{2+}]_i$ and blood pressure in essential hypertension has been noted in some studies[1-3] but not in others.[4,5] One investigative team has noted increased $[Ca^{2+}]_i$ responses to thrombin,[2] whereas others have not observed these increases.[3] More recently, a positive correlation between mean arterial pressure and basal platelet $[Ca^{2+}]_i$ has also been noted in normotensive individuals, suggesting a relationship between blood pressure and platelet $[Ca^{2+}]_i$.[6] Antihypertensive therapy with a calcium channel blocker, a β-blocker, and a diuretic in essential hypertensive patients was observed to reduce platelet $[Ca^{2+}]_i$, and this reduction was positively correlated with the decrease in blood pressure.[1] Other studies have produced variable results with respect to relationships between reductions in blood pressure and platelet $[Ca^{2+}]_i$. These results collectively suggest, however, that platelet $[Ca^{2+}]_i$ is correlated with blood pressure both prior to and following antihypertensive therapy.

It is generally assumed that increases in platelet $[Ca^{2+}]_i$ are reflective of similar increases in vascular smooth muscle cell Ca^{2+} levels.[1,7] Indeed, platelets have many similarities to vascular smooth muscle cells, such as the presence of Ca^{2+}-linked contractile mechanisms, adenylate cyclase–dependent α-adrenergic receptors,[7] and vasopressin-elicited elevation of $[Ca^{2+}]_i$.[8] However, there are some potential limitations in the use of platelets as surrogates for vascular smooth muscle $[Ca^{2+}]_i$ metabolism.[8] Several studies have documented that platelet $[Ca^{2+}]_i$ increases with age,[9] a phenomenon possibly related to increases in platelet aggregability with aging. There is considerable evidence that platelets from hypertensive individuals are hyperaggregable, a state possibly contributing to increased platelet $[Ca^{2+}]_i$.[7] Platelet $[Ca^{2+}]_i$ increases with platelet aggregation, and platelets may be activated, as evidenced by increased $[Ca^{2+}]_i$, simply by washing them and allowing them to sit over time.[8] Although vasopressin elicits transient rises in $[Ca^{2+}]_i$ in both platelets and vascular smooth muscle cells, the response to vasopressin in platelets was almost completely blocked by inhibitors of Ca^{2+} influx through voltage-operated Ca^{2+} channels,[8] whereas the response to vasopressin in vascular smooth muscle cells is only partly dependent on extracellular Ca^{2+}.[10] Thus, higher levels of platelet $[Ca^{2+}]_i$ associated with hypertension may be due to changes specific to platelet function, rather than reflecting a more generalized change in cell Ca^{2+} metabolism, including, for example, vascular smooth muscle cell Ca^{2+} metabolism.

Investigations evaluating cells other than platelets in essential hypertensive patients have yielded conflicting results. Increased Ca^{2+} content has been reported in erythrocytes[11] and adipocytes[12] in patients with essential hypertension compared with normotensive controls. In normotensive patients, leukocytes show a significant positive correlation between blood pressure and leukocyte $[Ca^{2+}]_i$, although, as a group, patients with essential hypertension do not differ in leukocyte $[Ca^{2+}]_i$ from normotensives.[13] These studies indicate that higher levels of $[Ca^{2+}]_i$ associated with hypertension are not present in all cells. With the caveats that platelets may not necessarily be representative of all cells and may have some differences from as well as similarities to vascular smooth muscle, the observations of an association of higher platelet $[Ca^{2+}]_i$ with hypertension nevertheless suggest that it may be worthwhile to inquire about mechanisms that may affect Ca^{2+} in many types of cells in hypertension.

Factors That May Regulate $[Ca^{2+}]_i$ in Essential Hypertension

Ouabainlike Factors

Circulating factors may cause an increase in $[Ca^{2+}]_i$. This was suggested by the observation that the $[Ca^{2+}]_i$ of platelets from normotensive subjects increased substantially when incubated in plasma from hypertensive subjects. In the same study, the $[Ca^{2+}]_i$ of platelets from hypertensive subjects decreased when incubated with control plasma.[14] It has been suggested that this increase in platelet $[Ca^{2+}]_i$ may be explained, in part, by a higher concentration of a Na^+ pump inhibitor in this plasma.[14,15] The presence of such a humoral pump inhibitor, in addition to causing natriuresis, increases vascular smooth muscle contractility to vasoactive agents. Recently, plasma ouabainlike activity, as evaluated by inhibition of Na^+/K^+ adenosine triphosphatase (ATPase) activity and ouabain binding, was found to be significantly correlated to platelet $[Ca^{2+}]_i$.[15] This relationship was independent of age and blood pressure. The investigators interpreted these results as indicating that a circulating ouabainlike factor may play a significant role in the regulation of $[Ca^{2+}]_i$. However, the precise role of this endogenous Na^+/K^+-ATPase inhibitor in the regulation of cell Ca^{2+} metabolism remains to be elucidated.

Changes in Calcitrophic Hormone in Essential Hypertension

Studies suggesting that the elevated $[Ca^{2+}]_i$ observed in essential hypertension may be linked to an alteration of Ca^{2+} metabolism, and resulting changes in calcitrophic hormones have recently been reviewed.[16] The major calcitrophic hormones, parathyroid hormone (PTH) and 1,25-dihydroxyvitamin D_3 (calcitriol), have been shown to be increased in some forms of essential hypertension. These increases in calcitrophic hormones appear to reflect decreased plasma ionized Ca^{2+} levels secondary to salt-induced Ca^{2+} excretion, a primary renal Ca^{2+} leak, or dietary Ca^{2+} deficiencies. PTH has been shown to stimulate the influx of free Ca^{2+} into isolated cardiac cells and osteoblastlike cells. However, in one study, PTH reduced Ca^{2+} uptake in vascular smooth muscle.[17] Therefore, the role of PTH in inducing increases in $[Ca^{2+}]_i$ and subsequently increasing vascular contraction is problematic. However, a potentially hypertensive circulating factor of parathyroid origin (but distinct from PTH), termed "parathyroid hypertensive factor" (PHF), recently has been identified.[18] PHF stimulates vascular smooth muscle Ca^{2+} uptake, increases blood pressure, and potentiates vasoconstrictor responses to other agonists.[18] As with PTH, PHF levels are increased in spontaneously hypertensive rats on a low-Ca^{2+} diet and suppressed in those rats on a high-Ca^{2+} diet.[18] Thus, although the effects of dietary calcium on PHF levels in humans have not yet been reported, it is possible that the antihypertensive effects of dietary Ca^{2+} may be attributed, in part, to suppression of circulating PHF.

Increased levels of circulating calcitriol may be related to increased cell $[Ca^{2+}]_i$. Brickman et al[3] observed elevated levels of calcitriol in untreated hypertensive male patients compared to age-matched normotensive male controls. These changes in calcitriol were accompanied by a significant rise in platelet $[Ca^{2+}]_i$ and a significant decrease in plasma ionized calcium. Similarly, Resnick et al[19] observed elevated calcitriol in essential hypertensive patients with low renin, compared with normotensive patients. It is known that calcitriol can stimulate Ca^{2+} influx into vascular myocytes.[20] Therefore, it appears that elevations in calcitrophic hormones, particularly calcitriol, may play a role in elevated cell $[Ca^{2+}]_i$, including that in cells regulating vascular tone.

Dietary Ca^{2+}

The idea that dietary Ca^{2+} intake may affect blood pressure has been derived from epidemiologic data as well as studies evaluating the effect of calcium supplementation in various hypertensive populations.[21] Blood pressure responses to dietary Ca^{2+} supplementation are very heterogeneous, with best responses occurring in "salt-sensitive" hypertensive individuals such as black, elderly, and insulin-resistant hypertensives.[21] Thus, dietary Ca^{2+} supplementation (to achieve daily levels of 800 to 1,000 mg/d of elemental Ca^{2+}) may help correct a subtle chronic deficiency of this cation and accompanying salt-induced alterations in Ca^{2+} homeostasis and blood pressure regulation in salt-sensitive persons. Specifically, salt-induced elevations in calcitriol, PTH, and/or PHF, which could potentially increase cell $[Ca^{2+}]_i$ levels, could be normalized by increasing dietary Ca^{2+} intake in salt-sensitive individuals.[21] This concept is extensively explored in a recent review.[21]

Factors Associated With Diabetes and/or Insulin Resistance

Insulin resistance appears to be a relatively common abnormality in essential hypertension as well as in hypertension associated with type II diabetes mellitus.[22] In studies by Berglund et al,[23] nondiabetic patients with essential hypertension had higher fasting insulin levels and higher blood glucose levels 1 hour after an oral glucose load than did nonhypertensive controls. In another study, Modan et al[24] reported greater postprandial insulin levels in hypertensive patients than in normotensive controls. More recently, Modan et al[25] found that hypertensive patients requiring greater amounts of antihypertensive medications exhibited greater glucose intolerance. These authors suggested that decreased responsiveness to antihypertensive medications might be a manifestation of the insulin resistance in these patients. In studies by Lucas et al,[26] diastolic and systolic blood pressure were positively correlated with fasting serum insulin levels in obese women, even after correcting for weight, age, and serum glucose. As reviewed recently by Ferrannini et al,[27] experiments using the euglycemic insulin clamp technique and the insulin suppression test to measure insulin sensitivity of patients with untreated essential hypertension have found that hypertension is associated with reduced insulin sensitivity. Natali et al[28] found that insulin-induced changes in glucose uptake in forearm tissues of patients with essential hypertension were significantly reduced compared to normotensive controls. These investigators further demonstrated that the abnormality in insulin response represents peripheral defects in nonoxidative glucose metabolism.

Abnormal insulin function in hypertensives may be due either to lack of insulin (eg, type I diabetes) or to inadequate insulin efficacy resulting from insulin resistance (type II diabetes and other insulin-resistant states). The measures of insulin function reviewed above mainly dealt with the effects of insulin on glucose metabolism, abnormalities of which would not necessarily have direct impact on blood pressure. Nevertheless, there is evidence that insulin can affect peripheral resistance as well. For example, Anderson et al[29] found that acute insulin infusions in the physiologic postprandial range cause decreased peripheral resistance even with increasing sympathetic nerve activity.

These effects of insulin and insulin resistance on peripheral resistance could be due to changes in Ca^{2+} transport mediated by insulin. Decreased activity of erythrocyte membrane Ca^{2+}-ATPase was apparent in black insulin-resistant hypertensive individuals.[30] This is consistent with observations by Cooper et al[4] showing that platelet $[Ca^{2+}]_i$ is increased in black hypertensives and with observations by Zemel et al[31] showing that vasopressin-induced rises in platelet $[Ca^{2+}]_i$ are increased in black women developing pregnancy-induced hypertension. Schaefer and colleagues[32] reported that Ca^{2+}-ATPase activity in erythrocytes from type I diabetics decreased compared to healthy controls. The level and distribution of calmodulin in erythrocytes from individuals with essential hypertension is normal.[16] Thus, the reported reduction in Ca^{2+}-ATPase activity may reflect either impaired calmodulin binding kinetics, with a subsequent failure to activate the pump, or an intrinsic defect in the pump itself, leading to reduced calmodulin activation of Ca^{2+}-ATPase.

As reviewed recently by Levy et al,[33] insulin can stimulate Ca^{2+}-ATPase activity in a variety of tissues, including kidney, heart, liver, and adipocytes. The lack of insulin activity in both insulin-resistant and insulinopenic diabetes might therefore result in a generalized reduction of Ca^{2+}-ATPase activity. Reduction of erythrocyte Ca^{2+}-ATPase in association with diabetes, reviewed in the previous paragraph, is consistent with this suggestion. If similar reductions in Ca^{2+}-ATPase activity also are found in vascular smooth muscle of diabetics, this might provide a mechanism by which increased peripheral resistance and high blood pressure could come about. A reduction in Ca^{2+}-ATPase could lead to a rise in resting $[Ca^{2+}]_i$ and exaggerated agonist responses without the "brake" of Ca^{2+}-ATPase activity during and after the agonist activity. Studies on vascular smooth muscle Ca^{2+} regulation in humans would be ideal to examine these possibilities. However, until now, the interactions of diabetes and hypertension with cellular aspects of vascular smooth muscle function have been studied mainly in animal models and tissues derived from them. As described below, such experiments support the hypothesis that insulin can have direct effects on vascular smooth muscle function by affecting the regulation of vascular smooth muscle Ca^{2+}.

Animal Hypertensive Models, Insulin Function, and Calcium

A general conclusion from the previous section is that cellular Ca^{2+} metabolism is abnormal in human hypertension. A variety of mechanisms may play a role in mediating the changes in Ca^{2+} metabolism and associated rises in blood pressure, including changes in ouabainlike plasma factors, calcitrophic hormones, dietary Ca^{2+}, and insulin function. It is not expected that any one mechanism will explain all forms of hypertension. However, given the focus of this volume on diabetes, we turn our attention in the remainder of this chapter to animal models and mechanisms in which insulin function and its disruption may be related to hypertension. Several animal models have abnormalities of insulin function, and, as also occurs in human diabetes, many of them exhibit abnormalities of blood pressure. These models include the spontaneously hypertensive rat (SHR), the fructose-fed rat, the streptozotocin-induced diabetic rat, and the Zucker obese rat.

Spontaneously Hypertensive Rat

SHRs become moderately hypertensive by 4 weeks of age and markedly hypertensive by 9 weeks.[34] They are hyperinsulinemic but euglycemic, indicating insulin resistance.[34,35] Further evidence of insulin resistance in SHRs is that insulin-stimulated glucose uptake into adipocytes from SHRs is decreased relative to Wistar-Kyoto normotensive control rats.[36] Adipocyte insulin resistance is already well established early in the development of hypertension in SHRs (at 6 weeks) and does not further increase as the animals become more hypertensive.[36] These findings indicate that the development of insulin resistance is probably not secondary to the development of hypertension.

Hypertension and insulin resistance in SHRs also appear to be accompanied by abnormalities in Ca^{2+} function. For example, there is less integral membrane Ca^{2+}-binding protein in cell membranes of SHRs than in controls.[37] Sugiyama et al[38] and Aqel et al[39] have demonstrated that intracellular Ca^{2+} pools in vascular smooth muscle cells of SHRs release more Ca^{2+} in response to caffeine than do such pools in controls. Rusch and Hermsmeyer[40] found that voltage-dependent Ca^{2+} currents are altered in SHRs. These studies showed relatively more Ca^{2+} current in L than in T channels in azygous vein cells in SHRs, compared to the predominance of T channel current in cells from normotensive controls. These and other changes in Ca^{2+} handling in SHRs have been reviewed recently.[41]

Fructose-Fed Rat

The association of insulin resistance and hypertension in the fructose-fed rat has been reviewed recently by Reaven.[42] Rats fed a high-fructose diet exhibit a rise in blood pressure of 20 to 30 mm Hg. This hypertensive response is accompanied by insulin resistance and hyperinsulinemia. Studies on changes in calcium regulation in this animal model would be quite interesting but have not been reported.

Streptozotocin-Induced Diabetic Rat

Streptozotocin injection into rats causes long-lasting decreases in plasma insulin levels, resulting in severely diabetic animals.[43,44] Blood pressure is significantly elevated 2 to 6 weeks after streptozotocin treatment.[43,344] These changes in insulin function and blood pressure are accompanied by changes in calcium handling by vascular tissues. Aortic $^{45}Ca^{2+}$ efflux was significantly slower in diabetic rats than it was in controls.[43] Furthermore, norepinephrine-induced contractions of aortic rings from diabetic rats showed a greater dependency on extracellular calcium than did aortic rings from controls.[45]

Zucker Obese Rat

The gene "fatty" (fa) in the Zucker obese rat causes extreme obesity of juvenile onset.[46] The *fa* allele is recessive, and therefore enables well-controlled experiments to be done by comparing *fa/fa* obese homozygotes to lean controls of similar genetic background (*fa/+* and *+/+* littermates). Obesity in the homozygotes is apparent at 4 weeks of age. Obesity in these animals is accompanied by hyperinsulinemia when compared to their lean littermates.[47] Liver preparations from obese rats exhibit age-related decreases in insulin-receptor regulation as a result of decreased receptor number with no change in insulin receptor affinity. No such changes are apparent in preparations from lean controls. Obese rats develop insulin resistance, as shown by impaired glucose tolerance and decreased insulin-stimulated glucose uptake. Insulin resistance develops earliest in skeletal muscle, then in adipose tissue, and finally in liver.[48] Thus, two important considerations in evaluating experiments in this rat model are (1) the age of the rats, and (2) the fact that the degree of insulin resistance varies with the tissue being studied.

Shemer et al[49] investigated the relationship of insulin resistance to insulin receptor binding and postreceptor events in the obese rat. These investigators showed that, although insulin binding in hepatocytes from obese rats was decreased compared to that in hepatocytes from lean rats, tyrosine kinase activity was higher in the obese rat preparations. These alterations in insulin receptor function are partially corrected by a 72-hour fast. Thus, despite the genetic cause for obesity in the Zucker obese rat model, the liver insulin receptor and its tyrosine kinase activity seem to be regulated by environmental factors that include circulating plasma insulin levels.

As with humans and several other animal models showing insulin resistance, the Zucker obese rat also exhibits hypertension. Mean arterial blood pressure measured in 5-week-old unanesthetized, unrestrained Zucker animals, using intra-arterial catheters, was significantly higher in obese animals (130 mm Hg) compared to lean controls (112 mm Hg)[50] (similar results were also obtained by Shehin et al[47]).

To evaluate a possible role of abnormal Ca^{2+} handling in the hypertension and insulin resistance exhibited by Zucker obese animals, Shehin et al[47] compared $^{45}Ca^{2+}$ efflux from vascular strips from Zucker hypertensive obese and normotensive lean rats. Efflux of $^{45}Ca^{2+}$ was delayed in preparations from obese animals compared to lean controls. These results correlated well with glucose-stimulated insulin levels and increased mean arterial pressures in these rats. These findings are in agreement with the hypothesis that increases in vascular resistance in this hypertensive model may be a consequence of abnormalities in Ca^{2+} regulation, concomitant with the insulin-resistant state.

Analysis of Putative Defective Mechanisms at the Cellular Level

The previous sections reviewed evidence that abnormalities in insulin function and abnormalities in Ca^{2+} metabolism frequently occur in human hypertensives and in hypertensive animal models. In this final section we explore what cellular mechanisms, if any, might be a common link explaining the coexistence of these phenomena. It has been suggested that abnormal cellular Ca^{2+} homeostasis links insulin resistance and high blood pressure.[22] In adipocytes from humans[51] and rats,[52,53] elevated $[Ca^{2+}]_i$ was found to be associated with decreased insulin-stimulated glucose uptake. Diabetes frequently appears to be accompanied by exaggerated pressor responses to norepinephrine and perhaps other pressor agents.[54] As reviewed below, several hypertensive animal models also exhibit enhanced vascular smooth muscle contractility and abnormal insulin function. Furthermore, insulin appears to be capable of regulating vascular smooth muscle contractility. Because Ca^{2+} is the critical regulator of excitation–contraction coupling in all muscle cells, a reasonable hypothesis is that abnormalities in insulin function in hypertensive states might cause changes in smooth muscle contractility by modifying Ca^{2+} handling in vascular smooth muscle cells. Recent evidence that insulin has such effects is reviewed.

Enhanced Blood Vessel Contractility in Animal Models of Hypertension

Mulvany et al[55] showed that norepinephrine-induced contractions of mesenteric resistance vessels in SHRs were more sensitive to Ca^{2+} than was the case in normotensive controls. Ca^{2+} sensitivity was measured as the amount of Ca^{2+} required to achieve a half-maximal response to 10-μM norepinephrine. As noted by Mulvaney et al,[55] these differences were apparent prior to full development of the hypertensive state and were not affected by antihypertensive therapy, suggesting that they were not caused by hypertension but may be involved in its development. Using aortic vascular preparations from Zucker hypertensive obese and normotensive lean rats, it has been reported that vascular reactivity to phenylephrine, serotonin, and potassium was significantly elevated without a change in endothelium-dependent relaxation between the two groups.[56] These studies in Zucker rats showed no change in maximal agonist-induced vasoconstrictive responses of isolated vessels. However, the ED_{50} values for all three agonists were shifted to lower concentrations in the obese rats.

Similarly, contractile responses to norepinephrine of aortic vessels isolated from streptozotocin-diabetic (insulinopenic) rats were increased compared to those in preparations from nondiabetic controls.[45,57,58] Furthermore, MacLeod and McNeill[58] found that increases in both sensitivity and maximal responses to serotonin and potassium also occurred in streptozotocin-diabetic rats. Consistent with the enhanced vascular reactivity of isolated vessels, Reddy et al[43] found that streptozotocin-diabetic rats exhibited greater stress-induced rises in intra-arterial blood pressure than did nondiabetic controls. Thus, vascular contractile responses from both insulin-resistant and insulinopenic animal models having both hypertension and abnormal insulin function appear to be exaggerated.

Regulation of Smooth Muscle Contractility by Insulin

One possible explanation of the enhanced contractility in the above animal models is that insulin normally regulates smooth muscle contractility, and that insulin function abnormalities remove this normal regulatory mechanism. Evidence that insulin can regulate vascular smooth muscle contractility comes from a number of laboratories. Yagi et al[59] have shown that insulin reduces vasoconstrictive responses of rabbit femoral artery and vein to norepinephrine and angiotensin II. Insulin treatment of blood vessel segments of normal rats resulted in a shift in the ED_{50} for phenylephrine and serotonin to higher concentrations without changing the maximal responses.[22,56] Similarly, Wambach and Liu[60] reported that insulin reduced the increment in tension of mesenteric resistance arteries caused by noradrenaline, serotonin, and potassium.

Because insulin appears normally to be able to reduce vascular smooth muscle contractility to certain vasoactive stimuli, we suggest the hypothesis, illustrated in Figure 16.1, that vascular reactivity is held in check by normal levels of insulin. When insulin action on vascular muscle is reduced either by lower insulin levels (insulinopenic states) or by insulin resistance (eg, in non-insulin-dependent diabetes), vascular reactivity increases and a hypertensive disease state ensues.

Role of Calcium in Insulin Effects on Vascular Reactivity

Changes in vascular reactivity brought about by insulin could be due to insulin acting at many different points in the excitation–contraction coupling mechanisms of vascular muscle (Figure 16.1). Although a complete investigation of the mechanisms of insulin action on contraction would necessitate evaluation of all points in the excitation–contraction coupling sequence, most studies have concentrated on the central role of Ca^{2+}: the increase of $[Ca^{2+}]_i$ in response to agonists, the release of Ca^{2+} from sarcoplasmic reticulum, the entry of Ca^{2+} through the plasma membrane, and the removal of Ca^{2+} by ATPases and Na^+-Ca^{2+} exchange.

Standley et al[10] and Hori et al[61] have both reported that agonist-induced transient rises in $[Ca^{2+}]_i$ in cultured vascular smooth muscle cells are reduced by insulin treatment. Standley et al[10] studied $[Ca^{2+}]_i$ transient responses to vasopressin of a7r5 cells, a vascular smooth muscle cell line originally derived from DB1X rat thoracic aorta. Treatment of a7r5 cells with insulin caused no change in baseline $[Ca^{2+}]_i$ but produced a decline in the peak $[Ca^{2+}]_i$ response to 10-nM vasopressin by 55% within 90 minutes. Furthermore, Standley et al[10] showed that insulin shifted the dose–response curve for vasopressin-induced rises in $[Ca^{2+}]_i$ to the right without a change in the maximally elicited vasopressin response, in agreement with in vitro vascular contractility studies[22,56] described above. In more recent experiments from our laboratory, illustrated in Figure 16.2, insulin was shown to reduce the vasopressin-induced $[Ca^{2+}]_i$ transient observed in vascular smooth muscle cells derived from Zucker lean rats. Similarly, Hori et al[61] found that insulin decreased $[Ca^{2+}]_i$ transients induced by angiotensin II in cultured rat vascular smooth muscle cells by more than 60% within 20 minutes.

The decrease in the $[Ca^{2+}]_i$ transient caused by insulin could be due to attenuation of Ca^{2+} entry into cell cytoplasm either from sarcoplasmic reticulum or from outside the cell through the plasma membrane. Potassium-elicited contractions are thought to be due largely to Ca^{2+} entering cells via voltage-dependent Ca^{2+} channels (eg, as demonstrated by Kannan et al[62]). Insulin attenuation of potassium-elicited contractions[60] may be due to disruption of the operation of these voltage-dependent Ca^{2+} channels. Consistent with this hypothesis is the fact that enhanced noradrenergic reactivity of vessels isolated from streptozotocin-diabetic rats appears to be due largely to a component of

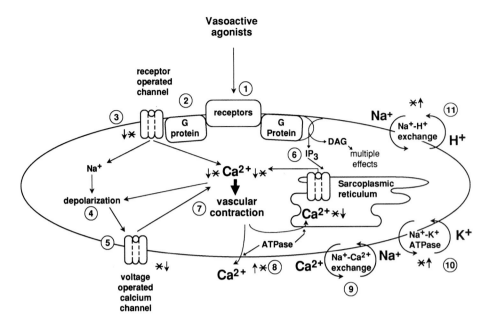

Figure 16.1 Schematic diagram depicting mechanisms regulating contraction in vascular smooth muscle cells and proposed targets of insulin action. Key steps in regulation of contraction are indicated by circled numbers. Agonists affecting smooth muscle tension would typically (1) bind to receptors; (2) activate receptor-coupled mechanisms, usually via a G protein coupled mechanism; (3) cause the opening of receptor-operated channels permeable to calcium and sodium, leading to (4) depolarization and the resultant activation of voltage-operated channels for (5) calcium and potassium (not shown); and (6) activate the production of inositol trisphosphate (IP$_3$), which triggers release of calcium from sarcoplasmic reticulum, and diacylglycerol (DAG), which activates protein kinase C and the opening of plasma membrane ion channels. (7) The rise in intracellular calcium triggered by these processes activates contraction by binding to calmodulin, which subsequently activates myosin kinase, leading to phosphorylation of myosin, the final step needed to trigger cross-bridge cycling with actin to elicit contraction. Relaxation of smooth muscle fibers and possibly some regulation of the rising phase of calcium during contraction come about as a result of removal of free calcium by (8) Ca^{2+}-ATPases in the sarcoplasmic reticulum and plasma membranes and by (9) Na^+-Ca^{2+} exchange. Ca^{2+} function, and hence contraction, is also indirectly regulated by (10) Na^+/K^+-ATPase and (11) Na^+-H^+ exchange. Mechanisms that previous experiments have shown to be affected by insulin in various tissues, although in most cases in vascular smooth muscle (see text), are indicated by *, and the direction of previously observed effects are indicated by an adjacent arrow. These previously demonstrated targets of insulin action are suggested to be sites at which insulin acts physiologically to hold vascular contractility in check in normotensive individuals.

the noradrenergic response that is nifedipine sensitive[57] and dependent on extracellular calcium.[45] To examine this hypothesis directly, Standley et al[10] used whole-cell voltage clamping to measure a voltage- and Ca^{2+}-dependent inward current and found that the voltage needed to activate inward current in a7r5 cells was shifted approximately 15 mV to the right, without changing the maximum current elicited. Thus, a greater depolarization is needed to activate this current in insulin-treated cells.

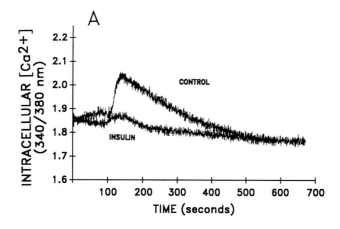

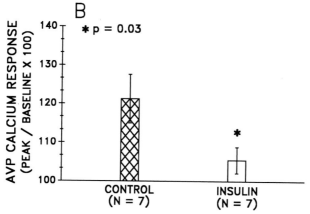

Figure 16.2 Insulin reduces arginine vasopressin (AVP, 10 nM)–stimulated Ca^{2+} transient in cultured vascular smooth muscle cells derived from aorta of Zucker lean rats. $[Ca^{2+}]_i$ was measured in confluent cells on cover slips by spectrofluorometry using Fura-2, as described by Standley et al[10] (A) Representative fluorometric records illustrating the AVP responses in insulin-treated (100 mU/mL, 60 minutes) and untreated cells (control). (B) Summary of AVP responses from seven insulin-treated cover slips and seven control cover slips, showing mean response ± S.E.

A second source of Ca^{2+} for the agonist-induced Ca^{2+} transient is through receptor-operated channels. As reviewed recently,[41] many smooth muscle agonists activate nonselective cation channels that are permeable to Ca^{2+} as well as other ions. The vasopressin-activated nonspecific cation inward current in a7r5 smooth muscle cells, first described by van Renterghem et al,[63] was studied by Standley et al,[10] who found that insulin reduced the vasopressin-elicited current by 65%.

Smooth muscle agonists also increase $[Ca^{2+}]_i$ by triggering the release of Ca^{2+} stored in sarcoplasmic reticulum. The proportion of Ca^{2+} released from this source appears to vary from agonist to agonist. For example, virtually the entire rise in $[Ca^{2+}]_i$ in response to angiotensin II appears to be dependent on intracellular stored Ca^{2+}.[64] In contrast, vasopressin-elicited $[Ca^{2+}]_i$ responses have a significant contribution from extracellular Ca^{2+} sources (more than 50%

in the studies of Standley et al[10]; similar dependence of vasopressin responses on extracellular Ca^{2+} was also reported by Nabika et al[64]). Accordingly, Hori et al[61] analyzed the effect of insulin on mechanisms regulating the release of Ca^{2+} from sarcoplasmic reticulum in response to angiotensin II. Insulin had no effect on inositol trisphosphate production activated by angiotensin II; however, insulin significantly reduced inositol trisphosphate–triggered release of Ca^{2+} from intracellular Ca^{2+} stores.[61]

Another aspect of intracellular Ca^{2+} regulation that is apparently affected by insulin is its removal mechanisms. Johnson et al[65] found that insulin stimulated efflux of radioactive Ca^{2+} from rat aortic strips. Insulin-mediated stimulation of calcium efflux required exposure to insulin for more than 60 minutes and could be blocked by cycloheximide, an inhibitor of protein synthesis.

Conclusions

The general conclusion from the above cellular analyses is that several aspects of Ca^{2+} regulation in vascular smooth muscle cells are affected by insulin. Insulin has other effects at the cellular level that also may influence Ca^{2+} metabolism and even may mediate some of the above changes. For example, in nonvascular cells (adipocytes), it has been shown that insulin activates one isoform of Na^+/K^+-ATPase,[66] a response that could affect intracellular sodium levels. Intracellular sodium can affect Ca^{2+} function, via Na^+-Ca^{2+} exchange and less directly by changing cell pH via Na^+-H^+ exchange. Insulin has also been shown to have effects on Na^+-H^+ exchange in another cell type (erythrocytes).[67] Effects of insulin on sodium regulation in vascular smooth muscle cells would be worth investigating, both in their own right and also because of their possible interactions with Ca^{2+} function and contractility. Although abnormalities in insulin function are unlikely to account completely for all forms of hypertension, the association of hypertension with insulin-resistant and insulinopenic states in both humans and animal models suggests that understanding the cellular mechanisms of insulin action on smooth muscle cells may be important in understanding the underlying causes of many forms of hypertension. Furthermore, the existence of animal models in which this association of abnormal insulin function and hypertension is present should enable analysis of causal mechanisms in these interactions.

References

1. Erne P, Bolli P, Burgisser E, et al: Correlation of platelet calcium with blood pressure: Effect of antihypertensive therapy. *N Engl J Med* 1984;310:1084–1088.
2. Lechi A, Lechi C, Bonadonna G, et al: Increased basal and thrombin-induced free calcium in platelets of essential hypertensive patients. *Hypertension* 1987;9:230–235.
3. Brickman AS, Nyby MD, von Hungen K, et al: Calcitropic hormones, platelet calcium, and blood pressure in essential hypertension. *Hypertension* 1990;16:515–522.
4. Cooper RS, Shamsi N, Katz S: Intracellular calcium and sodium in hypertensive patients. *Hypertension* 1987;9:224–229.
5. Hvarfner A, Larsson R, Morlin C, et al: Cytosolic free calcium in platelets: Relation-

ships to blood pressure and indices of systemic calcium metabolism. *J Hypertens* 1988;6:71–77.

6. Brickman A, Nyby M, von Hungen K, et al: Parathyroid hormone, platelet calcium, and blood pressure in normotensive subjects. *Hypertension* 1991;18:176–182.

7. Buhler FR, Resink TJ: Platelet membrane and calcium control abnormalities in essential hypertension. *Am J Hypertens* 1988;1:42–46.

8. Standley PR, Gangasani S, Prakash R, et al: Human platelet calcium measurements: Methodological considerations and comparisons with calcium mobilization in vascular smooth muscle cells. *Am J Hypertens* 1991;4:546–549.

9. Duggan J, Kilfeather S, Sheridan J, et al: The effects of age on platelet intracellular free calcium concentration in normotensives and hypertensives. *J Hypertens* 1991; 9:845–850.

10. Standley, PR, Zhang F, Ram JL, et al: Insulin attenuates vasopressin-induced calcium transients and a voltage-dependent calcium response in rat vascular smooth muscle cells. *J Clin Invest* 1991;88:1230–1236.

11. Zidek W, Spieker C, Vetter H: Ca^{2+}_i:K^+_i ratio and total intracellular calcium in essential and renal hypertension. *J Hypertens* 1986;4:507–510.

12. Postnov YV, Orlov SN, Pokudin NI: Alteration of intracellular calcium distribution in the adipose tissue of patients with essential hypertension. *Pflugers Arch* 1980;388: 89–91.

13. Bing RF, Heagerty AM, Jackson JA, et al: Leukocyte ionized calcium and sodium content and blood pressure in humans. *Hypertension* 1986;8:483–488.

14. Lindner A, Kenny M, Meacham AJ: Effects of a circulating factor in patients with essential hypertension on intracellular free calcium in normal platelets. *N Engl J Med* 1987;316:509–513.

15. LeQuan Sang KH, Pernollet MG, Meyer P, et al: Plasma digitalis-like activity and cytosolic Ca^{2+} in essential hypertension. *Am J Hypertens* 1990;3:171–175.

16. Sowers JR, Zemel MB, Standley PR, et al: Calcium and hypertension. *J Lab Clin Med* 1989;114:338–348.

17. Pang PK, Yang MC, Sham JS: Parathyroid hormone and calcium entry blockade in a vascular tissue. *Life Sci* 1988;42:1395–1400.

18. Lewanczuk RZ, Chen A, Pang PKT: The effects of dietary calcium on blood pressure in spontaneously hypertensive rats may be mediated by parathyroid hypertensive factor. *Am J Hypertens* 1990;3:349–353.

19. Resnick LM, Muller FB, Laragh JH: Calcium-regulating hormones in essential hypertension. *Ann Intern Med* 1986;105:649–654.

20. Xue H, McCarron DA, Bukoski RD: 1,25(OH)$_2$ vitamin D$_3$-induced ^{45}Ca uptake in vascular myocytes cultured from spontaneously hypertensive and normotensive rats. *Life Sci* 1991;49:651–659.

21. Sowers JR: Dietary calcium effects in salt-sensitive hypertension. *Clin Nutr* 1989;8: 158–163.

22. Sowers, JR, Khoury S, Standley P, et al: Mechanisms of hypertension in diabetes. *Am J Hypertens* 1991;4:177–182.

23. Berglund G, Larsson B, Anderson O, et al: Body composition and glucose metabolism in hypertensive middle-aged males. *Acta Med Scand* 1976;200:163–169.

24. Modan M, Halkin H, Almog S, et al: Hyperinsulinemia: A link between hypertension, obesity, and glucose intolerance. *J Clin Invest* 1985;75:809–817.

25. Modan M, Almog S, Fuchs Z, et al: Obesity, glucose intolerance, hyperinsulinemia, and response to antihypertensive drugs. *Hypertension* 1991;17:565–573.

26. Lucas CP, Estigarribia JA, Darga LL, et al: Insulin and blood pressure in obesity. *Hypertension* 1985;7:702–706.

27. Ferrannini E, Haffner SM, Stern MP: Insulin sensitivity and hypertension. *J Hypertens* 1990;8(suppl 7):S169–S174.

28. Natali A, Santoro D, Palombo C, et al: Impaired insulin action on skeletal muscle metabolism in essential hypertension. *Hypertension* 1991;17:170–178.

29. Anderson EA, Hoffman RP, Balon TW, et al: Hyperinsulinemia produces both sympathetic neural activation and vasodilation in normal humans. *J Clin Invest* 1991;87: 2246–2252.

30. Zemel MB, Bedford BA, Zemel PC, et al: Altered cation transport in non-insulin dependent diabetic hypertension: Effects of dietary calcium. *J Hypertens* 1988;6:S228–S230.

31. Zemel MB, Zemel PC, Berry S, et al: Altered platelet calcium metabolism as an early predictor of increased peripheral vascular resistance and preeclampsia in urban black women. *N Engl J Med* 1990;323:434–438.

32. Schaefer W, Priessen J, Mannhold R, et al: Ca^{2+}-Mg^{2+}-ATPase activity of human red blood cells in healthy and diabetic volunteers. *Klin Wochenschr* 1987;65:17–21.

33. Levy J, Zemel MB, Sowers JR: Role of cellular calcium metabolism in abnormal glucose metabolism and diabetic hypertension. *Am J Med* 1989;87(suppl 6A):7S–16S.

34. Michaelis OE IV, Ellwood KC, Judge JM, et al: Effect of dietary sucrose on the SHR/ N-corpulent rat: A new model for insulin-independent diabetes. *Am J Clin Nutr* 1984; 39:612–618.

35. Mondon CE, Reaven GM: Evidence of abnormalities of insulin metabolism in rats with spontaneous hypertension. *Metabolism* 1988;37:303–305.

36. Reaven GM, Chang H, Hoffman BB, et al: Resistance to insulin-stimulated glucose uptake in adipocytes isolated from spontaneously hypertensive rats. *Diabetes* 1989; 38:1155–1160.

37. Robinson BF: Altered calcium handling as a cause of primary hypertension. *J Hypertens* 1984;2:453–460.

38. Sugiyama T, Yoshizumi M, Takaku F, et al: Abnormal calcium handling in vascular smooth muscle cells of spontaneously hypertensive rats. *J Hypertens* 1990;8:369–375.

39. Aqel MB, Sharma RV, Bhalla RC: Increased norepinephrine sensitive intracellular Ca^{2+} pool in the caudal artery of spontaneously hypertensive rats. *J Hypertens* 1987;5:249–253.

40. Rusch NJ, Hermsmeyer K: Calcium currents are altered in the vascular muscle cell membrane of spontaneously hypertensive rats. *Circ Res* 63:997–1002.

41. Ram JL, Standley PR, Sowers JR: Calcium function in vascular smooth muscle and its relationship to hypertension, in Epstein M (ed): *Calcium Antagonists in Clinical Medicine*, 2. Philadelphia, Hanley & Belfus, Inc. 1992, pp 29–48.

42. Reaven GM: Insulin resistance, hyperinsulinemia, hypertriglyceridemia, and hypertension. Parallels between human disease and rodent models. *Diabetes Care* 1991; 14:195–202.

43. Reddy S, Shehin S, Sowers JR, et al: Aortic calcium-45 flux and blood pressure regulation in streptozotocin-induced diabetic rats. *J Vasc Med Biol* 1990;2:46–51.

44. Dunbar JC, Ergene E, Anderson GF, et al: Decreased cardiorespiratory effects of neuropeptide Y in the nucleus tractus solitarius in diabetes. *Am J Physiol* 1992;262:R865–R871.

45. Owen MP, Carrier GO: Calcium dependence of norepinephrine-induced vascular contraction in experimental diabetes. *J Pharmacol Exp Ther* 1980;212:253–258.

46. Zucker LM, Zucker TF: Fatty, a new mutation in the rat. *J Hered* 1961;52:275–278.

47. Shehin SE, Sowers JR, Zemel MB: Impaired vascular smooth muscle ^{45}Ca efflux and hypertension in Zucker obese rats. *J Vasc Med Biol* 1989;1:278–282.

48. Clark JB, Clark CM Jr: Age-related changes in insulin receptor regulation in liver membranes from Zucker fatty rats. *Endocrinology* 1982;111:964–969.

49. Shemer J, Ota A, Adamo M, et al: Insulin-sensitive tyrosine kinase is increased in livers in adult obese Zucker rats: Correction with prolonged fasting. *Endocrinology* 1988;123:140–148.

50. Kurtz TW, Morris RC, Pershadsingh HA: The Zucker fatty rat as a genetic model of obesity and hypertension. *Hypertension* 1989;13:896–901.

51. Segal S, Lloyd S, Sherman N, et al: Postprandial changes in cytosolic free calcium

and glucose uptake in adipocytes in obesity and non-insulin-dependent diabetes mellitus. *Horm Res* 1990;34:39–44.

52. Draznin B, Lewis D, Houlder N, et al: Mechanism of insulin resistance induced by sustained levels of cytosolic free calcium in rat adipocytes. *Endocrinology* 1989;125: 2341–2349.

53. Draznin B, Sussman K, Kao M, et al: The existence of an optimal range of cytosolic free calcium for insulin-stimulated glucose transport in rat adipocytes. *J Biol Chem* 1987;262:14385–14388.

54. Weidmann P, Trost BN: Pathogenesis and treatment of hypertension associated with diabetes. *Horm Metab Res Suppl* 1985;15:51–58.

55. Mulvany MJ, Korsgaard N, Nyborg N: Evidence that the increased calcium sensitivity of resistance vessels in spontaneously hypertensive rats is an intrinsic defect of their vascular smooth muscle. *Clin Exp Hypertens* 1981;3:749–761.

56. Zemel MB, Reddy S, Shehin SE, et al: Vascular reactivity in Zucker obese rats: Role of insulin resistance. *J Vasc Med Biol* 1990;2:81–85.

57. Scarborough NL, Carrier GO: Nifedipine and alpha adrenoceptors in rat aorta. II. Role of extracellular calcium in enhanced alpha-2 adrenoceptor-mediated contraction in diabetes. *J Pharmacol Exp Ther* 1984;231:603–609.

58. MacLeod KM, McNeill JH: The influence of chronic experimental diabetes on contractile responses of rat isolated blood vessels. *Can J Physiol Pharmacol* 1985;63:52–57.

59. Yagi S, Takata S, Kiyokawa H, et al: Effects of insulin on vasoconstrictive responses to norepinephrine and angiotensin II in rabbit femoral artery and vein. *Diabetes* 1988; 37:1064–1067.

60. Wambach G, Liu D: Insulin attenuates vasoconstriction by noradrenaline, serotonin, and potassium in rat mesenteric resistance arteries in vitro. *Blood Vessels* 1991;28: 342.

61. Hori M, Saito F, Fittengoff M, et al: Insulin attenuates angiotensin II mediated calcium mobilization in cultured rat vascular smooth muscle by depletion of intracellular calcium stores. *Clin Res* 1991;39:270A.

62. Kannan MS, Seip AE, Crankshaw DJ: Effect of nifedipine on calcium-induced contractions to potassium in the aorta and mesenteric arteries of spontaneously hypertensive and normotensive rats. *Can J Physiol Pharmacol* 1986;64:310–314.

63. van Renterghem C, Romey G, Lazdunski M: Vasopressin modulates the spontaneous electrical activity in aorta cells (line A7r5) by acting on three different types of ionic channels. *Proc Natl Acad Sci USA* 1988;85:9365–9369.

64. Nabika T, Velletri PA, Lovenberg W, et al: Increase in cytosolic calcium and phosphoinositide metabolism induced by angiotensin II and [Arg] vasopressin in vascular smooth muscle cells. *J Biol Chem* 1985;260:4661–4670.

65. Johnson BAB, Patel K, Sowers JR, et al: Possible mechanisms of insulin attenuation of vascular reactivity. *FASEB J* 1990;4:A857.

66. Lytton J, Lin JC, Guidotti G: Identification of two molecular forms of (Na^+, K^+)-ATPase in rat adipocytes: Relation to insulin stimulation of the enzyme. *J Biol Chem* 1985;260:1177–1184.

67. Pontremoli R, Rivera A, Canessa M: Insulin and cytosolic Ca^{++} (Ca_1) modulate the human red cell Na/H exchanger (EXC). *Clin Res* 1991;39:192A.

Chapter 17

Vascular Smooth Muscle in Diabetes: Function and Relevance to Hypertension

Michael L. Tuck, MD

Vascular Reactivity in Diabetes Mellitus

Several lines of evidence point to major abnormalities in the vasculature of subjects with diabetes mellitus. Numerous studies have demonstrated that the sensitivity of blood pressure responses to various stress situations and to pressor hormone infusions are enhanced in diabetic animals and humans.[1] In the human studies, exaggerated vascular responses occur in patients with both insulin-dependent diabetes mellitus (IDDM) and non-insulin-dependent diabetes mellitus (NIDDM). Vascular hyperreactivity is seen not only in the presence of microvascular complications but also in patients free of those complications and, in the presence or absence of hypertension. Also, despite differences in age, duration of disease, and control of sodium intake, studies have found a consistent increase in blood pressure responses to angiotensin II (A II) and norepinephrine in diabetic subjects.[2,3]

Christlieb et al[4] first examined the dose of A II required to elevated pressure by 20 mm Hg, and observed that the dose required was 40% lower in diabetic than control subjects. Weidmann and co-workers[2,3,5] have performed extensive studies on vascular reactivity in humans, finding that significantly lower doses of pressor agents such as A II are needed to attain pressor responses in diabetics compared to controls. They noted enhanced vascular reactivity in both normotensive and hypertensive diabetics with or without microvascular complications. Enhanced blood pressure responses to A II infusions are not secondary to low circulating levels of A II that might be expected to up-regulate vascular A II receptors, rendering them more responsive.[3] Drury et al[6] observed that normotensive IDDM patients who had no clinical evidence of microvascular complications had enhanced blood pressure responses to graded doses of infused A II. These early studies, especially in normotensive diabetics free of microvascular complications, offered evidence that enhanced blood pressure responses may be more a consequence of the metabolic changes of diabetes mellitus than secondary to prolonged hypertension or vascular damage.

Exaggerated blood pressure responses to the infusion of norepinephrine are also found in subjects with diabetes mellitus.[2] Because these subjects have normal circulating levels of norepinephrine, the enhanced blood pressure responses are not secondary to norepinephrine receptor changes on blood vessels. Similar to A II, enhanced blood pressure reactivity to norepinephrine is found in normotensive and hypertensive diabetics with or without microvascular complications. The abnormal blood pressure reactivity in diabetes mellitus is not confined to pressor agents, because generalized vascular stress such as heavy exercise (bicycle ergometry) and mental stress produce exaggerated blood pressure responses similar to observations in essential hypertension.[1,7,8] There also may be basic vascular defects in diabetes leading to enhanced responses to pressor agents on various vascular beds, because retinal and other vessels in patients with microvascular disease show decreased passive distensibility.[9]

Although the exact mechanism for exaggerated blood pressure responses in diabetes mellitus is not known, one appealing explanation is that insulin resistance and hyperinsulinemia could activate sympathetic activity and sodium retention. Either of these factors can contribute to a state of elevated vascular tone, as demonstrated in obesity and essential hypertension. Our laboratory has investigated the interaction between sodium balance and vascular reactivity to A II in NIDDM subjects under conditions of controlled sodium balance on high- and low-salt diets.[10] Under normal conditions sodium restriction leads to increased circulating levels of A II with down-regulation of vascular A II receptors and reduced vascular responses to A II, whereas sodium loading has the opposite effect. It was demonstrated in hypertensive NIDDM subjects that, on both sodium diets, there were enhanced blood pressure responses to A II but, more importantly, there was a failure to down-regulate these responses with sodium restriction (Figure 17.1). These findings suggest defective vascular A II receptor or postreceptor function in NIDDM subjects that prevents the normal attenuation of pressor responses with low sodium intake. Hyperinsulinemia and insulin resistance as part of NIDDM could be a factor in the abnormal interaction between

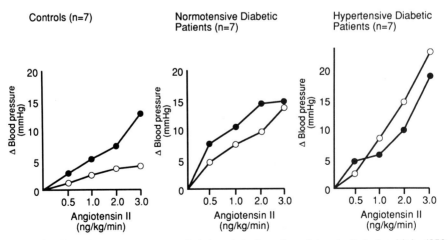

Figure 17.1 Vascular response to graded-dose infusion of angiotensin II during high- (250 mmol) (●) and low- (20 mmol) (○) sodium diet in controls and in normotensive and hypertensive subjects with non-insulin-dependent diabetes mellitus. (*Reprinted by permission, from Tuck ML, Corry D, Trujillo A: Salt-sensitive blood pressure and exaggerated vascular reactivity in the hypertension of diabetes mellitus. Am J Med 1990;88:210–216.*)

sodium and vascular A II responses. Insulin could indirectly alter vascular reactivity by increasing sodium retention or may have a direct effect on altering A II receptor number or function in the vasculature.

Studies have attempted to examine the acute interaction between insulin and pressor agents on blood pressure responses. Vierhapper[11] studied the effect of insulin on A II pressor responses in controls and IDDM patients by simultaneously infusing insulin and A II. There were no differences in blood pressure responses to infused A II with or without insulin infusion, suggesting no acute interaction between insulin and A II in blood pressure control. This study, however, may not exclude a more chronic effect of insulin on vascular responses to A II or norepinephrine in diabetes mellitus, but at present such chronic studies examining this interaction have not been performed in humans. Glucose levels may also influence blood pressure responses in diabetes. There is a positive correlation between blood glucose and systolic blood pressure both in basal states and after oral glucose tolerance testing.[12] In addition, studies have shown significant reductions in blood pressure after improved glycemic control or reductions in insulin levels in diabetic hypertensive patients on no antihypertensive agents.[13,14]

An alternative explanation for enhanced vascular responses in diabetes focuses on vascular structural changes related to the diabetic condition, because insulin's mitogenic properties could render the resistance vessels more responsive to agonist hormones. Decreased passive distensibility of the vascular bed is found in diabetes mellitus[9] and is consistent with the notion of altered structure of blood vessels. Insulin in excessive amounts is both atherogenic[15,16] and mitogenic,[15,16] so that its effect on the vasculature could be direct through altering vascular wall function. As documented by Folkow[17] in animal models of hypertension and in hypertensive humans, functional and structural abnormalities in the arterial bed may be the major contributing factor to the development of hypertension. Changes in microvascular collagen content have been demonstrated in cultured bovine retinal capillary endothelium[18] in response to changes in glucose and insulin concentration, and in rat mesangial matrix[19] in streptozotocin-induced diabetic rats. These studies might suggest changes in the elasticity of the resistance beds under conditions of hyperglycemia and/or hyperinsulinemia.

The finding that vascular responses to A II in patients with diabetes mellitus do not normally modulate with dietary sodium changes is similar to the abnormal renal and adrenal responses described by Hollenberg and Williams in nonmodulating essential hypertension.[20] In a substantial percentage of patients with essential hypertension (30% to 40%), renal vascular responses to A II do not normally modulate in response to dietary sodium restriction and loading. These patients may have abnormalities in vascular A II receptor function and their recognition of changes in sodium balance. Further studies will be needed to determine if a similar case can be made for the abnormal vascular responses in diabetes mellitus. A II is also the major determinant of aldosterone control, and aldosterone responses to A II are also impaired in nonmodulating essential hypertension. Abnormal aldosterone levels are also noted in some patients with diabetes mellitus, most notably in those with renal impairment as part of the hyporeninemic hypoaldosterone syndrome. In diabetic subjects without complications, aldosterone responses to A II can be normal[10,21] or slightly reduced.[21]

Individual sensitivity of blood pressure to high salt intake is another issue in the role of salt in the etiology of hypertension. Despite early studies showing correlations between salt intake in different societies and level of blood pressure, the recent INTERSALT Study[22] did not confirm this relationship. An alternate explanation is that, within given populations with high salt intake, there are genetic and environmental factors that predispose certain individuals to salt-induced rises in blood pressure. Salt-sensitive blood pressure responses may occur in up to 50% of the hypertensive population, influenced by such factors as genes, age, and body weight.[23]

The fixed, high blood pressure responses to A II despite very low sodium intake in patients with diabetes mellitus may explain their high incidence of salt-sensitive blood pressure responses to a high sodium intake.[10] Up to 60% of these patients had salt-sensitive blood pressure responses, based on a current definition of salt sensitivity wherein a greater-than-10–mm Hg increment in mean arterial pressure between low- and high-salt diets equals salt sensitivity.[10] These studies indicate a very high incidence of salt sensitivity in the diabetic population. In essential hypertension, body weight and age are important determinants of salt sensitivity of blood pressure.[23] NIDDM patients are frequently older and above ideal body weight, so they would be more prone to salt-sensitive blood pressure responses.

Salt-sensitive blood pressure responses in diabetes mellitus may be secondary to sodium retention. During high sodium (250 mEq/d) intake in controlled metabolic studies, patients with NIDDM have lower sodium excretion rates than control subjects, indicating net sodium retention.[10] Numerous reports have found that total exchangeable body sodium is approximately 10% to 15% higher in both normotensive and hypertensive diabetic patients with and without nephropathy.[24,25] Impaired sodium excretion has also been reported during volume

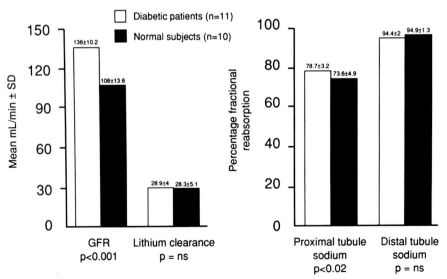

Figure 17.2 Comparison of glomerular filtration rate (GFR), renal plasma clearance of lithium, and tubular fractional resorption rates between diabetic and healthy subjects. (*Reprinted by permission, from Brochner-Mortensen J, Stockel M, Sorensen PJ, et al: Proximal glomerulotubular balance in patients with type I (insulin dependent) diabetes mellitus. Diabetologia 1984;27:189–192.*)

expansion induced by head-out water immersion in diabetic patients when compared to nondiabetic subjects.[26] Studies of tubular function in diabetes have revealed significant reductions in fractional sodium excretion in the proximal tubule, perhaps leading to net sodium resorption[27] (Figure 17.2). Thus, several abnormalities, such as enhanced vascular reactivity, increased body weight, and sodium retention, could act in concert to determine salt-sensitive blood pressure responses in the hypertension of diabetes mellitus.

Relationship Between Hyperinsulinemia and Hypertension

Numerous epidemiologic and clinical studies have shown a positive relationship between levels of insulin and blood pressure.[28–36]Insulin may have a role in blood pressure regulation because it has effects on systems that regulate volume and cardiovascular function, such as renal sodium transport, renal hemodynamics, renal cell growth, and sympathetic nervous system activity (Figure 17.3). In clinical conditions of hyperinsulinemia, such as obesity, NIDDM, and essential hypertension, the increased insulin levels develop in response to diminished insulin action for glucose disposal. Insulin resistance in these conditions is secondary to abnormal insulin receptor function or, more commonly, to abnormal postreceptor function in cell signal transduction.[37] Because receptors for insulin action have also been identified in vascular smooth muscle and endothelial cells,[38] a physiologic role for insulin in regulation of vascular tone has been proposed, and a possible resistance to insulin's normal actions on blood vessels could occur in states of generalized insulin resistance.

Insulin may be a factor in obesity-associated hypertension because circulating levels of insulin are high in obesity and, with weight reduction, there is a correlation between decreases in blood pressure and serum insulin.[8] Increased sympathetic nervous system activity and high plasma norepinephrine levels have been reported in obesity.[8] During weight reduction there are significant

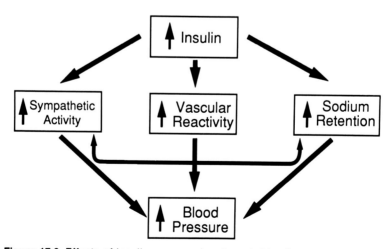

Figure 17.3 Effects of insulin on several systems in blood pressure regulation.

correlations between falls in blood pressure and plasma norepinephrine[8] that may be related to reduced insulin levels.

Insulin resistance with increased basal and insulin responses are also found in subjects with essential hypertension.[30] Reduced insulin sensitivity (insulin resistance) occurs in both obese and nonobese essential hypertensive subjects, suggesting that hypertension per se can be associated with hyperinsulinemia. In several studies, insulin levels correlated with blood pressure in normotensive as well as hypertensive subjects. Thus essential hypertensive subjects as well as NIDDM and obese subjects are characterized by a significant reduction in insulin-mediated whole-body glucose utilization.[30]

Some studies have found no association between insulinemia and blood pressure or have noted only weak correlations.[33] Other variables such as age and race also may determine the association of insulin and blood pressure.

Effects of Insulin on Blood Vessels and Other Blood Pressure Regulating Mechanisms

Insulin has several biologic effects with possible impact on blood pressure regulation, such as effects on renal sodium handling, interactions with the sympathetic nervous system, effects on vascular growth, and lipid plaque formation.

Sodium Handling

Using the glucose clamp technique, studies have shown that insulin decreases sodium clearance in the absence of changes in filtered load of glucose, glomerular filtration rate (GFR), renal plasma flow (RPF), and plasma aldosterone concentration.[39,40] In vitro studies have shown that insulin can directly act on the proximal and distal segments of the tubule,[40–42] enhancing sodium resorption and decreasing free water clearance. In human studies, insulin also appears to have direct effects on renal vascular and hemodynamic function.[42] Mogensen et al[43] reported a decrease in GFR and RPF in IDDM patients after intravenous insulin infusion at doses chosen to normalize serum glucose. Christiansen et al[44] also observed decreased renal hemodynamics with insulin administration. The effects of insulin on the kidney to increase sodium resorption may have physiologic relevance. In contrast, its effects on renal hemodynamics are less well established, because blood glucose and hyperglycemia also can change GFR and RPF.

Sympathetic Activity

The infusion of insulin into normal subjects has been shown to increase plasma norepinephrine levels[45,46] and neural outflow as studied by the method of microneurography.[47] Insulin stimulation of neural outflow could lead to vasoconstriction and a neurogenic form of hypertension. During the euglycemic hyperinsulinemic clamp, norepinephrine levels as well as mean arterial blood pressure have been found to increase in dogs.[48] In this study, simultaneous blood flow was also measured and was increased in skeletal muscles, whereas it was shown to be decreased in splanchnic and renal beds. Therefore, insulin seems to have different effects on various vascular beds, causing vasodilation in skeletal muscle that may actually antagonize the predicted vasoconstrictive effects of the insulin-induced rise in catecholamines. In elderly subjects, infusion of insulin during the euglycemic clamp does not stimulate norepinephrine release and therefore produces hypotension rather than vasoconstriction.[49] The same hemodynamic changes with a fall in blood pressure have been found in diabetic patients with autonomic neuropathy.[50] Thus, in these acute studies insulin appears to act on the vasculature as a vasodilator and may offset the vasoconstrictor effects of norepinephrine.

Laakso et al[51] compared insulin-mediated glucose uptake and blood flow in skeletal muscle of obese and lean subjects. Using the euglycemic clamp and leg blood flow and glucose balance techniques over a large range of induced elevations in plasma insulin levels, they demonstrated that, in both groups, insulin-mediated glucose uptake in the leg, as well as blood flow, increased in a dose-dependent fashion. However, in obese subjects, the dose–response curve was shifted to the right, suggesting resistance to the vascular action of insulin in states of insulin resistance, such as obesity.

Electrolyte Transport

Insulin has acute effects on several ion transport pathways, such as the Na^+-K^+ pump and the Na^+-H^+ antiport. Most of the information on insulin's effect on transport pathways has been determined under in vitro conditions, and less is known about its in vivo effects as a regulator of cell sodium transport. Addition of insulin to various cells types in vitro stimulates Na^+ and K^+ transport through the Na^+-K^+ pump[52] and increases the activity of the Na^+-H^+ antiport system.[53] This effect on ion transport theoretically could lead to intracellular sodium accumulation in cardiovascular and other tissues. Based on the hypothesis of Blaustein,[54] wherein cell sodium accumulation should lead to cell calcium accumulation, the net result would be an increase in vascular reactivity. The rise in intracellular calcium would constitute a hypertensive mechanism by increasing peripheral resistance in arterioles and precapillary sphincters. Whether insulin could raise blood pressure through this mechanism is far from being proven. It is interesting to note, however, that insulin can raise cytosolic calcium levels in rat adipocytes.[55]

Insulin excess may also be associated with other electrolyte disturbances, because research has linked both hypertension and diabetes to defects in calcium and magnesium metabolism. Hypercalciuria is found in insulin-deficient, streptozotocin-induced diabetic rats as a result of a specific defect in renal tubular calcium resorption.[56] In humans, hypercalciuric responses to induced hyperinsulinemia have also been demonstrated.[57] Hypercalciuria in diabetes mellitus is associated with low to normal serum ionized calcium levels and with decreased duodenal calcium transport.[57] The same renal and gastrointestinal defects in calcium and magnesium also have been reported in patients with essential hypertension and in experimental hypertension.[57] In diabetes and essential hypertension, higher levels of parathyroid hormone could increase calcium uptake in both cardiac tissue and vascular smooth muscle, leading to enhanced vascular tone.[57] Recent experiments from our laboratory show that parathyroid hormone can attenuate the A II–induced rises in cytosolic calcium in cultured vascular smooth muscle cells by an adenylate cylase–dependent mechanism.[58]

Insulin and the Vascular Bed

A basic model for the initiating event in the evolution of the atherosclerotic plaque has been proposed by Ross and Glomset.[59] A variety of adverse processes, such as hypertension, hyperglycemia, hyperlipidemia, or immune reactions, may accelerate endothelial cell injury and atherosclerosis in diabetes mellitus.[15,60,61] Exposure of subendothelial collagen as a result of disruption of the normal endothelial lining may precipitate platelet aggregation, which, in turn, results in the release of platelet-derived vasoconstrictor and vasodilatory prostaglandins as well as growth factors. Released growth factors can enhance macrophage migration as well as smooth muscle and fibroblast proliferation, effects that are further abetted by circulating insulin. Local deposition of lipids is facilitated by (1) distortion of the normal vascular surface, (2) the lipotrophic effect of insulin, and (3) hyperlipidemia. The process of vascular damage is further accentuated by hyperglycemia, hyperinsulinemia, and perhaps other determinants prevailing in hypertension and diabetes, as depicted in Figure 17.4).

The production of prostacyclin, a platelet-derived vasodilator that is also a potent antiaggregant, is diminished in human and experimental diabetes.[62,63] In contrast, the synthesis of thromboxane, which promotes aggregation and vasoconstriction, is increased.[64–66] Correction of hyperglycemia may normalize the imbalance between prostacyclin and thromboxane.[67–69] The biosynthesis of von Willebrand factor (a component of factor VIII) by endothelial cells is enhanced in type II diabetics with microangiopathy.[70] Plasminogen activator, the platelet-derived enzyme that promotes thrombolysis via the generation of plasmin, can be depressed in diabetes mellitus,[71] whereas plasmin inhibitors are increased.[72] Collectively, these multiple abnormalities could promote local hypercoagulability and platelet aggregation,[15,60,61] thus leading to increased release of en-

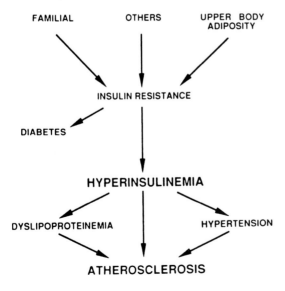

Figure 17.4 The proposed relationship between insulin and atherosclerosis in conditions associated with insulin resistance and hyperinsulinemia.

dothelial-derived growth factors,[73] which could facilitate cell growth and replication and ultimately result in arterial wall thickening.[74]

Of particular interest is the diabetic serum growth factor, a potent platelet-derived promoter of smooth muscle cell proliferation and migration that is enhanced during poor diabetic control, with levels normalizing with improved glucose concentration.[75,76] Insulin itself can enhance proliferation of cultured smooth muscle cells,[77,78] so that hyperinsulinemia could contribute to subendothelial vascular smooth muscle cell replication. In addition, supernatant obtained from platelets of insulin-treated patients was 83% more active in promoting growth of rat vascular smooth muscle cells than was the platelet-derived supernatant from normal subjects.[79] Finally, vascular wall lipid deposition is enhanced, especially in poorly controlled diabetics, because of elevations in low-density lipoprotein (LDL) cholesterol and reductions in high-density lipoprotein (HDL) cholesterol; this enhancement is secondary to increases in apoproteins B and E. Systemic hyperinsulinemia may further accelerate fat deposition into the vasculature via the lipogenic effect of insulin.[15,16]

Hemodynamic Factors in Diabetes and Hypertension

Alterations in the peripheral microcirculation in diabetes could play a role in the initiating events for hypertension and other complications in this disorder. Brenner and coworkers[80,81] have provided evidence for a state of generalized peripheral hyperperfusion in diabetic subjects, similar to that described for the diabetic glomerular capillary circulation. During poor metabolic control, patients with IDDM have increased blood flow in the muscular and cutaneous tissues of the forearm and in abdominal fat tissue;[82–84] this increased flow is normalized with improved glycemic control. Resting forearm blood flow was shown to be 50% to 100% higher in IDDM patients, and insulin treatment significantly reduced the increased flow toward the normal range. Morphologic studies have demonstrated capillary dilation, congestion, or tortuosity in the toe nailfold, facial skin,[85,86] and cheek mucosa[85–87] of diabetic individuals. Vasodilation of high-order arterioles and venules has also been described in rats with streptozotocin-induced diabetes.[88] The systemic vasodilation in the microcirculation in diabetes mellitus may be related to expansion of extracellular and plasma volume, local overproduction of vasodilatory substances such as prostaglandin E and prostacyclin, or the effects of systemic hormones such as atrial natriuretic peptide. Atrial natriuretic peptide is a potent vasodilator, and the circulating levels of this peptide are elevated in experimental and human diabetes.[89]

Insulin deficiency or ineffective insulin action may also result in a generalized vasodilation in the microcirculation by inducing relative tissue hypoxia in the presence of an enhanced demand for oxygen in the diabetic state.[90,91] The contractile state of the microvasculature is inversely related to variations in oxygen tension.[92] Oxygen consumption is higher in diabetic subjects, and increases in erythrocyte 2,3-diphosphoglycerate and hemoglobin are adaptive mechanisms to counteract tissue hypoxia.[93]

This vasodilatory state of the microcirculation may have relevance to the early occurrence of hypertension. Increased flow and pressure may contribute to peripheral microangiopathy in resistance vessels by mechanisms similar to those outlined for the glomerular and retinal microcirculation. Furthermore, the increased peripheral flow might initiate a chain of hemodynamic responses, including early increases in cardiac output, as observed in some patients with early essential hypertension.[94] Reduced duration of the cardiac pre-ejection interval in diabetic individuals without overt cardiomyopathy is consistent with early changes in cardiac function in this disorder.[95,96] However, these possibilities remain speculative because no prospective studies assessing the microcirculation in relation to the subsequent development of increased peripheral resistance and hypertension are available.

Direct Vascular Effects of Insulin

One problem with implicating a direct role for insulin in the pathogenesis of hypertension is that most studies have shown a predominantly vasodilatory action of insulin on blood vessels.[97,98] In patients with diabetes mellitus and autonomic neuropathy, insulin administration causes a fall in blood pressure and an increase in heart rate.[50] Insulin may directly stimulate sympathetic activity in blood vessels to offset its vasodilatory action, and this response is absent in diabetic neuropathy. In the streptozotocin-diabetic rat, insulin therapy by continuous subcutaneous infusion lowers systolic blood pressure, suggesting a hypotensive effect of this agent.[99,100] In other animal studies, insulin also has been shown to have a vasodilatory effect on the skeletal muscle vasculature[101] and on the coronary arteries.[102,103]

However, in certain rodent models of metabolic dysfunction, either genetic or by experimental induction, significant increases in blood pressure have been reported. Sprague-Dawley rats fed a fructose-enriched diet develop insulin resistance, hyperinsulinemia, and hypertriglyceridemia and also show significant increments in systolic blood pressure over a 10-day period. This effect lasts for as long as 3 months on the diet and disappears when the diet is removed.[104] Methods to attenuate insulin resistance and hyperinsulinemia, such as exercise or somatostatin, also reduce blood pressure. Shargill et al[105] have reported rises in blood pressure in normotensive Sprague-Dawley rats implanted with mini-osmotic pumps to release a constant amount of insulin with development of significant hyperinsulinemia. Whether insulin is acting directly on blood vessel responses to pressor hormones in its hypertensive effect or through sodium retention in this insulin-infused model remains to be elucidated.

Spontaneously hypertensive rats (SHRs) have recently been shown to be hyperinsulinemic and have insulin resistance in addition to being hypertriglyceridemic.[106] Glucose transport by insulin-stimulated adipocytes is also reduced in cells from SHRs compared to Wistar Kyoto rats. Recent studies using the hyperinsulinemic euglycemic clamp methodology in SHRs failed to document insulin resistance, showing actual enhanced insulin sensitivity.[107] An alternative argument is that prolonged hypertension may cause defective insulin action. To examine this hypothesis, hypertension was induced in the 2-kidney–1-clip model of renovascular hypertension. The significant rise in blood pressure over 3 weeks in these rats was not accompanied by changes in insulin action as measured by the euglycemic hyperinsulinemic clamp method for insulin sensitivity.[108] Hall and colleagues[109] have provided extensive data showing that prolonged insulin infusion in dogs does not alter blood pressure even under the most extreme conditions of uninephrectomy, high salt intake, and simultaneous infusion of pressor agents. Thus, examination of these animal models of hyperinsulinemia has yet to firmly establish a positive relationship of insulin to blood pressure, and it remains to be determined if these experiments will shed any light on the human state of insulin resistance and hypertension.

Insulin has been shown in in vitro studies to decrease the contractile response to norepinephrine in cardiac and vascular smooth muscle tissue. Alexander and Oake[97] found that insulin attenuated the vasoconstrictive response to norepinephrine in the resistance bed of isolated perfused rat tail vessels. Further evidence of the vasorelaxant properties of insulin comes from Yagi et al,[98] who found a dose-dependent inhibitory effect of insulin on norepinephrine- and A II–induced contractions as studied in vitro in isolated rabbit femoral arteries and veins (Figure 17.5). This vasorelaxant effect was seen at insulin doses as low as 120 μU/mL, suggesting that this effect can occur at physiologic levels. Recently, Standley et al[110] investigated the mechanism of insulin action on arginine vasopressin (AVP)–induced $[Ca^{2+}]_i$ responses and membrane potential in cultured vascular smooth muscle cells (VSMCs), showing significant attenuation by insulin of AVP-induced increments in $[Ca^{2+}]_i$ and a shift in current voltage. These data support an interaction of insulin to offset pressor hormone contractility and second messenger responses in vascular tissue. Certain actions of pressor hormones, such as vascular reactivity and Ca^{2+} fluxes, are abnormal in animal models of hyperinsulinemia and insulin resistance, such as the Zucker obese rat.[111]

Despite significant in vitro evidence for a direct action of insulin on blood vessels, the in vivo significance of insulin as a physiologic regulator of vascular tone has not been established. However, recent studies by Baron and associates[51,112] using the hyperinsulinemic euglycemic clamp have provided

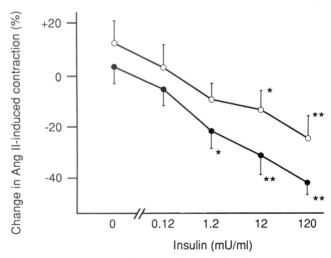

Figure 17.5 Changes in angiotensin II–induced contraction in response to increasing concentrations of insulin in isolated femoral artery (●) and vein (○) from rabbit blood vessels. (*Reprinted by permission, from Yagi S, Takata S, Kiyokawa H: Effects of insulin on vasoconstrictive responses to norepinephrine and angiotensin II in rabbit femoral artery and vein. Diabetes 1988;37:1064–1067.*)

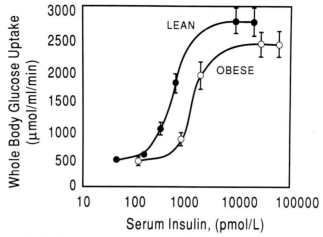

Figure 17.6 The effect of increasing doses of insulin during insulin infusion using the euglycemic insulin clamp on leg blood flow in normal controls and obese subjects. (*Reprinted, by permission, from Laakso M, Edelman SV, Brechtel G, et al: Decreased effect of insulin to stimulate skeletal muscle blood flow in obese man. J Clin Invest 1990;85:1844–1852.*)

evidence in humans that insulin can have significant hemodynamic actions both systemically and at the level of the skeletal muscle. Graded-dose infusion of insulin in normal subjects significantly increased leg blood flow, and this vascular effect of insulin was reduced in obese subjects with insulin resistance (Figure 17.6). These data suggest that, in conditions in which there is insulin resistance to glucose uptake, there may also be resistance to other actions of insulin, such as relaxation of tone in vascular tissue. These investigators have gone on to show that there are reduced effects of insulin to stimulate skeletal muscle blood flow in vivo, and have proposed a novel mechanism for insulin resistance for glucose disposal whereby reductions in insulin's hemodynamic action may lead to reduced blood flow and delivery of insulin to insulin-sensitive tissues.[112]

Table 17.1 Insulin Actions in Vascular Tissues

Vasoconstrictor Actions of Insulin

Stimulation of Na^+-H^+ exchange
Stimulation of Na^+-K^+ ATPase
Inhibition of Ca^{2+}-Mg^{2+} ATPase
Increase in phosphoinositide synthesis
Increase in inositide-specific phospholipase activity

Vasodilating Actions of Insulin

Stimulation of guanylate cyclase
Production of vasodilating prostaglandins
Phosphorylation of caldesmon
Phosphorylation of calmodulin
Hyperpolarization of vascular cells
Activation of specific phosphoprotein phosphatase(s)

Based on evidence that insulin has some effects on vascular tissue, it is reasonable to propose that insulin may be contributing to vasomotion in the balance between factors favoring vasoconstriction and vasodilation to determine vascular tone. Specific receptors for insulin have been identified in bovine aortic VSMCs, and these receptors demonstrate properties such as internalization and degradation similar to receptors on established target tissues for insulin.[38,113,114] The vascular insulin receptor may mediate some metabolic and mitogenic effects of insulin in vascular cells, and the presence of these receptors offer support of a role for insulin in regulation of vascular tone. Insulin receptors have also been described in vascular endothelial cells,[113] and insulin has been proposed as a regulator of endothelial cell proliferation. Table 17.1 summarizes the current findings on the cellular actions of insulin and their potential effects on vascular tone.

Factors in Normal Control of Vascular Tone

In order to understand the significance of the interaction of insulin with factors that regulate vascular contractility, it is important to summarize the mechanisms of vascular contraction and relaxation. Changes in cytosolic $[Ca^{2+}]_i$ have been strongly linked to pressor-induced contraction in vascular smooth muscle cells. The early events following pressor hormone–receptor coupling (ie, A II, endothelin, and vasopressin) in VSMCs involve the activation of phospholipase C (PLC).[115] This results in the hydrolysis of phosphatidylinositol biphosphate (PIP_2) and formation of inositol 1,4,5-triphosphate (IP_3) and 1,2-diacylglycerol.[116] IP_3 causes rapid calcium mobilization from the sarcoplasmic reticulum, leading to elevations in $[Ca^{2+}]_i$. The formation of IP_3 is rapid and transient, and leads directly to activation of myosin light chain (MLC) kinase, phosphorylation of MLC, activation of Mg^{2+} adenosine triphosphatase (ATPase), and contraction. The turnover of diacylglycerol is sustained, activating the calcium- and phospholipid-sensitive enzyme, protein kinase C (PKC). PKC in turn is involved with the maintenance of sustained contraction in response to calcium influx from the extracellular space. Okamura and co-workers[117] have recently demonstrated alterations in aortic diacylglycerol content and composition following norepinephrine stimulation in streptozotocin-induced diabetic rats. Specifically, they found that diacylglycerol content was reduced in diabetic rats compared with control rats and that the arachidonic acid content of the diacylglycerol, as a percentage of total eicosanoid content, was also reduced. Because hydrolysis of membrane phospholipids is the initial response to many hormone–receptor coupled events, alterations in structure of these compounds by shifts in their fatty acid content may be associated with abnormal responses to hormonal stimulation.

Perhaps the most significant systems of interaction between insulin and vascular tone regulation occur in the control of cyclic nucleotide levels and their effects on both contraction and relaxation.[118] Activation of guanylate cyclase and the increase in cyclic guanosine monophosphate (cGMP) has long been recognized as an important factor in vascular relaxation. Stimulation of isolated vessels with vasodilators such as actylcholine, histamine, and endothelial-derived relaxing factor (EDRF) causes an increase in the activity of the soluble form of guanylate cyclase, whereas atrial natriuretic factor (ANF) stimulates the particulate form of the enzyme. In both cases, relaxation is preceded by an increase in cGMP levels. Other stimulators of cGMP formation, such as ATP and sodium nitroprusside, can mimic the effects of ANF and acetylcholine, whereas inhibitors of guanylate cyclase, such as methylene blue, block their effects. There are several theories for the mechanism of cGMP-induced relaxation, including effects on Ca^{2+} metabolism, inhibition of phosphoinositide metabolism, and inhibition of MLC phosphorylation. Increases in cGMP levels also cause activation of cGMP-activated cyclic adenosine monophosphate (cAMP) phosphodiesterase. Both cAMP-dependent protein kinase (AK), which is necessary for the loading of calcium into intracellular storage sites, and cGMP-dependent protein kinase (GK), which exhibits effects on MLC phosphorylation and on Ca^{2+}-ATPase activity, consequently act both to move calcium across the cell membrane and load Ca^{2+} ions into intracellular storage sites, functions that serve as important modulators of calcium metabolism.

The effects of insulin on these intracellular modulators of vascular reactivity are currently the focus of increased investigation. Insulin could affect hormone receptor kinetics or could act through any one of several postreceptor second messenger pathways. Our laboratory has demonstrated that the mechanism whereby insulin attenuates the pressor effects of A II is by blocking the A II–induced increments in $[Ca^{2+}]_i$ as studied in cultured rat VSMCS (F. Saito, M. T. Hori, M. Fittingoff, et al, unpublished data) (Figure 17.7). In the studies of blood vessels (cultured VSMCS), the effect of insulin to attenuate A II action was not secondary to changes in A II receptor affinity or density. Most studies on insulin action in the vasculature have been acute, and we have proposed that more long-term insulin exposure in states of insulin resistance and chronic insulinemia could alter the attenuating action of insulin on A II contractility. This sequence of events would lead to a more vasoconstrictive state as a result of a "resistance" to insulin's actions to attenuate $[Ca^{2+}]_i$ responses to A II and other pressor agents.

Studies have been devised to probe the interaction between insulin and A II by examining an established model of A II–dependent mechanisms, aldosterone production in isolated rat zona glomerulosa cells.[119] In vitro aldosterone production can be determined in adrenal glomerulosa cells during incubation

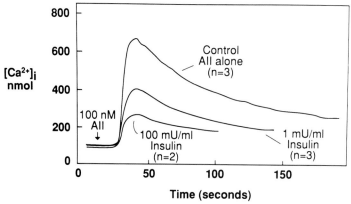

Figure 17.7 Cytosolic calcium response to angiotensin II in cultured vascular smooth muscle cells is attenuated in the presence of insulin at two concentrations.

in the presence of A II (10^{-10} to 10^{-8} M) alone or with insulin (5 ng/mL). These studies have shown a marked attenuation of A II–stimulated aldosterone production after acute or long-term exposure to insulin. Since adrenal glomerulosa cell A II receptor numbers and binding kinetics were not altered by insulin, this effect is best explained by insulin and A II converging on common intracellular pathways such as the IP_3/diacylglycerol/$[Ca^{2+}]_i$ systems. This information then can be used to examine the effects of A II on the vasculature, where the early intracellular events in A II action are similar to those in adrenal glomerulosa cells.

Insulin interactions with pressor agonists also have been examined in vascular segments using in vitro contractile preparations. In these vascular contractility preparations there is normally a vasodilatory response to potassium added to femoral vessels precontracted with norepinephrine as studied in a zero-potassium incubation medium. This effect of potassium can be totally blocked by addition of 1-mM ouabain, suggesting that contractility in this preparation is dependent on vascular Na^+-K^+ pump activity. Addition of insulin substituted for potassium mimics the vasodilatory effects of potassium, suggesting a direct vasodilatory action of insulin perhaps mediated in part by an effect on Na^+/K^+-ATPase activity in blood vessels.

Although the vasocative properties of insulin have been demonstrated in vascular tissue, its overall action may differ in vessels from different vascular beds and may differ depending on animal species. The role of the endothelium in the interaction of insulin with pressor agonists also may be important in its vascular actions, and study of this possibility is in its infancy regarding information on insulin's vascular effects. Insulin action in human pulmonary and coronary arteries on prostaglandin-induced contraction requires an intact endothelium.[120] The effect of insulin on canine carotid arteries has been reported to be endothelium independent.[121]

Studies from our laboratory also have examined A II–stimulated $[Ca^{2+}]_i$ in VSMCs cultured from rat thoracic aortas using the fluorescent dye Fura 2/AM and monitoring $[Ca^{2+}]_i$ by spectrofluorometric methods. Neither acute (20 minutes) nor long-term (24 hours) exposure to insulin alone alters basal $[Ca^{2+}]_i$; however, as previously stated, mean peak increments in $[Ca^{2+}]_i$ after A II addition were dose-dependently reduced in the presence of insulin. Similar to findings of insulin's attenuation of A II–stimualted aldosterone in adrenal glomerulosa cells, insulin also appears to reduce A II-mediated vascular contractility, and this interaction is at the A II postreceptor level of intracellular second messenger effects in VSMCs.

Mechanisms of Insulin-Mediated Attenuation of A II–Induced Calcium Transients

Further investigation into the mechanisms involved in the observations of insulin's effect on A II–induced calcium transients in VSMCs revealed that the reduction of A II–induced calcium mobilization with acute insulin exposure was not due to changes in (1) A II receptor density or affinity, (2) crossover reactions with insulin like growth factor receptors, or (3) attenuation of PLC activity or IP_3 release (F. Saito, M. T. Hori, M. Fittingoff, et al, unpublished data). In contrast,

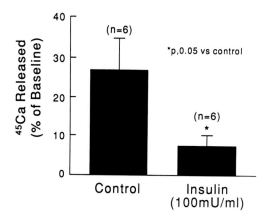

Figure 17.8 The effect of insulin to attenuate inositide triphosphate–mediated release of calcium ($^{45}Ca^{2+}$) from intracellular storage sites in vascular smooth muscle cells in culture.

studies indicate that the primary effect of insulin on A II–mediated signal transduction occurs in the IP_3-mediated release of calcium from intracellular calcium stores (Figure 17.8). In addition, there is an increase in lanthanum-insensitive calcium flux, and/or an increase in cGMP-dependent protein kinase activity in cultured VSMCs on exposure to insulin.

Conclusion

The multiple effects of insulin on the vascular system, either by direct actions or indirectly through sodium and neural mechanisms, point to a potential role for this hormone in regulation of vasomotor tone. Even more provoking is the potential for insulin as a mitogen to chronically alter vascular structures, thereby changing vascular tone. It should be noted, however, that the direct proof linking insulin to vascular control and hypertension is still lacking.

References

1. Stern N, Tuck ML: Mechanisms of hypertension in diabetes mellitus, in Laragh JH, Brenner BM (eds): *Hypertension: Pathophysiology, Diagnosis, and Management.* New York, Raven Press, 1990, pp 1689–1702.
2. Beretta-Piccoli C, Weidmann P: Exaggerated pressor responsiveness to norepinephrine in non-azotemic diabetes mellitus. *Am J Med* 1981;71:829–835.
3. Weidmann P, Beretta-Piccoli C, Trost BN: Pressor factors and responsiveness in hypertension accompanying diabetes mellitus. *Hypertension* 1985;7(suppl II):II-33–II-42.
4. Christlieb AR, Janka HU, Kruas B: Vascular reactivity to angiotensin II and norepinephrine in diabetic subjects. *Diabetes* 1976;25:268–274.
5. Weidmann P, Ferrari P: Central role of sodium in hypertension in diabetic subjects. *Diabetes Care* 1991;14:220–232.
6. Drury PL, Smith GM, Ferris JB: Increased vasopressor responsiveness to angiotensin II in type I (insulin-dependent) diabetic patients without complications. *Diabetologia* 1983;27:174–179.

7. Hollenberg NK, Williams, GH, Adams DF: Essential hypertension: Abnormal renal vascular responses to mild psychological stimulus. *Hypertension* 1981;3:11–19.
8. Tuck ML: Obesity, the sympathetic nervous system and essential hypertension. *Hypertension* 1992;19(suppl I):I-67–I-77.
9. Faris I, Agerskov K, Henrikenson O: Decreased distensibility of a passive vascular bed in diabetes mellitus: An indicator of microangiopathy. *Diabetologia* 1982;23:411–414.
10. Tuck ML, Corry D, Trujillo A: Salt-sensitive blood pressure and exaggerated vascular reactivity in the hypertension of diabetes mellitus. *Am J Med* 1990;88:210–216.
11. Vierhapper H: Effects of exogenous insulin on blood pressure regulation in healthy diabetic subjects. *Hypertension* 1985;7(suppl II):II-49–II-53.
12. Tuck ML: Glucose, insulin and insulin resistance as biochemical predictors of hypertension. *Am J Hypertens* 1991;4:638s–641s.
13. Ferris JB, O'Hare JA, Kelleher CCM: Diabetic control and the renin angiotensin system, catecholamines and blood pressure. *Hypertension* 1985;7(suppl II):II-58–II-63.
14. Tedde R, Sechi LA, Marigliano A, et al: Antihypertensive effect of insulin reduction in diabetic hypertensive patients. *Am J Hypertens* 1989;2:163–170.
15. Stolar MW: Atherosclerosis in diabetes: The role of hyperinsulinemia. *Metabolism* 1988;34:S1–S9.
16. Stout RW: Insulin and atheroma: A 20 year perspective. *Diabetes Care* 1990;13:631–654.
17. Folkow B: Cardiovascular structural adaptation: Its role in the initiation and maintenance of primary hypertension. The fourth Volhard lecture. *Clin Sci Mol Med* 1978;55(suppl):3s–22s.
18. Hayakawa K, Walker L, Constable IJ: The effect of glucose and insulin concentration on type IV collagen by bovine retinal capillary endothelial cells in vitro. *Jpn J Ophthalmol* 1990;341:463–471.
19. Abrass CK, Peterson CV, Raugi GJ: Phenotype expression of collagen types in mesangial matrix of diabetic and nondiabetic rats. *Diabetes* 1988;37:1695–1702.
20. Hollenberg NK, Williams GH: Abnormal renal function, sodium-volume homeostasis and renin system behavior in normal-renin essential hypertension, in Laragh JH, Brenner BM (eds): *Hypertension: Pathophysiology, Diagnosis and Management.* New York, Raven Press, 1990, pp 1349–1370.
21. Beretta-Piccoli C, Weidmann P, Fraser R: Responsiveness of plasma 18-hydroxycorticosterone and aldosterone to angiotensin II or corticotropin in nonazotemic diabetes mellitus. *Diabetes* 1983;32:105.
22. Mancilha JJ, Baruzzi RG, Howard PF, et al: Blood pressure in four remote populations in the INTERSALT study. *Hypertension* 1989;14:238–246.
23. Sullivan JM: Salt sensitivity: Definition, conception, methodology and long-term issues. *Hypertension* 1991;17(suppl I):I-61–I-68.
24. Weidmann P, Beretta-Piccoli C, Keusch G: Sodium-volume factor, cardiovascular reactivity and hypotensive mechanism of diuretic therapy in mild hypertension associated with diabetes mellitus. *Am J Med* 1979;67:779–784.
25. O'Hare JA, Ferriss JB, Brady D, et al: Exchangeable sodium and renin in hypertensive diabetic patients with and without nephropathy. *Hypertension* 1985;7(6, part 2):II-43–II-48.
26. O'Hare JA, Roland JM, Walters G, et al: Imparied sodium excretion in response to volume expansion induced by water immersion in insulin-dependent diabetes mellitus. *Clin Sci* 1986;71:403–409.
27. Brochner-Mortensen J, Stockel M, Sorensen PJ, et al: Proximal glomerulo-tubular balance in patients with type I (insulin dependent) diabetes mellitus. *Diabetologia* 1984;27:189–192.
28. Modan M, Halkin H, Almog S, et al: Hyperinsulinemia: A link between hypertension, obesity and glucose intolerance. *J Clin Invest* 1985;75:809–817.

29. Manicardi V, Camellini L, Bellodi G, et al: Evidence for an association of high blood pressure and hyperinsulinemia in obese man. *J Clin Endocrinol Metab* 1986;62:1302–1304.

30. Ferrannini E, Buzzigoli G, Bonadonna R, et al: Insulin resistance in essential hypertension. *N Engl J Med* 1987;317:350–357.

31. Pollare T, Lithell H, Berne C: Insulin resistance is a characteristic feature of primary hypertension independent of obesity. *Metabolism* 1990;39:167–174.

32. Singer P, Godicke W, Voigt S, et al: Postprandial hyperinsulinemia in patients with mild essential hypertension. *Hypertension* 1985;7:182–186.

33. Saad MF, Lillioja S, Nyomba BL, et al: Racial differences in the relation between blood pressure and insulin resistance. *N Engl J Med* 1991;324:733–739.

34. Falkner B, Hulman S, Tannenbaum J, et al: Insulin resistance and blood pressure in young black men. *Hypertension* 1990;16:706–711.

35. Shen DC, Shieh SM, Fuh MT: Resistance to insulin-stimulated glucose uptake in patients with hypertension. *J Clin Endocrinol Metab* 1988;66:580–583.

36. Mbanya J-CN, Thomas TH, Wilkinson R, et al: Hypertension and hyperinsulinemia: A relation in diabetes but not essential hypertension. *Lancet* 1988;1:733–734.

37. Moller DE, Flier JS: Insulin-resistance—mechanisms, syndromes and implications. *N Engl J Med* 1991;32S:938–948.

38. Pfeifle B, Ditschuneit H: Two separate receptors for insulin and insulin-like growth factors on arterial smooth muscle cells. *Exp Clin Endocrinol* 1983;81:280–286.

39. DeFronzo RA, Cooke CR, Andres R, et al: The effect of insulin on renal handling of sodium, potassium, calcium, and phosphate in man. *J Clin Invest* 1975;55:845–855.

40. DeFronzo RA: Insulin and renal sodium handling: Clinical implications. *Int J Obes* 1981;5(suppl 1):93–104.

41. Baum M: Insulin stimulates volume absorption in the rabbit proximal convoluted tubule. *J Clin Invest* 1987;79:1104–1109.

42. Skott P, Hother-Nielsen, Bruun NE, et al: Effects of insulin on kidney function and sodium excretion in healthy subjects. *Diabetologia* 1989;32:694–699.

43. Mogensen CE, Christensen NJ, Gundersen HJG: The acute effect of insulin on renal hemodynamics and protein excretion in diabetics. *Diabetologia* 1978;15:153–157.

44. Christiansen JS, Frandsen M, Parving HH: The effect of intravenous insulin infusion on kidney function in insulin-dependent diabetes mellitus. *Diabetologia* 1981;20:199–204.

45. Rowe JW, Young JB, Minaker KL, et al: Effect of insulin and glucose infusions on sympathetic nervous activity. *Diabetes* 1981;30:219–225.

46. Kribben A, Philipp TH: The contribution of the sympathetic nervous system to hypertension in diabetes mellitus. *Diabetes Metab* 1989;15:313–317.

47. Anderson EA, Hoffman RP, Balon TW, et al: Hyperinsulinemia in humans increases muscle sympathetic nerve activity but reduces forearm vascular resistance. *Hypertension* 1992;19(suppl I):I-130.

48. Rocchini AP: Cardiovascular regulation in obesity-induced hypertension. *Hypertension* 1992;19(suppl I):I-56–I-60.

49. Minaker KL, Rowe JW, Young JB, et al: Effect of age on insulin stimulation of sympathetic nervous system activity in man. *Metabolism* 1982;12:1181–1184.

50. Page M, Watkins PJ: Provocation of postural hypotension by insulin in diabetic autonomic neuropathy. *Diabetes* 1976;25:90–95.

51. Laakso M, Edelman SV, Brechtel G, et al: Decreased effect of insulin to stimulate skeletal muscle blood flow in obese man. *J Clin Invest* 1990;85:1844–1852.

52. Rosic NK, Strandaert ML, Pollet RF: The mechanism of insulin stimulation of Na^+/K^+ ATPase activity in muscle. *J Biol Chem* 1985;260:6202–6212.

53. Hernandez H, Spencer BA, Arsenis G: Stimulation of Na^+/H^+ exchange by insulin and isoproterenol in rat adipocytes. *Diabetes* 1989;38(suppl 2):182A.

54. Blaustein MP: Sodium ions, calcium ions, blood pressure regulation and hypertension: A reassessment and a hypothesis. *Am J Physiol* 1977;323:C165–C173.

55. Draznin B, Kao M, Sussman KE: Insulin and glyburide increase cytosolic free Ca^{2+} concentrations in isolated rat adipocytes. *Diabetes* 1987;36:174–178.

56. Guruprakash GA, Krothapalli RK, Rouse D, et al: The mechanism of hypercalciuria in streptozotocin-induced diabetic rats. *Metabolism* 1988;37:306–311.

57. Resnick LM: Hypertension and abnormal glucose homeostasis. Possible role of divalent ion metabolism. *Am J Med* 1989;87(6A):17s–22s.

58. Hino T, Hori M, Nyby M, et al: Parathyroid hormone attenuates angiotensin II-induced rises in cytosolic calcium in cultured vascular smooth muscle cells. *Clin Res* 1992;38:A109.

59. Ross R, Glomset JA: The pathogenesis of atherosclerosis. *N Engl J Med* 1976;295: 369–377.

60. Ruderman NA, Haudenschild C: Diabetes as an atherogenic factor. *Prog Cardiovasc Dis* 1984;26:373–412.

61. Colwell JA, Halushka PV, Sarji KE, et al: Diabetic vascular disease. Pathophysiological mechanisms and therapy. *Arch Intern Med* 1979;139:225–230.

62. Schernthaner G, Sinizinger H, Silberbauer K, et al: Vascular prostacyclin and platelet-specific proteins in diabetes mellitus. *Horm Metab Res* 1981;13(suppl 11):33–43.

63. Harrison HE, Reece AH, Johnson M: Decreased vascular prostacyclin in experimental diabetes. *Life Sci* 1978;23:351–355.

64. Halushka PV, Mayfield R, Colwell JA: Insulin and arachidonic acid metabolism in diabetes mellitus. *Metabolism* 1985;34(suppl 1):32–36.

65. Halushka PV, Roger RC, Loadholt CB, et al: Increased platelet thromboxane sythesis in diabetes mellitus. *J Lab Clin Med* 1981;97:87–96.

66. Roth DM, Reibel DK, Lefer AM: Vascular responsiveness and eicosanoid production in diabetic rats. *Diabetologia* 1983;24:372–376.

67. Colwell JA, Winocour PD, Halushka PV: Do platelets have anything to do with diabetic microvascular disease? *Diabetes* 1983;32(suppl 2):14–19.

68. Gerrard JM, Stuart MJ, Rao GHR, et al: Alteration in the balance of prostaglandin and thromboxane sythesis in diabetic rats. *J Lab Clin Med* 1980;95:950–958.

69. Valentovic M, Lubawy W: Impact of insulin or tolbutamide on ^{14}C-arachidonic acid conversion to prostacyclin and/or thromboxane in lungs, aortas and platelets of streptozotozin induced diabetic rats. *Diabetes* 1983;32:846–851.

70. Rak K, Beck P, Udvardy M, et al: Plasma levels of beta thromboglobulin and factor VIII-related antigen in diabetic children and adults. *Thromb Res* 1983;29:155–162.

71. Almer LO, Pandolfi M, Nilson IM: Diabetic retinopathy and the fibrinolytic system. *Diabetes* 1975;24:529–534.

72. Almer LO: Vascular fibrinolytic activity in long term treatment with second generation sulfonylurea compounds. *Acta Endocrinol* 1980;239(suppl):53–55.

73. Koschinsky T, Buntin CE, Rutter R, et al: Vascular growth factors and the development of macrovascular disease in diabetes mellitus. *Horm Metab Res* 1985; 17(suppl):23–27.

74. King GL: Cell biology as an approach to the study of the vascular complications of diabetes. *Metabolism* 1985;34(suppl 1):17–24.

75. Koschinsky T, Bunting CE, Schuippert B, et al: Increased growth stimulation of fibroblasts from diabetics by diabetic serum factors of low molecular weight. *Atherosclerosis* 1980;37:311–317.

76. Koschinsky T, Bunting CE, Schuippert B, et al: Regulation of diabetic serum growth factors for human vascular cells by the metabolic control of diabetes mellitus. *Atherosclerosis* 1981;39:313–319.

77. King GL, Goodman AD, Buzngy S, et al: Receptors and growth promoting effects of insulin and insulin-like growth factors on cells from bovine retinal capillaries and aorta. *J Clin Invest* 1985;75:1028–1036.

78. Pfefile B, Ditschuneit H: Effects of insulin on growth of cultured human arterial smooth muscle cells. *Diabetologia* 1981;20:155–158.

79. Hamet P, Sugimoto H, Umeda T, et al: Abnormalities of platelet-derived growth factors in insulin-dependent diabetes. *Metabolism* 1985;34(suppl 1):25–31.

80. Zatz R, Brenner BM: Pathogenesis of diabetic microangiopathy: The hemodynamic view. *Am J Med* 1986;80:443–453.

81. Hostetter TH, Rennke HB, Brenner BM: The case for intrarenal hypertension in the initiation and progression of diabetic and other glomerulopathies. *Am J Med* 1982; 72:375–380.

82. Butterfield WJH, Wichelow MJ: Peripheral glucose metabolism in control subjects and diabetic patients during glucose, glucose-insulin and insulin sensitivity tests. *Diabetologia* 1965;1:42–53.

83. Gunderson HJG: Peripheral blood flow and metabolic control in juvenile diabetes. *Diabetologia* 1974;10:225–231.

84. Christensen NJ: A reversible vascular abnormality associated with diabetic ketosis. *Clin Sci* 1970;39:539–548.

85. Chazan BI, Balodimos MC, Lavine RL, et al: Capillaries of the nailbed of the toe in diabetes mellitus. *Microvasc Res* 1970;2:504–507.

86. Landau J, Davis E: The small blood vessels of the conjunctiva and nailbed in diabetes mellitus. *Lancet* 1960;2:731–734.

87. Gitelson S, Wertheimer-Kaplinski N: Color of the face in diabetes mellitus. *Diabetes* 1965;14:201–208.

88. Bohlen HG, Hankins KD: Early arteriolar and capillary changes in streptozotocin-induced diabetic rats and in intraperiotneal hyperglycemic rats. *Diabetologia* 1982; 22:344–348.

89. de Chatel R, Toth M, Barna I: Exchangeable sodium: Its relationship with blood pressure and ANP in patients with diabetes mellitus. *J Hypertens* 1986;4(suppl 6): S526–S528.

90. Horstman P: The oxygen consumption in diabetes mellitus. *Acta Med Scand* 1951; 139:326–330.

91. Nair KS, Halliday D, Garrow JS: Increased energy expenditure in poorly controlled type I (insulin-dependent) diabetic patients. *Diabetologia* 1984;27:13–16.

92. Ross JM, Fairchild HM, Weldy S, et al: Autoregulation of blood flow by oxygen lack. *Am J Physiol* 1962;202:21–24.

93. Ditzel J, Standl E: The problem of tissue oxygenation in diabetes mellitus II. Evidence of disordered oxygen release from the erythrocytes of diabetics in various conditions of metabolic control. *Acta Med Scand* 1975;578(suppl):59–68.

94. Tarazi RC: The hemodynamics of hypertension, in Genest J, Kuchel O, Hamet P, et al (eds): *Hypertension,* ed 2. New York, McGraw-Hill, 1983, pp 15–42.

95. DeiCas L, Zuliani J, Manca C, et al: Noninvasive evaluation of left ventricular performance in 294 diabetic patients without clinical heart disease. *Acta Diabetol Lat* 1980;17:145–152.

96. Sykes CA, Wright AD, Malins JM, et al: Changes in systolic time intervals during treatment of diabetes mellitus. *Br Heart J* 1977;39:255–259.

97. Alexander WD, Oake RJ: The effect of insulin on vascular reactivity to norepinephrine. *Diabetes* 1977;26:611–614.

98. Yagi S, Takata S, Kiyokawa H: Effects of insulin on vasoconstrictive responses to norepinephrine and angiotensin II in rabbit femoral artery and vein. *Diabetes* 1988; 37:1064–1067.

99. Head RJ, Longhurst PA, Panek RL, et al: A contrasting effect of the diabetic state upon the contractile responses of aortic preparations from the rat and rabbit. *Br J Pharmacol* 1987;91:275–286.

100. Pfaffman MA, Ball CR, Darby A, et al: Insulin reversal of diabetes-induced inhibition of vascular contractility in the rat. *Am J Physiol* 1982;242:H490–H495.

101. Flatman JA, Clausen T: Combined effects of adrenaline and insulin on active electrogenic Na^+-K^+ transport in rat soleus muscle. *Nature* 1979;281:580–581.

102. Yanagisawa-Miwa A, Ito H, Sugimoto T: Effects of insulin on vasoconstriction induced by thromboxane A2 in porcine coronary artery. *Circulation* 1990;81:1645–1659.

103. Downing SE, Lee JC, Matisoff DN: Coronary blood flow in the diabetic lamb with metabolic acidosis. *Am J Physiol* 1980;238:H263–H268.

104. Hwang IS, Ho H, Hoffman BB, et al: Fructose-induced insulin resistance and hypertension in rats. *Hypertension* 1987;10:512–516.

105. Shargill NS, Chan TM, Buchanan TA, et al: Chronic hyperinsulinemia elevates blood pressure in rats. *Clin Res* 1990;38:110A.

106. Reaven GM: Insulin resistance, hyperinsulinemia and hypertension: Parallels between human disease and rodent models. *Diabetes Care* 1991;14:195–202.

107. Buchanan T, Sipos G, Liu C, et al: Hyperinsulinemia in spontaneously hypertensive rats. *Clin Res* 1990;38:109A.

108. Buchanan TA, Sipos GF, Gadalah S, et al: Glucose tolerance and insulin action in rats with renovascular hypertension. *Hypertension* 1991;18:341–347.

109. Hall JE, Brandi MW, Hildebrandt DA, et al: Obesity-associated hypertension: Hyperinsulinemia and renal mechanisms. *Hypertension* 1992;19(suppl I):I-45–I-55.

110. Standley PR, Zhang F, Ram JL, et al: Insulin attenuates vasopressin-induced calcium transients and a voltage-dependent calcium response in rat vascular smooth muscle cells. *J Clin Invest* 1991;88:1230–1236.

111. Zemel MB, Shehin S, Reddy S, et al: Increased vascular reactivity and blood pressure associated with delayed calcium efflux in Zucker obese rats. *Am J Hypertens* 1989;2:30A.

112. Baron AD, Laakso M, Brechtel G, et al: Reduced capacity and affinity of skeletal muscle for insulin-mediated glucose uptake in noninsulin-dependent diabetic subjects. *J Clin Invest* 1991;87:1186–1194.

113. Bar RS, Boes M, Dake BL, et al: Insulin, insulin-like growth factors, and vascular endothelium. *Am J Med* 1988;85(suppl 5A):59–70.

114. King GL, Goodman AD, Buzngy S: Receptors and growth promoting effects of insulin and insulin-like growth factors in cells from bovine retinal capillaries and aorta. *J Clin Invest* 1985;75:1028–1036.

115. Rasmussen H: The calcium messenger system. *N Engl J Med* 1986;314:1094–1101.

116. Somlyo AV, Bond M, Somlyo AP, et al: Inositol trisphosphate-induced calcium release and contraction in vascular smooth muscle. *Proc Natl Acad Sci USA* 1985;82:5231–5235.

117. Okamura K, Nishiura T, Awaji Y, et al: 1,2-diacylglycerol content and its fatty acid composition in thoracic aortas of diabetic rats. *Diabetes* 1991;40:820–824.

118. Exton JH: Some thoughts on the mechanism of action of insulin. *Diabetes* 1991;40:521–526.

119. Petrasek D, Jensen G, Tuck ML, et al: In vitro effects of insulin on aldosterone production in rat zona glomerulosa cells. *Life Sci* 1992;50:1781–1788.

120. Thom S, Hughes A, Sever P: Endothelium dependent responses in human arteries, in Vanhoutte PM (ed): *The Endothelium, Relaxing and Contracting Factors*. NJ, Humana Press, 1988, pp 511–528.

121. D'Orleans-Juste P, Dion D, Mizrahi J, et al: Effects of peptides and non-peptides on isolated arterial smooth muscles: Role of endothelium. *Eur J Pharmacol* 1985;114:9–21.

Chapter 18

Insulin Resistance and Hypertension

Boris Draznin, MD, PhD

Epidemiologic studies and clinical observations provide strong evidence in favor of an association among obesity, impaired glucose tolerance, non-insulin-dependent diabetes mellitus (NIDDM), hypertension, and dyslipidemia.[1-12] The epidemiology of this relatedness is reviewed in detail elsewhere in this volume. Suffice it to say that the San Antonio Heart Study, a large epidemiologic survey, has estimated that by the fifth decade of life, more than 80% of diabetic individuals are hypertensive and obese. Over 80% of obese subjects have abnormal glucose tolerance and are hypertensive, and approximately 70% of hypertensive subjects are both diabetic and obese.[13]

The frequency with which these associations occur may lead one to believe that there exists a common pathogenetic mechanism connecting these disorders. The initial epidemiologic data suggested that hyperinsulinemia may be a linking factor between hypertension and NIDDM with and without associated obesity.[1-12] In fact, some investigators went even further, postulating that hyperinsulinemia, in and of itself, may be a significant factor participating in the pathogenesis of essential hypertension.[14] That is, it was proposed that high levels of circulating insulin could induce hypertension by promoting Na^+ retention by the kidney, by stimulating the sympathetic nervous system, and by affecting the intracellular ion concentrations and thereby contractility of vascular smooth muscle cells.[15-21]

However, subsequent numerous studies designed to examine this possibility under various experimental conditions failed to support the role of hyperinsulinemia as a causative factor for essential hypertension.[22-24] There are at least four lines of evidence refuting the causative role of hyperinsulinemia in the pathogenesis of hypertension. First, experimental insulin infusions failed to produce hypertension.[22-24] Second, the cause-and-effect relationship between hyperinsulinemia and hypertension appears to be holding for white men only. The same relationship was either weak or absent completely in blacks, Hispanics, and Pacific Island populations.[25-28] Third, the majority of patients with insulinoma are not hypertensive.[29] Finally, there is no evidence that exogenously administered insulin (which commonly exceeds physiologic concentrations of circulating insulin) induces hypertension in patients with diabetes. Because most of the experimental studies examined the role of hyperinsulinemia in the relatively short-term setting, there is still an outside possibility that chronic hyperinsulinemia, lasting for months or even years, may be important in the pathogenesis of essential hypertension.

Nevertheless, the focus of attention has shifted from hyperinsulinemia per se to the presence and role of insulin resistance as a major factor linking NIDDM and hypertension.[6,9,16,19,30-34] Under this scenario, hyperinsulinemia is regarded merely as a marker of the underlying insulin resistance. This theory is much more plausible, but the molecular mechanism(s) bridging insulin resistance with essential hypertension remain(s) poorly understood.

If one assumes, as epidemiologic studies imply, that these two conditions coexist in a "cause-and-effect" relationship, then the old question "which one comes first, the chicken or the egg?" must be addressed relative to an association between hypertension and insulin resistance. If insulin resistance comes first, then what is the mechanism whereby it causes hypertension? If the reverse situation is true and hypertension comes first, what is the mechanism of insulin resistance in this case? Alternatively, one can envision hypertension and insulin resistance as independently arising entities that then cross-talk by changing the intracellular milieu, resulting in the appearance of a second entity. In other words, either of these conditions can appear first and create a favorable environment for the other, suggesting that both the first and the second possibilities are correct. Such an interrelationship assumes that hypertension can diminish cellular sensitivity to insulin as well as the presence of insulin resistance can impose conditions favorable for the development of hypertension. In this chapter, I attempt to summarize the evidence that the latter possibility is the most appropriate answer to this multiple-choice question.

Possibility #1: Insulin Resistance is a Pathogenetic Factor in the Development of Hypertension

How can insulin resistance participate in the development of hypertension? What is the biochemical mechanism that links an inability of cells to respond to insulin with the changes responsible for hypertension? Strictly speaking, there are only two distinct possibilities: selective insulin resistance or total insulin resistance.

Selective Insulin Resistance

"Selective" insulin resistance implies that not all cells in the body are created equal in terms of their responsiveness to insulin.[13,15,16,35,36] For example, muscle cells may be resistant to insulin action, whereas kidney cells or sympathetic nervous system cells may remain very sensitive to this hormone. If this were the case, then hyperinsulinemia, which would appear as a result of muscular resistance to insulin, would stimulate excessive retention of sodium by the kidney[15,16,37] and activate the sympathetic nervous system.[17,18,38,39] Both sodium retention and activation of the sympathetic nervous system are extremely important in the pathogenesis of hypertension.[5,8,16,32] This selective insulin resistance may express itself not only in terms of organ specificity (eg, muscle versus kidney) but also in terms of the specificity of a given action of insulin. For example, the cells may be resistant to insulin as far as glucose transport and utilization are concerned, but still be fairly sensitive to insulin relative to inhibition of lipolysis.

The hypothesis of selective insulin resistance appears to be a valid working hypothesis. Although it is attractive, this hypothesis still fails to account for the inability of insulin infusions to modulate blood pressure in experimental animals.[22,23] One would think that experimentally produced hyperinsulinemia should impact in a manner similar to that of endogenous hyperinsulinemia resulting from insulin resistance. Unfortunately, this does not occur. Furthermore, patients with insulinoma, an experiment of nature, do not develop hypertension,[29] again casting doubts on the ability of hyperinsulinemia to elevate blood pressure.

Total Insulin Resistance

The second possible mechanism whereby insulin resistance can influence the development of hypertension is that *all* cells are resistant to insulin (ie, there exists a state of *total insulin resistance*). Under this paradigm, the cells are not influenced by insulin appropriately even though the levels of circulating insulin are high. In fact, the tissues and the cells are in the same condition as they would have been in a hypoinsulinemic environment. Under these circumstances, there appears to be a "circuit break" in the process of transmittal of the insulin-generated signal intracellularly. As a result, the intracellular milieu of insulin-resistant cells would be altered in a manner similar to that observed in the absence of insulin. If one takes into consideration the fact the insulin influences ion fluxes across the cell membrane, one would anticipate that the lack of this influence would severely disrupt normal ionic balance and transmembrane fluxes. In particular, there are three major enzymes (Na^+/K^+ adenosine triphosphatase [ATPase], Ca^{2+}-ATPase, and Na^+-H^+ antiport) that are activated by insulin.[12,19,21,32,40-46] Under the circumstances in which influence of insulin dissipates, these enzymes are no longer activated appropriately. The results are not difficult to predict. There will be an accumulation of intracellular Na^+ and Ca^{2+} and a shift in the intracellular pH.

In the absence of insulin (ie, insulinopenic diabetes) or in the absence of adequate insulin action, as could be observed in the state of insulin resistance, the cell would not be able to extrude Na^+ (low activity of Na^+/K^+-ATPase) or Ca^{2+} (diminished Ca^{2+}-ATPase activity), resulting in an inappropriate accumulation of these ions intracellularly. If one further assumes that an accumulation of intracellular Ca^{2+} in vascular smooth muscle cells leads to increased contractility of these cells,[47] then one can easily envision an impact of insulin resistance on the development of hypertension.

Under normal circumstances, it is exceedingly difficult to maintain high levels of cytosolic Ca^{2+}. Calcium efflux is ordinarily an extremely efficient mechanism compensating for any increases in the intracellular concentration of this ion. Plasma membrane Ca^{2+}-ATPase is one of the main enzymes that controls calcium efflux. This enzyme has been shown to be sensitive to insulin.[44] Moreover, it has been demonstrated that, in the state of insulin resistance, the activity of Ca^{2+}-ATPase was impaired and the enzyme was no longer influenced by insulin.[44,48] Inability of insulin to stimulate Ca^{2+}-ATPase may contribute significantly to an accumulation of cytosolic Ca^{2+}.

At the same time, if insulin resistance is accompanied by hyperglycemia, the latter can also participate in inducing increases in the intracellular Ca^{2+} concentrations. Glucose may be rapidly converted into diacylglycerol,[49,50] with the subsequent stimulation of protein kinase C–dependent system and a profound effect on cellular handling of Ca^{2+}. We have previously shown that isolated normal adipocytes incubated for 24 hours in the presence of high concentrations of glucose and insulin become insulin resistant and display elevated levels of cytosolic calcium.[51] These effects of hyperglycemia and hyperinsulinemia were effectively blocked by the calcium channel blocker verapamil, suggesting that, regardless of the initial mechanism, Ca^{2+} influx via voltage-dependent calcium channels is an important pathogenetic link. Further work is needed to evaluate whether the effect of hyperglycemia and hyperinsulinemia on calcium influx is direct or is mediated via the protein kinase C–dependent system.

Accumulations of intracellular Na^+ can also predispose to the development of hypertension. Blaustein's theory[52] suggests that elevations in cytosolic Na^+ secondary to a diminution in Na^+/K^+-ATPase activity may lead to an enhancement in the concentrations of cytosolic Ca^{2+}. The stimulatory effect of insulin on Na^+/K^+-ATPase may be lacking in the state of insulin resistance. This would result in a decrease in Na^+/K^+-ATPase activity and accumulation of intracellular Na^+, which in turn can lead to increases in cytosolic Ca^{2+}. The influence of high levels of cytosolic Ca^{2+} on vascular contractility[47] may account for the development of hypertension under these circumstances.

Thus, the overall data are supportive of the fact that insulin resistance rather than hyperinsulinemia may be an important pathogenetic factor in the development of hypertension. Conceivably, the influence of hyperinsulinemia on Na^+ retention and the sympathetic nervous system may supplement the impact of insulin resistance, amplifying the odds for the appearance of hypertension.

Possibility #2: Development of Insulin Resistance in Patients With Hypertension

Can hypertensive patients develop insulin resistance as a consequence of metabolic abnormalities seen in hypertension? The answer appears to be affirmative, but with one important caveat. Not all hypertensive patients are insulin resistant,[16] suggesting that there might exist a subgroup of patients with essential hypertension in whom an association between these two conditions is more likely to exist. This is not an unexpected conclusion. Hypertension is a syndrome, a phenotypic expression of various etiologic and pathogenetic mechanisms. It is likely that only certain types of hypertension may lead to the development of insulin resistance. Recent studies in this area have indeed indicated that the patients with salt-sensitive hypertension are those who display this association.[53] If we further assume that some patients with essential hypertension possess high levels of cytosolic Ca^{2+} in various tissues, including insulin target tissues, then we ought to be cognizant of the possibility that increased levels of cytosolic Ca^{2+} in insulin target tissues might render these tissues insulin resistant.

The increases in the levels of cytosolic Ca^{2+} in various tissues of hypertensive patients have been demonstrated in numerous studies.[54–59] The most commonly studied tissue in these patients was platelets. However, cytosolic Ca^{2+} was found to be increased also in aortas, lymphocytes, erythrocytes, and adipocytes.[12,19,20,38,40,60–64] For the purposes of this discussion, it is important to assume that other insulin-sensitive tissues of some patients with essential hypertension also contain high levels of cytosolic Ca^{2+}. Keeping in mind that only those hypertensive individuals (salt sensitive?) who have high levels of cytosolic Ca^{2+} in their insulin-sensitive tissues will go on to develop insulin resistance, the following questions must be addressed. How can the presence of elevated levels of cytosolic Ca^{2+} in insulin-sensitive tissues diminish the magnitude of insulin action? What is the mechanism whereby high intracellular Ca^{2+} can interfere with the insulin-generated signal?

The initial observations indicated that insulin action in adipocytes was optimal when cytosolic Ca^{2+} concentration ranged between 140 and 340 nmol/L. When the level of intracellular Ca^{2+} exceeded this range, the insulin-stimulated glucose transport was diminished.[65] Kelly and co-workers[66] did not observe an obligatory relationship between the cytosolic Ca^{2+} and insulin action, but found a highly significant correlation ($r = .92$) between the rate of Ca^{2+} influx and an inhibition of insulin action (glucose oxidation).

The subsequent investigations directed at the mechanism of Ca^{2+} action showed that sustained elevations of cytosolic Ca^{2+} did not affect insulin binding to its cell surface receptor or the tyrosine kinase activity of the insulin receptor.[67] Furthermore, the cells with high levels of cytosolic Ca^{2+} possessed normal amounts of glucose transporters, whose cellular distribution between the membranous and low-density microsomal pools remained intact.[67] These observations, coupled with a significant decrease in the overall glucose uptake, implied that high levels of cytosolic Ca^{2+} may impair intrinsic activity of glucose transporters.

The nature of the intrinsic activity of glucose transporter remains elusive. We still do not know what regulates the ability of the insulin-sensitive glucose transporters to increase or decrease their transporting capacity. Recently obtained evidence hinted that the state of phosphorylation of glucose transporters may be involved in regulation of their intrinsic activity.[68-71] Thus, an exposure of adipocytes to isoproterenol or parathyroid hormone (PTH) or depolarizing concentrations of K^+ enhanced phosphorylation of the insulin-regulatable glucose transporter GLUT-4, and decreased the rate of glucose uptake.[71] In experiments with PTH or K^+, the presence of either a calcium channel blocker (nitrendipine) or a cyclic adenosine monophosphate (cAMP) antagonist (RpcAMP) reversed excessive phosphorylation of GLUT-4 and improved the overall glucose uptake.[71] Furthermore, when the adipocytes were exposed to okadaic acid, a potent inhibitor of phosphoprotein phosphatases of classes 1 and 2A, the basal glucose uptake was increased but the insulin-stimulated glucose transport was significantly inhibited.[72-76] Taken together, these data imply that there might exist a relationship between the state of phosphorylation of GLUT-4 and its intrinsic activity. Alternatively, the excessive phosphorylation of GLUT-4 may impair other properties of this transporter, such as its ability to translocate to the plasma membrane or to recycle back into the cell interior. Further studies are urgently needed to dissect the role of phosphorylation of GLUT-4 in regulating its function.

It appears that high levels of cytosolic Ca^{2+} affect the state of phosphorylation of intracellular proteins not only by promoting the rate of phosphorylation, but also by inhibiting cellular phosphatases responsible for normal dephosphorylation of these proteins.[77] Many insulin-sensitive enzymes are active in their dephosphorylated form. This fact suggests that the insulin-generated signal that initially stimulates cellular kinases must flip-flop somewhere downstream in the cascade of insulin action to activate phosphatases.[78,79] Recent studies suggested that insulin activates phosphoserine phosphatase 1 (PP-1) by stimulating its phosphorylation in the site-specific manner.[78] The activated PP-1 in turn dephosphorylates and thereby activates many insulin-sensitive enzymes. Therefore, if high levels of cytosolic Ca^{2+} inhibit the PP-1 activity, they may interfere with the insulin-generated signal at distal postreceptor steps of insulin action. We have recently demonstrated that this may indeed be the case in certain states of insulin resistance. We found that, in adipocytes, sustained levels of cytosolic Ca^{2+} induced by various mechanisms inhibited PP-1 activity and dephosphorylation of glycogen synthase and GLUT-4.[71,77] These proteins remained in their phosphorylated state, which accompanied their lower metabolic activity.

The precise mechanism of the calcium-induced inhibition of PP-1 activity is only partially understood. It appears that high levels of cytosolic Ca^{2+} stimulate phosphorylation and activity of inhibitor 1.[80] Inhibitor 1 that has been activated by phosphorylation binds to the catalytic subunit of PP-1, thereby decreasing PP-1 activity.[72,81] In addition to the activation of inhibitor 1, high levels of cytosolic Ca^{2+} appear to be affecting PP-1 directly or via cAMP- and protein kinase A–dependent mechanisms. The cAMP-dependent pathway promotes phosphorylation of PP-1 on a site distinct from that phosphorylated by insulin.[78] This cAMP-induced phosphorylation diminishes PP-1 activity.[78] We found that approximately 90% of the detrimental effect of high levels of cytosolic Ca^{2+} could be reversed by cAMP antagonists (ie, RpcAMP), suggesting that the bulk of Ca^{2+} influence is mediated by the cAMP-dependent mechanism.

The data accumulated to date indicate that insulin target cells containing high levels of cytosolic Ca^{2+} may become resistant to insulin, and that the mechanism of insulin resistance involves postreceptor steps of insulin action. An impairment in the rate of dephosphorylation of certain insulin-sensitive enzymes and proteins appears to be responsible for the development of insulin resistance. If one accepts the postulate that increases in the levels of cytosolic Ca^{2+} are the integral component of hypertension in selected group of patients, then one can envision how these alterations in the intracellular milieu may lead to the development of insulin resistance.

Conclusion

Based on the data presented in this chapter, one might conclude that either hypertension or insulin resistance can appear to be an initial abnormality (Figure 18.1). Either one of these two conditions may lead to the development of the second entity. The connecting point between hypertension and insulin resistance appears to be an increase in cytosolic Ca^{2+}. If this increase involves vascular smooth muscle cells in patients with insulin resistance, these patients are likely to develop hypertension. Conversely, if patients with essential hypertension display an increase in cytosolic Ca^{2+} in the insulin target cells, these patients are likely to demonstrate insulin resistance as well. Finally, if there exists a pathophysiologic process that increases cytosolic Ca^{2+} concentrations in insulin-sensitive cells and vascular smooth muscle cells (eg, primary hyperparathyroidism, insulin-dependent diabetes mellitus), this might lead to a simultaneous development of both hypertension and insulin resistance.

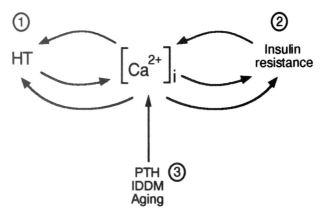

Figure 18.1 The relationship between hypertension and insulin resistance involves elevations in cytosolic calcium in the vascular smooth muscle cells (VSMCs) and insulin target cells. (1) Hypertension (HT) appears first and is accompanied by elevations in the cytosolic free calcium concentration ($[Ca^{2+}]_i$) in the insulin target cells, thereby promoting insulin resistance. (2) Insulin resistance is a primary abnormality. It may lead to increases in the cytosolic free calcium concentration and hypertension. (3) Other pathophysiologic conditions, such as hyperparathyroidism (PTH) or insulin-dependent diabetes mellitus (IDDM), may increase the levels of cytosolic free calcium simultaneously in VSMCs and insulin target cells, promoting both hypertension and insulin resistance.

References

1. Modan M, Halkin H, Almog S, et al: Hyperinsulinemia: A link between hypertension, obesity and glucose intolerance. *J Clin Invest* 1985;75:809–817.
2. Ferrannini E, Buzzigoli G, Bonadonna R, et al: Insulin resistance in essential hypertension. *N Engl J Med* 1987;317:350–357.
3. Sowers JR, Levy J, Zemel MB: Hypertension and diabetes. *Med Clin North Am* 1988; 72:1399–1413.
4. Ferrannini E, Natali A, Cerri M, et al: Hypertension: A metabolic disorder? *Diabete Metab* 1989;15:284–291.
5. Ferrannini E, DeFronzo RA: The assocaition of hypertension, diabetes, and obesity: A review. *J Nephrol* 1989;1:3–15.
6. Berne C: Insulin resistance in hypertension—a relationship with consequences? *J Int Med* 1991;229:65–73.
7. Ferrannini E, Haffner SM, Mitchell BD, Hyperinsulinaemia: The key feature of a cardiovascular and metabolic syndrome. *Diabetologia* 1991;34:416–422.
8. Ferrari P, Weidmann P: Editorial review: Insulin, insulin sensitivity and hypertension. *J Hypertens* 1990;8:491–500.
9. Flack JM, Sowers JR: Epidemiologic and clinical aspects of insulin resistance and hyperinsulinemia. *Am J Med* 1991;91:11S–21S.
10. Jarrett RJ: Hypertension in glucose intolerance and diabetes. *J Int Med* 1991;229:85–88.
11. Reaven GM: Insulin resistance, hyperinsulinemia, and hypertriglyceridemia in the etiology and clinical course of hypertension. *Am J Med* 1991;90:7S–12S.
12. Resnick LM: Calcium metabolism in hypertension and allied metabolic disorders. *Diabetes Care* 1991;14:505–520.
13. Ferrannini E, Haffner SM, Stern MP: Essential hypertension: An insulin-resistant state. *J Cardiovasc Pharmacol* 1990;15(suppl 5):S18–S25.
14. Reaven GM, Hoffman BB: A role for insulin in the aetiology and course of hypertension? *Lancet* 1987;2:435–437.

15. Rocchini AP, Katch V, Kveselis D, et al: Insulin and renal sodium retention in obese adolescents. *Hypertension* 1989;14:367–374.

16. Rocchini AP: Insulin resistance and blood pressure regulation in obese and nonobese subjects. *Hypertension* 1991;17:837–842.

17. Landsberg L: Diet, obesity and hypertension: An hypothesis involving insulin, the sympathetic nervous system, and adaptive thermogenesis. *Q J Med* 1986;61:1081–1090.

18. Landsberg L, Krieger DR: Obesity, metabolism and the sympathetic nervous system. *Am J Hypertens* 1989;2:125S–132S.

19. Sowers JR: At the cutting edge: Insulin resistance and hypertension. *Mol Cell Endocrinol* 1990;74:C87–C89.

20. Standley PR, Zhang F, Ram JL, et al: Insulin attenuates vasopressin-induced calcium transients and a voltage-dependent calcium response in rat vascular smooth muscle cells. *J Clin Invest* 1991;88:1230–1236.

21. Aviv A, Lasker N: A common pathway for essential hypertension and non-insulin-dependent diabetes mellitus in blacks: The central role of cytosolic free calcium and the sodium-proton exchange. *J Vascul Med Biol* 1990;2:91–93.

22. Brands MW, Mizelle HL, Gaillard CA, et al: The hemodynamic response to chronic hyperinsulinemia in conscious dogs. *Am J Hypertens* 1991;4:164–168.

23. Hall JE, Brands MW, Kivlighn SD, et al: Chronic hyperinsulinemia and blood pressure: Interaction with catecholamines? *Hypertension* 1990;15:519–527.

24. Anderson EA, Hoffman RP, Balon TW, et al: Hyperinsulinemia produces both sympathetic neural activation and vasodilation in normal humans. *J Clin Invest* 1991;87:2246–2252.

25. Saad MF, Lillioja S, Nyomba BL, et al: Racial differences in the relation between blood pressure and insulin resistance. *N Engl J Med* 1991;324:733–739.

26. Falkner B, Hulman S, Tannenbaum J, et al: Insulin resistance and blood pressure in young black men. *Hypertension* 1990;16:706–711.

27. Haffner S, Mitchell B, Stern M, et al: Decreased prevalence of hypertension in Mexican-Americans. *Hypertension* 1990;16:225–232.

28. Collins VR, Dowse GK, Finch CF, et al: An inconsistent relationship between insulin and blood pressure in three pacific island populations. *J Clin Epidemiol* 1990;43:1369–1378.

29. Tsutsu N, Nunoi K, Kodama T, et al: Lack of association between blood pressure and insulin in patients with insulinoma. *J Hypertens* 1990;8:479–482.

30. Reaven GM: Role of insulin resistance in human disease. *Diabetes* 1988;37:1595–1607.

31. Pollare T, Lithell H, Berne C: Insulin resistance is a characteirstic feature of primary hypertension independent of obesity. *Metabolism* 1990;39:167–174.

32. Sowers JR, Standley PR, Ram JL, et al: Insulin resistance, carbohydrate metabolism, and hypertension. *Am J Hypertens* 1991;4:466S–472S.

33. DeFronzo RA, Ferrannini E: Insulin resistance: A multifaceted syndrome responsible forn IDDM, obesity, hypertension, dyslipidemia, and atherosclerotic cardiovascular disease. *Diabetes Care* 1991;14:173–194.

34. Reaven GM: Insulin resistance, hyperinsulinemia, hypertriglyceridemia, and hypertension: Parallels between human disease and rodent models. *Diabetes Care* 1991;14:195–202.

35. Newman WP, Brodows RG: Insulin action during acute starvation: Evidence for selective insulin resistance in normal man. *Metabolism* 1983;32:590–596.

36. Cohen P, Barzilai N, Lerman A, et al: Insulin effects on glucose and potassium metabolism in vivo: Evidence for selective insulin resistance in humans. *J Clin Endocrinol Metab* 1991;73:564–568.

37. DeFronzo RA: The effect of insulin on renal sodium metabolism. A review with clinical implications. *Diabetologia* 1981;21:165–171.

38. Landsberg L, Young JB: Fasting, feeding and regulation of the sympathetic nervous ssytem. *N Engl J Med* 1978;298:1295–1301.

39. Rowe JW, Young BY, Minaker KL, et al: Effect of insulin and glucose infusions on sympathetic nervous system activity in normal man. *Diabetes* 1981;30:219–225.

40. Lytton J: Insulin affects the sodium affinity of the rat adipocyte (Na^+-K^+)-ATPase. *J Biol Chem* 1985;260:10075–10080.

41. Rosic NK, Standaert ML, Pollet RJ: The mechanism of insulin stimulation of (Na^+,K^+)-ATPase transport activity in muscle. *J Biol Chem* 1985;260:6202–6212.

42. Nishida K, Ohara T, Johnson J, et al: Na^+/K^+-ATPase activity and its αII subunit gene expression in rat skeletal muscle: Influence of diabetes, fasting, and refeeding. *Metabolism* 1992;41:56–63.

43. Aviv A: Prospective review: The link between cytosolic Ca^{2+} and the Na^+-H^+ antiport: A unifying factor for essential hypertension. *J Hypertens* 1988;6:685–691.

44. Levy J, Gavin JR III, Hammerman MR, et al: Ca^{2+}-Mg^{2+}-ATPase activity in kidney basolateral membrane in non-insulin-dependent diabetic rats: Effects of insulin. *Diabetes* 1986;35:899–905.

45. Zemel MB, Bedford BA, Zemel PC, et al: Altered cation transport in non-insulin-dependent diabetic hypertension: Effects of dietary calcium. *J Hypertens* 1988;6:S228–S230.

46. Resnick LM, Gupta RK, Gruenspan H, et al: Hypertension and peripheral insulin resistance: Possible mediating role of intracellular free magnesium. *Am J Hypertens* 1990;3:373–379.

47. Stull JT, Gallagher PJ, Herring BP, et al: Vascular smooth muscle contractile elements: Cellular regulation. *Hypertension* 1991;17:723–732.

48. Levy J, Gavin JR III, Fausto A, et al: Impaired insulin action in rats with non-insulin dependent diabetes. *Diabetes* 1984;33:901–906.

49. Draznin B, Leitner JW, Sussman KE, et al: Insulin and glucose modulate protein kinase C activity in rat adipocytes. *Biochem Biophys Res Commun* 1988;156:570–575.

50. Hoffman JM, Ishizuka T, Farese RV: Interrelated effects of insulin and glucose on diacylglycerol–protein kinase-C signalling in rat adipocytes and solei muscle in vitro and in vivo in diabetic rats. *Endocrinology* 1991;128:2937–2948.

51. Draznin B, Sussman KE, Eckel RH, et al: Possible role of cytosolic free calcium concentrations in mediating insulin resistance of obesity and hyperinsulinemia. *J Clin Invest* 1988;82:1848–1852.

52. Blaustein MP: Sodium ions, calcium ions, blood pressure regulation, and hypertension: A reassessment and a hypothesis. *Am J Physiol* 1977;232:C165–C173.

53. Rocchini AP: The influence of obesity in hypertension. *News Physiol Sci* 1990;5:245–249.

54. Bruschi G, Bruschi ME, Caroppo M, et al: Cytoplasmic free [Ca^{2+}] is increased in the platelets of spontaneously hypertensive rats and essential hypertensive patients. *Clin Sci* 1985;68:179–184.

55. Lechi A, Lechi C, Bonadonna G, et al: Increased basal and thrombin-induced free calcium in platelets of essential hypertensive patients. *Hypertension* 1987;9:230–235.

56. Erne P, Bolli P, Bürgisser E, et al: Correlation of platelet calcium with blood pressure. *N Engl J Med* 1984;310:1084–1088.

57. Lindner A, Kenny M, Meacham AJ: Effects of a circulating factor in patients with essential hypertension of intracellular free calcium in normal paltelets. *N Engl J Med* 1987;316:509–513.

58. Haller H, Lenz T, Thiede M, et al: Platelet intracellular free calcium and hypertension. *J Clin Hypertens* 1987;3:12–19.

59. Bühler FR, Resink TJ: Platelet membrane and calcium control abnormalities in essential hypertension. *Am J Hypertens* 1988;1:42–46.

60. Jelicks LA, Gupta RK: NMR measurement of cytosolic free calcium, free magnesium, and intracellular sodium in the aorta of the normal and spontaneously hypertensive rat. *J Biol Chem* 1990;265:1395–1400.

61. Sada T, Koike H, Ikeda M, et al: Cytosolic free calcium of aorta in hypertensive rats: Chronic inhibition of angiotensin converting enzyme. *Hypertension* 1990;16:245–251.

62. Resnick LM, Gupta RK, Bhargava KK, et al: Cellular ions in hypertension, diabetes, and obesity: A nuclear magnetic resonance spectroscopic study. *Hypertension* 1991; 17:951–957.

63. Oshima T, Matsuura M, Kido K, et al: Intralymphocytic sodium and free calcium and palsma renin in essential hypertension. *Hypertension* 1988;12:26–21.

64. Draznin B, Reusch J, Begum N, et al: Calcium, insulin action and insulin resistance. *Excerpta Medica, International Congress Series* 1991;980:225–245.

65. Draznin B, Sussman KE, Kao M, et al: The existence of an optimal range of cytosolic free calcium for insulin-stimulated glucose transport in rat adipocytes. *J Biol Chem* 1987;262:14385–14388.

66. Kelly KL, Deeney JT, Corkey BE: Cytosolic free calcium in adipocyte. *J Biol Chem* 1989;264:12754–12757.

67. Draznin B, Lewis D, Houlder N, et al: Mechanism of insulin resistance induced by sustained levels of cytosolic free calcium in rat adipocytes. *Endocrinology* 1989;125: 2341–2349.

68. James DE, Hiken J, Lawrence JC Jr: Isoproterenol stimulates phosphorylation of IRGT in rat adipocytes. *Proc Natl Acad Sci USA* 1989;86:8368–8372.

69. Gibbs ME, Allard WJ, Leinhard GE: The glucose transporter in 3T3-L1 adipocytes is phosphorylated in resposne to phorbol ester but not in response to insulin. *J Biol Chem* 1986;261:16597–16603.

70. Joost HC, Weber TM, Cushman SW, et al: Activity and phosphorylation state of glucose transporters in plasma membranes from insulin-, isoproterenol-, and phorbol ester-treated rat adipose cells. *J Biol Chem* 1987;262:11261–11267.

71. Reusch J, Begum N, Sussman KE, et al: Regulation of GLUT-4 phosphorylation by intracellular calcium in adipocytes. *Endocrinology* 1991;129:3269–3273.

72. Cohen P, Cohen PTW: Protein phosphatases come of age. *J Biol Chem* 1989;264: 21435–21438.

73. Lawrence JC, Hiken JF, James DE: Stimulation of glucose transport and glucose transporter phosphorylation by okadaic acid in rat adipocytes. *J Biol Chem* 1990;265: 19768–19776.

74. Shibata H, Robinson FW, Soderling TR, et al: Effect of okadaic acid on insulin-sensitive cAMP phosphodiesterase in rat adipocytes. Evidence that insulin may stimulate the enzyme by phosphorylation. *J Biol Chem* 1991;266:17948–17953.

75. Tanti JF, Gremeaux T, VanObberghen E, et al: Effect of okadaic acid, an inhibitor of protein phosphatase -1 and 2A, on glucose transport and metabolism in skeletal muscle. *J Biol Chem* 1991;266:2099–2103.

76. Corvera S, Jaspers S, Pasceri M: Acute inhibition of insulin-stimulated transport by the phosphatase inhibitor—okadaic acid. *J Biol Chem* 1991;266:9271–9275.

77. Begum N, Sussman KE, Draznin B: High levels of cytosolic free calcium inhibit dephosphorylation of insulin receptor and glycogen synthease. *Cell Calcium* 1991;12: 423–430.

78. Dent P, Lavoinne A, Nakielny S, et al: The molecular mechanism by which insulin stimulates glycogen synthesis in mammalian skeletal muscle. *Nature* 1990;348:302–308.

79. Moller DE, Flier JS: Insulin resistance—mechanisms, syndromes, and implications. *N Engl J Med* 1991;325:938–948.

80. Begum N, Sussman K, Draznin B: Calcium-induced inhibition of phosphoserine phosphatase in insulin target cells is mediated by the phosphorylation and activation of inhibitor 1. *J Biol Chem* 1992;267:5959–5963.

81. Cohen P: Protein phosphorylation and hormone action. *Proc R Soc Lond* 1988;234: 115–144.

Chapter 19

Epidemiology and Genetics of Hypertension in Diabetes Mellitus

Andrzej S. Krolewski, MD, PhD, and
James H. Warram, MD, ScD

This review of the epidemiology and genetics of hypertension in patients with type I and type II diabetes mellitus provides the basis for a discussion of future directions for etiologic studies of hypertension in diabetes. As will be seen, the factors leading to diabetes, as well as the metabolic abnormalities of diabetes mellitus itself, can be considered as modifiers of the evolution of essential hypertension in the general population. Thus, the occurrence of hypertension and its determinants in the general population are reviewed first.

Occurrence of Hypertension in the General Population

Arterial blood pressure is closely regulated to maintain tissue perfusion during a wide variety of physiologic conditions. The level of arterial blood pressure in different individuals varies quite widely, however. Determinants of this interindividual variability became a major focus of biomedical research after it was shown that the risks of stroke and coronary artery disease are related to high levels of arterial blood pressure.[1,2]

The Joint National Committee on Detection, Evaluation, and Treatment of High Blood Pressure (called JNC III) defines elevated blood pressure (hypertension) as a diastolic blood pressure equal to or greater than 90 mm Hg, a systolic blood pressure equal to or greater than 140 mm Hg, or prescription of treatment for hypertension.[3] The best estimates of the prevalence of hypertension as defined above came from the second National Health and Nutrition Examination Survey (NHANES II) conducted in 1976–1980.[4] A random sample of the US civilian, noninstitutionalized population ages 18 to 74 years (n = 12,504) had a standardized medical examination including blood pressure measurements. Age-specific prevalence of hypertension, defined according to JNC III criteria, in white participants in NHANES II is shown in Figure 19.1. The prevalence increased with age from 9% in the youngest age group to 63% in the 65 to 74 age category. The rates were slightly higher in men than women, and were

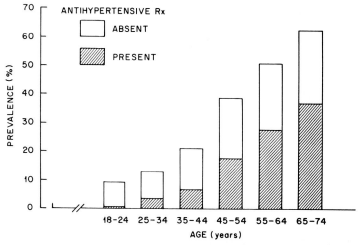

Figure 19.1 Age-specific prevalence of hypertension, defined according to JCN III criteria, in white participants of the National Health and Nutrition Examination Survey of a random sample of the US population in 1976–1980 (*National Center for Health Statistics, Drizd T, Dannenberg AL, et al: Blood pressure levels in persons 18–74 years of age in 1976–80, and trends in blood pressure from 1960 to 1980 in the United States. Series 11, No. 234 DHHS Pub (PHS) 86-1684. Hyattsville, MD, Public Health Service, 1986.*)

higher in blacks than whites (data not shown). As can be seen in Figure 19.1, about half of those with hypertension were on antihypertensive medication at the time of examination or in the past. Interestingly, the proportion with untreated hypertension was highest among young individuals.

Determinants of Hypertension

Despite intensive research, only modest progress has been made in identifying determinants of the variability in arterial blood pressure and, specifically, the factors responsible for hypertension. The findings can be grouped into three categories: (1) genetic factors, (2) environmental factors, and (3) personal risk indicators.

Genetic Factors

A substantial proportion of the observed interindividual variation in blood pressure is genetically determined, as evidenced by significant correlations between blood pressures obtained from relatives (Figure 19.2). On the basis of such data, an estimated 25% to 50% of the observed variation in blood pressure in a population is attributed to genetic factors.[5,6] Controversy exists, however, as to whether this reflects multifactorial inheritance[7] or a major gene effect modified by environmental factors.[8] While this debate continues,[6,9,10] many investigators are choosing a different approach; they select a particular physiologic characteristic that is involved in the pathogenesis of essential hypertension and then seek evidence that it is genetically determined (ie, a so-called intervening phenotype).[5,6] Basically, two approaches are applied. In one, segregation of the putative intervening phenotype in two- or three-generation families is examined

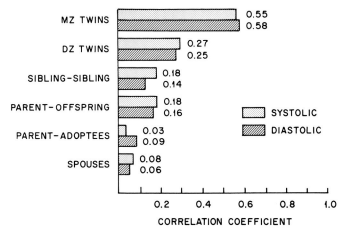

Figure 19.2 Familial correlation of blood pressures between specific types of family members. MZ = monozygotic, DZ = dizygotic. (*Reprinted, by permission, from Williams RR, Hunt SC, Haastedt SJ, et al: Inherited bimodal traits and susceptibility to hypertension in Utah pedigrees, in Rettig R, Ganten D, Luft FC (eds): Salt and Hypertension. Heidelberg, Springer-Verlag, 1989, pp 139–155.*)

by maximum likelihood methods with the goal of identifying the mode of inheritance of this predisposition to hypertension.[5,11] The other approach is to compare the distributions of the putative intervening phenotype in young offspring of hypertensive parents and young offspring of normotensive parents.[12–14] A difference in distributions is evidence that the phenotype is associated with genetic predisposition to hypertension. Several such abnormalities have been found and they are reviewed below.

Abnormalities in Renal Hemodynamics. In several studies, normotensive offspring of hypertensive parents exhibited abnormalities in renal hemodynamics and sodium handling in comparison with normotensive offspring of normotensive parents. The reported abnormalities represent a wide spectrum of changes, including increased glomerular filtration rate, decreased renal plasma flow, and exaggerated natriuresis in response to a sodium load.[12–16] It is notable that increased renal vascular resistance in normotensive offspring of hypertensive parents has been observed mainly in association with high dietary sodium intake.[15] These alterations in renal hemodynamics have been postulated to be inherited defects that predispose to the development of essential hypertension.[15] It is unclear, however, what genes may be involved in determining such defects and what would be the pathogenetic mechanisms leading from these defects to increased arterial blood pressure.

Abnormalities in Cation Transport Systems. Many abnormalities in cellular cation transport systems have been described in hypertensives as well as their relatives.[17,18] Some abnormalities could not be confirmed, and many varied according to race. An elevated maximal activity (V_{max}) of the lithium-sodium countertransport (Li^+-Na^+ CTT) in red blood cells is the most consistent finding in caucasian hypertensives.[19] The V_{max} of Li^+-Na^+ CTT is genetically determined, and at present is considered to be a marker of predisposition to hypertension.[20,21] One must realize, however, that although a large proportion of the general population has an elevated V_{max} of Li^+-Na^+ CTT in red blood cells, only a fraction of them are, or ever will be, hypertensive.[21] This implies that the predisposition to hypertension that is indicated by a high V_{max} of Li^+-Na^+ CTT must interact with other genetic or environmental factors to produce hypertension. The protein for Li^+-Na^+ CTT and its biologic function are unknown. A recent linkage study suggests that the gene for Li^+-Na^+ CTT may be localized to the long arm of chromosome 4.[22] Several authors, however, postulate that Li^+-Na^+ CTT represents an activity of the Na^+-H^+ exchanger.[23] Current findings point to the existence of at least two Na^+-H^+ exchangers: one blocked by amiloride and the other resistant to amiloride.[23,24] Whereas the former has been excluded as a possible candidate gene for Li^+-Na^+ CTT,[25] the latter needs to be examined once the human cDNA is known.

Insulin Resistance. Although several authors described impaired insulin-mediated glucose disposal (diminished insulin sensitivity) and compensatory hyperinsulinemia in patients with hypertension,[26–28] only recently has it been shown that their normotensive offspring also have impaired glucose disposal in comparison with normotensive offspring of normotensive parents.[29] Normotensive offspring of hypertensive parents also have elevated serum levels of lipids such as cholesterol and triglycerides.[29] Recently, a form of hypertension that is associated with hyperinsulinemia and lipid abnormalities has been described.[30] Based on these associations, a distinct familial trait for essential hypertension that coexists with defects in carbohydrate and lipid metabolism has been postulated.[29,30] The nature of this trait is unclear. Some authors postulate that this might be related to genetically determined abnormalities in Ca^{2+} metabolism.[31,32]

Environmental Factors

Interindividual variation in blood pressure is influenced by environmental factors as well. Blood pressure correlations between monozygotic twins (genetically identical) are only .50 (Figure 19.2). The remaining variability in blood pressure must be determined in large degree by environmental factors.[6] Despite intensive research, only a few such factors have been found to be associated with high blood pressure.

An association between dietary intake of salt and level of blood pressure was found in several multinational comparisons.[33,34] When countries were treated as the observational unit and arrayed across a broad range of sodium consumption, a positive correlation existed between the prevalence of hypertension and sodium intake or excretion. Lesser developed countries and tribal societies had low sodium intake and a low or negligible prevalence of hypertension. In contrast, industrialized countries had high levels of sodium intake and high prevalence of hypertension. The highest level of sodium intake and the greatest prevalence of hypertension were found in the Japanese, especially those residing in northern Japan. When one examines data within each of these populations, however, the relationships between dietary sodium intake and blood pressure are not consistent.[33–35] Moreover, no association was found between sodium intake and the development of hypertension in a large follow-up study.[36] Various explanations have been invoked to accommodate these findings.[33,35] Most frequently, authors point to the lack of precision in measurements of sodium intake as biasing the findings toward an absence of association.[33,36]

An emerging body of evidence supports an inverse relationship between dietary calcium intake and blood pressure. In several epidemiologic studies conducted within populations, low dietary calcium intake was associated with high blood pressure.[37-39] However, intervention studies that could confirm a causal role of high calcium intake in preventing hypertension have not been performed. Some authors postulate that the findings in these observational studies result from an association between low calcium intake and low income status, high exposure to stress, and high alcohol consumption, all being factors implicated in the development of hypertension.[36,40]

Personal Risk Indicators

In many epidemiologic studies, age-related increases in arterial blood pressure were strongly related to the level of blood pressure at the preceding age.[36,41-43] This is, perhaps, a proxy for the persistence of other risk factors that determined the level of blood pressure during the earlier time. Obesity is the second strongest correlate of elevated blood pressure in most cross-sectional as well as in follow-up studies.[36,41-43] The mechanisms underlying this association are not clear, but abnormalities in glucose disposal and hyperinsulinemia that are seen in obese individuals may contribute to it (see discussion below). In addition, high blood pressure is associated with low socioeconomic status.[36,44] Although this is a very reproducible observation, its meaning is unclear. It could be an indicator of environmental exposures such as diet or an indicator of stress.

Heterogeneous Etiology of Hypertension

The heterogeneous etiology of human hypertension has been recognized for some time.[45] In light of the preceding discussion, one must assume that the development of hypertension in humans must result from interactions between genetically determined susceptibilities and environmental factors or exposures.[5,6,46] There might be several different genetic defects that determine susceptibility to hypertension as well as several environmental factors that interact with these putative susceptibilities. As a result, the pathogenesis of hypertension in humans may be very heterogeneous.[45] This has been clearly shown to be the case in animal models.[47] In the general population, all possible combinations/interactions might take place, although with different frequencies. However, in considering the possible effects of diabetes on the development of hypertension, one can expect that certain predispositions might be favored (made manifest) more than others. In other words, the hypertension that occurs in types I and II diabetes may be more homogeneous than hypertension in the general population.

Occurrence of Hypertension in Insulin-Dependent Diabetes Mellitus

Insulin-dependent diabetes mellitus (IDDM; type I) results from immunologic destruction of beta cells and the consequent lack of endogenous insulin. Although replacement therapy with exogenous insulin prevents acute metabolic complications, it does not completely restore metabolic homeostasis. The result of this imperfect treatment is a "novel milieu" (exposure) that can include,

among other elements, various combinations of hyperinsulinemia, hyperglycemia, glucosuria, and ketonemia. These alterations may act independently, or,
more likely, they interact with certain genetic susceptibilities to produce late
complications of diabetes, including hypertension.[48] The lifetime risk of type I
diabetes is 1%, with a third of the cases having onset before age 30.[48]

Blood pressures in patients with newly diagnosed IDDM are similar to the
blood pressures of nondiabetic individuals of the same age and sex.[49] In juvenile-
onset IDDM patients, blood pressure increases with duration of diabetes. This
increase must, however, be compared to the age-related increase in blood pressure that is observed in nondiabetic populations (see Figure 19.1). In order to
assess how much might be due to diabetes itself, we conducted a retrospective
cohort study in which a group of 292 patients who came to the Joslin Clinic with
newly diagnosed juvenile-onset diabetes (before age 21) in 1939, 1949, and 1959
was followed until 1981.[50] Based on the 20- to 40-year follow-up data, we estimated the cumulative risk of hypertension as a function of duration of diabetes
and attained age. The latter was the dominant factor in the development of
hypertension in the study cohort. A diagnosis of hypertension was made if the
blood pressure criteria outlined above (90 mm Hg or greater diastolic, or 140
mm Hg or greater systolic) were fulfilled on two out of three consecutive visits
to the Joslin Clinic.

Using life-table analysis, we determined that about half of the cohort developed hypertension between ages 15 and 55 years. In the majority of patients
in the IDDM cohort, hypertension developed in conjunction with the appearance
of nephropathy. The cumulative incidence of each outcome increased with attained age until the fifth decade of life and then leveled off (Figure 19.3). It is
important to notice that, despite the development of renal complications in a
large proportion of this cohort of patients with IDDM, the cumulative risk of
hypertension was only slightly higher than the prevalence of hypertension in
the nondiabetic population, 39% in the age category 45 to 54 in Figure 19.1. This
conclusion is consistent with an earlier cross-sectional study in which the age-
specific prevalence of hypertension was found to be only slightly higher in IDDM
patients than in nondiabetic individuals.[51] Furthermore, studies of IDDM patients
who do not have renal complications despite a very long duration of diabetes
have found them to be normotensive.[52,53]

Susceptibility to Hypertension and Diabetic Nephropathy

The fact that hypertension in juvenile-onset IDDM patients develops mainly in
connection with the appearance of diabetic nephropathy suggested the possibility that predisposition to essential hypertension or elevated blood pressure
itself may underlie the development of renal complications in IDDM. To examine
this hypothesis, patients with newly diagnosed juvenile-onset IDDM who had
come to the Joslin Clinic between 1967 and 1972 were examined in 1986–1988
after 15 to 21 years of diabetes.[54,55] On average, the cohort was 13 years of age
at the first visit to the Joslin Clinic and 30 years of age at the time of the study.
A random sample of patients from this cohort underwent a special examination.
Using a case–control design, the following groups were compared: patients with
advanced nephropathy and hypertension, patients with hypertension only, and
patients who remained both normoalbuminuric and normotensive despite 15 to
21 years of IDDM.

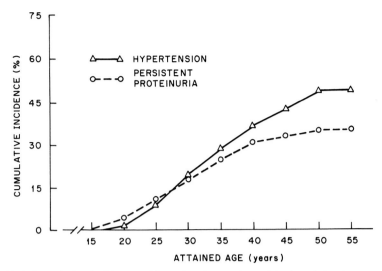

Figure 19.3 Cumulative incidence of hypertension and persistent proteinuria according to attained age in a cohort of 292 patients, with IDDM diagnosed before age 21, who were followed from the diagnosis of diabetes for 20 to 40 years. Persistent proteinuria was diagnosed if patients had protein levels of 30 mg/dL or greater in two or more out of three consecutive urinalyses. Hypertension was diagnosed if, on two or more out of three consecutive clinic visits, diastolic blood pressure was 90 mm Hg or greater, or systolic blood pressure was 140 mm Hg or greater. (*Adapted from Krolewski AS, Warram JH, Christlieb AR, et al: The changing natural history of nephropathy in Type I diabetes. Am J Med 1985;78:785–790.*)

The frequency of three different measures of predisposition to hypertension were more frequent in cases than controls (Table 19.1). All three measures followed the same pattern: in comparison with normoalbuminuric and normotensive controls, those with advanced nephropathy were more likely to have parents with hypertension, to have a high velocity of Na^+-Li^+ CTT in red cells, and to have had higher systemic blood pressures during adolescence and early adulthood.

During the last few years, several authors have reported on the association between predisposition to essential hypertension and diabetic nephropathy. Viberti and co-workers reported that parents of IDDM patients with proteinuria were more frequently hypertensive than parents of IDDM patients without renal complications.[56] The same investigators recently demonstrated that parents of patients with diabetic nephropathy have a significantly higher V_{max} of Na^+-Li^+ CTT than parents of normoalbuminuric IDDM patients.[57] Moreover, Semplicini et al showed that IDDM patients with isolated hypertension (without nephropathy) were more likely to have hypertensive parents and a high V_{max} of Na^+-Li^+ CTT than IDDM patients with normal blood pressure and albumin excretion.[58]

One report, however, is not in full agreement with these conclusions.[59] Although those authors, too, found an excess prevalence of parental hypertension and elevated V_{max} of Li^+-Na^+ CTT in patients with diabetic nephropathy as compared to patients without renal complications, the statistical significance of these differences was only borderline as a result of a bias in the selection of the study groups.[60] On this basis, the authors have erroneously concluded that

Table 19.1 Characteristics of Study Patients According to the Presence of Three Different Outcomes at Examination, 15 to 21 Years After the Diagnosis of Juvenile-Onset IDDM

Characteristics	No Nephropathy and Normal BP ($N = 61$)	Proteinuria and Hypertension[a] ($N = 43$)	Hypertension Only[a] ($N = 17$)
Hypertension[b] in:			
Mother (%)	26	47	47
Father (%)	21	39	30
One or both parents (%)	38	70	71
Mean arterial pressure during adolescence[c] (mm Hg, mean ± SD)	82 ± 4	85 ± 7	88 ± 7
V_{max} of Na^+-Li^+ CTT in RBC[d] at examination (mean ± SD)	0.36 ± 0.20	0.49 ± 0.24	0.46 ± 0.18
Hyperglycemic index[e] (first 12 yr of IDDM) (mean ± SD)	42 ± 18	52 ± 18	34 ± 21
Hemoglobin A_1 (%) at examination (mean ± SD)	10.9 ± 1.9	12.2 ± 2.0	10.5 ± 1.4

Adapted from Barzilay J, Warram JH, Bak M, et al: Predisposition to hypertension: a risk factor for nephropathy and hypertension in IDDM. Kidney Int, to be published.)

[a] Hypertension was diagnosed if diastolic blood pressure (BP) was 90 mm Hg or greater, or systolic BP was 140 mm Hg or greater, or antihypertensive treatment was prescribed.

[b] Hypertension diagnosed before age 60 and treated by medical doctor.

[c] Blood pressure readings between ages 13 and 20 were used for those with IDDM diagnosed before age 13; blood pressure reading during first 8 years of IDDM were used for those who had diabetes diagnosed between age 13 and 20.

[d] V_{max} of Na^+-Li^+ CTT in mmoles/liter of red blood cells/hour; it was measured in 34, 29, and 12 individuals in the group without nephropathy and normal BP, the group with proteinuria and hypertension, and the group with hypertension only, respectively.

[e] Proportion of clinic visits with severe hyperglycemia.[55]

there is no association between predisposition to hypertension and risk of diabetic nephropathy.

The occurrence of hypertension among individuals with adult-onset IDDM is unknown. It is unclear whether these patients have a risk of developing diabetic nephropathy and hypertension as high as those with IDDM diagnosed early in life. The major obstacle to the examination of these questions is the low prevalence of IDDM among patients with diabetes diagnosed after age 30.

Poor Glycemic Control and Susceptibility to Hypertension

The other finding that emerged from the recent studies in juvenile-onset IDDM patients is a demonstration of the importance of glycemic control in the development of diabetic nephropathy and hypertension as compared to the development of essential hypertension without nephropathy. Patients with proteinuria had poor glycemic control, whereas those with hypertension alone had the best glycemic control of all the study groups (Table 19.1). Because these two groups of cases were similar with regard to measures of predisposition to hypertension and differed only with regard to glycemic control, it follows that poor glycemic control interacts with elevated blood pressure or its predisposing abnormalities to produce diabetic nephropathy.

The specific component mechanisms of the predisposition to hypertension that can make these patients vulnerable to nephropathy are not known. As was reviewed earlier, offspring of hypertensive parents have significant abnormalities in renal hemodynamics when on a high-salt diet.[12-16] These abnormalities, perhaps, are magnified in the presence of poor glycemic control. Specifically, it has been shown that patients with poor glycemic control have higher filtration fractions than patients with good glycemic control.[61] Moreover, when IDDM patients were divided into low and high groups according to the V_{max} of Li^+-Na^+ CTT, the high group was characterized by low renal blood flow and high filtration fraction.[62]

Occurrence of Hypertension in Non-Insulin-Dependent Diabetes Mellitus

Non-insulin-dependent diabetes mellitus (NIDDM, type II) occurs because of impaired insulin action in peripheral tissues and failure of the beta cells to secret a sufficient amount of endogenous insulin to meet the extra requirement. A state of impaired glucose tolerance precedes the development of frank NIDDM, and, in most instances, it is characterized by impaired insulin action, hyperinsulinemia, and lipid abnormalities.

The best estimates of prevalence of impaired glucose tolerance (IGT) and NIDDM come from a random sample of the US population examined during the NHANES II in 1976–1980.[63,64] Age-specific prevalence rates for the white participants of the NHANES II are shown in Figure 19.4. Prevalence of NIDDM and IGT increased with age from 3.7% in the group ages 20 to 44 years to 26.4% in the group ages 65 to 74. The rates were slightly higher in men than women, and

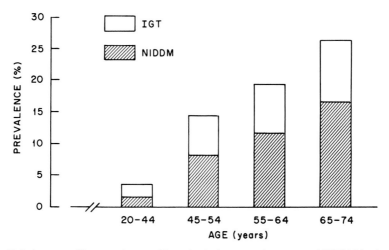

Figure 19.4 Age-specific prevalence of impaired glucose tolerance and NIDDM in the white participants of the National Health and Nutrition Examination Survey of a random sample of the US population in 1976–1980. (*Adapted from Harris MI, Hadden WC, Knowler WC, et al: Prevalence of diabetes and impaired glucose tolerance and plasma glucose levels in the US population aged 20–74 yr. Diabetes 1987;36:523–534, and Harris MI: Impaired glucose tolerance in the US population. Diabetes Care 1989;12:464–474.*)

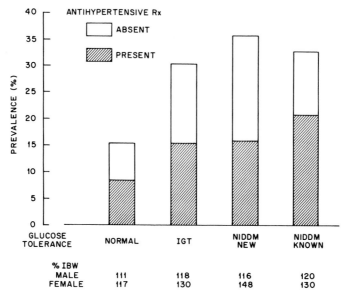

Figure 19.5 Age-adjusted prevalence of significant hypertension according to categories of glucose tolerance in the white participants of the National Health and Nutrition Examination Survey of a random sample of the US population in 1976–1980. Significant hypertension was diagnosed if diastolic blood pressure was 95 mm Hg or greater, or systolic blood pressure was 160 mm Hg or greater, or antihypertensive medication was prescribed. Impaired glucose tolerance (IGT) and "NIDDM new" were recognized during the survey. "NIDDM known" was diabetes diagnosed before the survey. (*Adapted from Harris MI, Hadden WC, Knowler WC, et al: Prevalence of diabetes and impaired glucose tolerance and plasma glucose levels in the US population aged 20–74 yr. Diabetes 1987;36:523–534, and Harris MI: Impaired glucose tolerance in the US population. Diabetes Care 1989;12:464–474.*)

were higher in blacks than whites. By contrasting Figure 19.4 with Figure 19.1, one can see that the prevalence of glucose intolerance (NIDDM plus IGT) is only 40% of that for hypertension but follows a similar age-dependent pattern.

Individuals with type II diabetes have elevated blood pressure in comparison with nondiabetics. This has been found in several studies[65–67] and is best illustrated in Figure 19.5. This figure shows the prevalence of hypertension according to four categories of glucose tolerance in the random sample of the white US population ages 20 to 74 that participated in the NHANES II.[64] The prevalence of significant hypertension (for a definition, see Figure 19.5) in all three groups with glucose intolerance (IGT, newly diagnosed NIDDM, and previously diagnosed NIDDM) is twice that in the normoglycemic group. This was true for treated hypertension as well as untreated hypertension. The excess prevalence of hypertension in individuals with IGT and NIDDM can be accounted for by several mechanisms, which are reviewed below.

NIDDM and Hypertension Share a Common Determinant

In a large population study, parents of patients with NIDDM were found to have an excess prevalence of diabetes and an excess, as well, of hypertension and coronary artery disease.[68] In another study, the offspring of patients with NIDDM had elevated blood pressure and lipid abnormalities more frequently than offspring of nondiabetic parents.[69] These findings suggest that hypertension and NIDDM cluster in the same families. This can be due to the shared familial environment or to shared genes that predispose to the development of both NIDDM and a certain type of hypertension.

At the individual level, the common risk factor for both disorders is the presence of obesity. As discussed earlier, obesity is one of the strongest predictors of the development of hypertension in nondiabetic individuals.[36,41–43] Also, obesity is the strongest risk factor for the development of NIDDM and IGT.[70,71] As shown in Figure 19.5, individuals with IGT and NIDDM had higher mean values of percentage of ideal body weight at the time of examination in comparison with individuals who had normal glucose tolerance. The same pattern was seen when weight at age 25 or maximum weight were compared among the four subgroups (data not shown).

Since obesity is a very complex disorder, it is not clear whether the aspects of obesity that predispose to the development of hypertension are the same as those that predispose to abnormalities in glucose tolerance and type II diabetes.[72] There are no data sets to examine these questions, and the existing literature provides only indirect answers.

A common characteristic of obesity is impaired glucose disposal and compensatory hyperinsulinemia.[71,72] Bergman has proposed a minimal model of glucose disposal that defines two components of glucose clearance, insulin-dependent glucose disposal (insulin sensitivity) and insulin-independent glucose disposal (glucose clearance at basal insulin). Estimates of these components can be derived for the glucose and insulin values obtained during a 3-hour intravenous glucose tolerance test, and these indices have been validated against comparable measures derived from clamp techniques.[73] In a recent follow-up study of 151 normoglycemic individuals with a strong family history of NIDDM, we found that all of the individuals who developed NIDDM during 10 to 20 years of follow-up had significantly impaired glucose disposal (insulin dependent or insulin independent) from the start in comparison with those who remained normoglycemic.[74] When other variables were taken into account in the analysis, only the two components of glucose disposal were significant and independent predictors of NIDDM. Obesity was not significant because there were lean individuals who were insensitive to insulin and obese individuals who were sensitive to insulin; thus, neither characteristic is necessary or sufficient for the other. Only the subset of obese individuals with coexistent insulin resistance was at high risk of developing NIDDM. We do not have follow-up data to examine in the same way the relationship between the development of hypertension and impaired glucose disposal. Cross-sectional comparisons, however, show similar findings.[75] Low insulin-independent glucose disposal was associated with higher diastolic blood pressure regardless of obesity, whereas low insulin-dependent glucose disposal as associated with higher blood pressure only in obese individuals.

Significant controversy has arisen as to whether the pathogenic mechanisms that underlie the association between impaired glucose disposal and hypertension operate through hyperinsulinemia.[76] Although this issue is not discussed further in this chapter, certain points should be made to help conceptualize alternative interpretations.

First of all, in several studies patients with insulinoma have been found not to have elevated blood pressure.[77] Furthermore, the population of Pima Indians, which has one of the highest prevalences of obesity and the highest risk of NIDDM in the world, has very high levels of serum insulin but does not have a high prevalence of hypertension. This population may have a very specific genetic defect in glucose disposal that does not have an impact on blood pressure. Also, unlike caucasians, the level of blood pressure in Pima Indians is unrelated to the level of serum insulin.[78] Findings similar to those in Pima Indians have been reported in US blacks.[78] Also, in a very recent study of a large family in which high insulin levels segregate as an autosomal dominant disorder, we did not find any association between insulin level and blood pressure (A. S. Krolewski et al, unpublished data). High insulin levels and frequent NIDDM in this family were due to a genetic defect in the insulin receptor. Pedigree members with very high fasting insulin levels had blood pressures in the normal range. If one considers all of these findings together, the only plausible interpretation is that a certain genetically determined type of insulin resistance (occurring mainly in caucasians) contributes to the development of hypertension as well as NIDDM. Characteristics that would distinguish this specific subtype of insulin resistance are not known at present.[31,32,79,80]

Antihypertensive Treatment May Increase the Risk of NIDDM

Whereas most of the studies showing that hypertensive patients have an excess risk of developing NIDDM or IGT can be explained by the mechanisms described above, a growing number of studies have demonstrated that antihypertensive treatment itself may contribute to the development of glucose intolerance and NIDDM.[81–84] In clinical trials it was shown that treatment with nonselective or selective β blockers as well as with diuretics was associated with an increased insulin resistance.[83] During 5 years of follow-up in the Medical Research Council Mild Hypertension Study, clinically important glucose intolerance developed in 2.5% of patients taking thiazides, whereas this abnormality occurred in only 1% of these treated with placebo.[84]

NIDDM May Cause the Development of Hypertension

The reverse type of interaction is also possible. The diabetic milieu may contribute to the development of hypertension. Few studies have examined this question, and one of them was conducted at the Joslin Clinic in the 1960s before treatment with antihypertensive drugs became commonplace.[85] Figure 19.6 compared mean blood pressures in NIDDM patients ages 65 to 74 according to duration of diabetes. Particularly high systolic and diastolic blood pressures were found in patients who had diabetes duration of 10 to 15 years, suggesting increasing blood pressure with duration of diabetes. Because the study was cross-sectional, a lower mean blood pressure among individuals with diabetes duration of 20 to 25 years is consistent with a poorer survival rate among those with the highest blood pressures. The mechanisms underlying the increase in blood pressure with increasing duration of NIDDM are unclear.

Summary

A precise accounting of the mechanisms responsible for the excess of hypertension in individuals with IGT and NIDDM (Figure 19.5) is not possible. Based on the discussion above, a plausible argument can be made that all of these

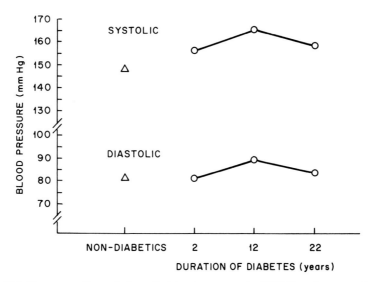

Figure 19.6 Mean systolic and diastolic blood pressure in NIDDM patients aged 65–74 at examination according to duration of diabetes. Relative to the values for non-diabetics, mean elevations in patients with diabetes duration 12 years (15 and 10, respectively) were significantly higher than those for the group with duration 2 years (5 and 0, respectively). (*Data adapted from Krolewski AS, Warram JH, Cupples A, et al: Hypertension, orthostatic hypotension and the microvascular complications of diabetes. J Chron Dis 1985;38:319–326.*)

mechanisms are involved, and that the excess of hypertension in NIDDM is due to factors that operate before manifestation of glucose intolerance as well as after the development of NIDDM.

Implications for Studies on Etiology of Hypertension in Diabetes

Although pharmacologic means of treating hypertension are expanding, it is important to unravel the etiology of hypertension in diabetes. This might make primary prevention possible or provide nonpharmacologic approaches to lowering blood pressure in established hypertension. Based on the review above, three areas can be outlined for future research on the etiology of hypertension in diabetes.

IDDM patients with certain type(s) of genetic predisposition to essential hypertension are at high risk of developing hypertension and renal complications. Identification of the genetic abnormalities that underlie this "susceptibility" to hypertension will permit identification of target groups for special preventive programs. These might include improvement in glycemic control or pharmacologic intervention to modify intrarenal hemodynamics, for example. Application of methods of molecular genetics will facilitate these aims.[86,87]

One approach is to examine the DNA sequences of specific candidate genes to identify sequence differences that are responsible for susceptibility to essential hypertension/diabetic nephropathy. Some of these candidate genes are listed in Table 19.2. A second approach is to screen specific parts of human

Table 19.2 Candidate Genes for Susceptibility to
Hypertension/Nephropathy in IDDM

Candidate Genes	Chromosomal Location
Renin	1q
Angiotensin-converting enzyme	17q
Kallikrein	19q
Na^+-H^+ exchanger (amiloride resistant)	unknown
Haptoglobin	16q
MN blood groups	3q

(Adapted from Krolewski AS, Doria A, Magre J, et al: Molecular genetic approaches to the identification of genes involved in the development of nephropathy in insulin-dependent diabetes mellitus. J Am Soc Nephrol 1992;3(suppl 4):S9–S17.)

chromosomes for evidence that they contain genes that contribute to the these disorders. There are two strategies for these studies. One is a comparison of alleles at a particular locus (usually the locus of a candidate gene) between groups of unrelated individuals (cases and controls). The other strategy is based on families, studies of either sib pairs or large families. Although the family studies are feasible now from the standpoint of the tools of molecular genetics, they cannot be conducted because of a lack of DNA from appropriate families.

It is clear that only a subset of the general population is at high risk of developing the cluster of conditions: obesity, hypertension, and NIDDM. A trait common to these outcomes is impaired glucose disposal. Although this impairment seems to have a significant genetic component, it is likely that several genetic factors play a role.[88–90] The challenge is to identify specific genetic defects that contribute to impaired glucose disposal and to the development of hypertension. To accomplish this, it may be particularly appropriate to study the families of caucasians with NIDDM and hypertension. The approaches and strategies are similar to those described above for identifying genes involved in predisposition to hypertension and diabetic nephropathy.[86,87]

Finally, the role of environmental factors in the development of hypertension in IDDM and NIDDM should be studied as well. There is growing evidence that low intake of dietary calcium may have significant impact on the development of hypertension in nondiabetics.[37–39] The same may be true in diabetic patients. Similarly, there is growing evidence that exercise can prevent the development of hypertension and NIDDM.[91–93] However, it is unknown whether this will have any impact on lowering blood pressure in diabetic patients.

References

1. Freis ED, and the Veterans Administration Cooperative Study Group on Antihypertensive Agents: Effects of treatment on morbidity in hypertension. I. Results in patients with diastolic blood pressure average 115 through 129 mm Hg. *JAMA* 1967;202: 1028–1034.
2. Kannel WB: Hypertension and the risk of cardiovascular disease, in Laragh JH, Brenner BM (eds): *Hypertension: Pathophysiology, Diagnosis and Management.* New York, Raven Press Ltd, 1990, pp 101–117.

3. The 1984 report of the Joint National Committee on Detection, Evaluation and Treatment of High Blood Pressure. *Arch Intern Med* 1984;144:1045–1057.

4. National Center for Health Statistics, Drizd T, Dannenberg AL, et al: Blood pressure levels in persons 18–74 years of age in 1976–80, and trends in blood pressure from 1960 to 1980 in the United States. Series 11, No. 234, DHHS Pub. (PHS) 86-1684. Hyattsville, MD, Public Health Service, 1986.

5. Williams RR, Hunt SC, Hasstedt SJ, et al: Inherited bimodal traits and susceptibility to hypertension in Utah pedigrees, in Rettig R, Ganten D, Luft FC (eds): *Salt and Hypertension.* Heidelberg, Springer-Verlag, 1989, pp 139–155.

6. Ward R: Familial aggregation and genetic epidemiology of blood pressure, in Laragh JH, Brenner BM (eds): *Hypertension: Pathophysiology, Diagnosis and Management.* New York, Raven Press Ltd, 1990, pp 81–100.

7. Hamilton M, Pickering GW, Roberts JAF, et al: The etiology of essential hypertension: IV. The role of inheritance. *Clin Sci* 1954;13:273–274.

8. Platt R: Heredity in hypertension. *Lancet* 1963;1:899–904.

9. Rice T, Bouchard C, Borecki IB, et al: Commingling and segregation analysis of blood pressure in a French-Canadian population. *Am J Hum Genet* 1990;46:37–44.

10. Schork NJ, Weder AB, Schork MA: On the asymmetry of biological frequency distributions. *Genet Epidemiol* 1990;7:427–446.

11. Williams RR, Hunt SC, Hasstedt SJ, et al: Definition of genetic factors in hypertension: A search for major genes, polygenes, and homogeneous subtypes. *J Cardiovasc Pharmacol* 1988;12(suppl 3):7–20.

12. Wiggins RC, Basar I, Slater JDH: Effect of arterial pressure and inheritance on the sodium excretory capacity of normal young men. *Clin Sci* 1978;54:639–647.

13. Bianchi G, Cusi D, Barlassina C, et al: Renal dysfunction as a possible cause of essential hypertension in predisposed subjects. *Kidney Int* 1983;23:870–875.

14. Uneda S, Fujishima S, Fujiki Y, et al: Renal hemodynamics and renin angiotensin system in adolescents genetically predisposed to essential hypertension. *J Hypertens* 1984;2(suppl 3):437–439.

15. Textor SC, Turner ST: Renal vascular response to sodium loading in sons of hypertensive parents. *Hypertension* 1991;17:982–988.

16. Hannedouche TP, Marques L-P, Guicheney P, et al: Predisposition to essential hypertension and renal hemodynamics in recent onset insulin-dependent diabetic patients. *J Am Soc Nephrol* 1992;3(suppl 4):S34–S40.

17. Hilton PJ: Cellular sodium transport in essential hypertension. *N Engl J Med* 1986; 314:222–229.

18. Weder AB: Cation transport markers as predictors of hypertension. *Am J Hypertens* 1991;4:633S–637S.

19. Canessa M, Adragna N, Solomon HS, et al: Increased sodium-lithium countertransport in red cells of patients with essential hypertension. *N Engl J Med* 1980;302:772–776.

20. Motulsky AG, Burke W, Billings PR, et al: Hypertension and genetics of red cell membrane abnormalities. *Ciba Found Symp* 1987;130:150–166.

21. Weder AB, Schork NJ, Krause L, et al: Red blood cell lithium-sodium countertransport in the Tecumseh blood pressure study. *Hypertension* 1991;17:652–660.

22. Weder AB, Schork NJ, Julius S: Linkage of MN locus and erythrocyte lithium-sodium countertransport in Tecumseh, Michigan. *Hypertension* 1991;17:977–981.

23. Huot SJ, Aronson PS: Na-H exchanger and its role in essential hypertension and diabetes mellitus. *Diabetes Care* 1991;14:521–535.

24. Biemesderfer D, Hildebrandt F, Exner M, et al: Cloning and immunolocalization of a Na/H exchanger in LLC-PK1 cells [abstract]. *J Am Soc Nephrol* 1990;1:743.

25. Lifton RP, Hunt SC, Williams RR, et al: Exclusion of the Na/H antiport as a candidate gene in human essential hypertension by genetic linkage analysis. *Hypertension* 1991; 17:8–14.

26. Modan M, Halkin H, Almog S, et al: Hyperinsulinemia: A link between hypertension, obesity and glucose intolerance. *J Clin Invest* 1985;75:809–817.

27. Christlieb AR, Krolewski AS, Warram JH, et al: Is insulin the link between hypertension and obesity? *Hypertension* 1985;7(suppl II):54–57.

28. Ferrannini E, Buzzigoli G, Bonadona R, et al: Insulin resistance in essential hypertension. *N Engl J Med* 1987;317:350–357.

29. Ferrari P, Weidmann P, Shaw S, et al: Altered insulin sensitivity, hyperinsulinemia, and dyslipidemia in individuals with a hypertensive parent. *Am J Med* 1991;91:589–596.

30. Hunt SC, Wu LL, Hopkins PN, et al: Apolipoprotein, low density lipoprotein subfraction, and insulin associations with familial combined hyperlipidemia: Study of Utah patients with familial dyslipidemic hypertension. *Arteriosclerosis* 1989;9:335–344.

31. Draznin B, Sussman KE, Eckel RH, et al: Possible role of cytosolic free calcium concentrations in mediating insulin resistance of obesity and hyperinsulinemia. *J Clin Invest* 1988;82:1848–1852.

32. Resnick LM: Calcium metabolism in hypertension and allied metabolic disorders. *Diabetes Care* 1991;14:505–520.

33. Elliott P: Observational studies of salt and blood pressure. *Hypertension* 1991;17(suppl I):3–8.

34. Stamler J, Rose G, Elliott P, et al: Findings of the international cooperative INTERSALT study. *Hypertension* 1991;17(suppl I):9–15.

35. Kotchen TA, Kotchen JM, Boegehold MA: Nutrition and hypertension prevention. *Hypertension* 1991;18(suppl I):115–120.

36. Ford ES, Cooper RS: Risk factors for hypertension in a national cohort study. *Hypertension* 1991;18:598–606.

37. Kesteloot H, Geboers J: Calcium and blood pressure. *Lancet* 1982;1:813–815.

38. McCarron D, Morris CD, Henry JH, et al: Blood pressure and nutrient intake in the United States. *Science* 1984;224:1392–1398.

39. Witteman JC, Willett WC, Stampfer MJ, et al: A prospective study of nutritional factors and hypertension among U.S. women. *Circulation* 1989;80:1320–1327.

40. Witteman JC, Willett WC, Stampfer MJ, et al: Relation of moderate alcohol consumption and risk of systemic hypertension in women. *Am J Cardiol* 1990;65:633–637.

41. Leitschuh M, Cupples LA, Kannel W, et al: High-normal blood pressure progression to hypertension in the Framingham Heart Study. *Hypertension* 1991;17:22–27.

42. Hunt SC, Stephenson SH, Hopkins PN, et al: Predictors of an increased risk of future hypertension in Utah. A screening analysis. *Hypertension* 1991;17:969–976.

43. Jamerson K, Julius S: Predictors of blood pressure and hypertension. General principles. *Am J Hypertens* 1991;4:598S–602S.

44. Sear AM, Weinrich M, Hersh JE, et al: The relationship between income, education and hypertension. *J Biosoc Sci* 1982;14:213–221.

45. Weinberger MH: Can essential hypertension be subclassified with respect to mechanisms? *Hypertension* 1991;18(suppl I):82–86.

46. Williams RR, Hunt SC, Hasstedt SJ, et al: Are there interactions and relations between genetic and environmental factors predisposing to high blood pressure? *Hypertension* 1991;18(suppl I):29–37.

47. Rapp JP: Dissecting the primary causes of genetic hypertension in rats. *Hypertension* 1991;18(suppl I):18–28.

48. Krolewski AS, Warram JH, Rand LI, et al: Epidemiologic approach to the etiology of type I diabetes mellitus and its complications. *N Engl J Med* 1987;317:1390–1398.

49. Kelleher C, Kingston SM, Barry DG, et al: Hypertension in diabetic clinic patients and their siblings. *Diabetologia* 1988;31:76–81.

50. Krolewski AS, Warram JH, Christlieb AR, et al: The changing natural history of nephropathy in type I diabetes. *Am J Med* 1985;78:785–790.

51. Keen H, Track NS, Sowry GCS: Arterial pressure in clinically apparent diabetics. *Diabete Metab* 1975;1:159–164.

52. Oakley WG, Pyke DA, Tattersall RB, et al: Long-term diabetes: A clinical study of 92 patients after 40 years. *Q J Med* 1974;43:145–156.
53. Borch-Johnson K, Nissen RN, Nerup J: Blood pressure after 40 years of insulin-dependent diabetes. *Diabetic Nephrop* 1985;4:11–12.
54. Krolewski AS, Canessa M, Warram JH, et al: Predisposition to hypertension and susceptibility to renal disease in insulin-dependent diabetes mellitus. *N Engl J Med* 1988; 318:140–145.
55. Barzilay J, Warram JH, Bak M, et al: Predisposition to hypertesnion: A risk factor for nephropathy and hypertension in IDDM. *Kidney Int* 1992;41:723–730.
56. Viberti GC, Keen H, Wiseman MJ: Raised arterial pressure in parents of proteinuric insulin-dependent diabetics. *BMJ* 1987;295:515–517.
57. Walker JD, Tariq T, Viberti GC: Sodium-lithium countertransport activity in red cells of patients with insulin-dependent diabetes and nephropathy and their parents. *BMJ* 1990;301:635–638.
58. Semplicini A, Mozzato MG, Sama B, et al: Na/H and Li/Na exchange in red blood cells of normotensive and hypertensive patients with insulin-dependent diabetes mellitus (IDDM). *Am J Hypertens* 1989;2:174–177.
59. Jensen JS, Mathiesen ER, Norgaard K, et al: Increased blood pressure and erythrocyte sodium/lithium countertransport activity are not inherited in diabetic nephropathy. *Diabetologia* 1990;33:619–624.
60. Laffel L, Warram JH, Krolewski AS: Letter to the Editor. *Diabetologia* 1991;34:452–453.
61. Jenkins DAS, Cowan P, Collier A, et al: Blood glucose control determines the renal haemodynamic response to angiotensin converting enzyme inhibition in type I diabetes. *Diabetic Med* 1990;7:252–257.
62. Wolpert HA, Lenhard MJ, Simonson DC: Renal hemodynamics in type I diabetic patients with elevated sodium/lithium countertransport activity [abstract]. *Diabetologia* 1991;34(suppl 2):A31.
63. Harris MI, Hadden WC, Knowler WC, et al: Prevalence of diabetes and impaired glucose tolerance and plasma glucose levels in the U.S. population aged 20–74 yr. *Diabetes* 1987;36:523–534.
64. Harris MI: Impaired glucose tolerance in the U.S. population. *Diabetes Care* 1989;12:464–474.
65. Jarrett RJ, Keen H, McCartney M, et al: Glucose tolerance and blood pressure in two populations samples: Their relation to diabetes mellitus and hypertension. *Int J Epidemiol* 1978;7:15–24.
66. Barrett-Connor E, Criqui MH, Klauber MR, et al: Diabetes and hypertension in a community of older adults. *Am J Epidemiol* 1981;113:276–284.
67. Teuscher A, Egger M, Herman JB: Blood pressure in clinical diabetic patients and a control population. *Arch Intern Med* 1989;149:1942–1945.
68. Krolewski AS, Czyzyk A, Kopczynski J, et al: Prevalence of diabetes mellitus, coronary heart disease and hypertension in the families of insulin dependent and insulin independent diabetics. *Diabetologia* 1981;21:520–524.
69. Haffner SM, Stern MP, Hazuda HP, et al: Parental history of diabetes is associated with increased cardiovascular risk factors. *Arteriosclerosis* 1989;9:928–933.
70. Colditz GA, Willett WC, Stampfer MJ, et al: Weight as a risk factor for clinical diabetes in women. *Am J Epidemiol* 1990;132:501–513.
71. Reaven GM: Role of insulin resistance in human disease. *Diabetes* 1988;37:1595–1607.
72. Ferrannini E, Natali A, Cerri M, et al: Hypertension: A metabolic disorder? *Diabete Metab* 1989;15:284–291.
73. Bergman RN: Toward physiological understanding of glucose intolerance: Minimal model approach. *Diabetes* 1989;38:1512–1527.
74. Martin BC, Warram JH, Krolewski AS, et al: Glucose and insulin resistance precede and predict the development of type II diabetes mellitus. *Lancet* 1992;340:925–929.

75. Ganda OP, El-Hashimy M, Soeldner JS: Insulin-independent glucose disposal as well as insulin-sensitivity are determinants of blood pressure variability in offspring of type II diabetic parents. [abstract] *Diabetes* 1992;41(suppl 1):125A.
76. Hall JE, Brands MW, Hildebrandt DA, et al: Obesity-associated hypertension: Hyperinsulinemia and renal mechanisms. *Hypertension* 1992;19(suppl I):45–55.
77. Sawicki PT, Baba T, Berger M, et al: Normal blood pressure in patients with insulinoma despite hyperinsulinemia and insulin resistance. *J Am Soc Nephrol* 1992;3(suppl 4): S64–S68.
78. Saad MF, Lillioja S, Nyomba BL, et al: Racial differences in the relation between blood pressure and insulin resistance. *N Engl J Med* 1991;324:733–739.
79. Natali A, Santoro D, Palombo C, et al: Impaired insulin action on skeletal muscle metabolism in essential hypertension. *Hypertension* 1991;17:170–178.
80. Kahn CR, Saad M: Alterations in insulin receptor and substrate phosphorylation in hypertension rats. *J Am Soc Nephrol* 1992;3(suppl 4):S69–S77.
81. Bengtsson C, Blohme G, Lapidus L, et al: Diabetes in hypertensive: An effect of antihypertensive drugs or the hypertensive state per se? *Diabetic Med* 1988;5:261–264.
82. Skarfors ET, Selinus KI, Lithell HO: Risk factors for developing non-insulin dependent diabetes: A 10 year follow-up of men in Uppsala. *BMJ* 1991;303:755–760.
83. Pollare T, Lithell H, Berne C: A comparison of the effects of hydrochlorothiazide and captopril on glucose and lipid metabolism in patients with hypertension. *N Engl J Med* 1989;321:868–871.
84. Medical Research Council Working Party: MRC trial of treatment of mild hypertension: Principal results. *BMJ* 1985;291:97–104.
85. Krolewski AS, Warram JH, Cupples A, et al: Hypertension, orthostatic hypotension and the microvascular complications of diabetes. *J Chron Dis* 1985;38:319–326.
86. Dudley CRK, Giuffra LA, Reeders ST: Identifying genetic determinants in human essential hypertension. *J Am Soc Nephrol* 1992;3(suppl 4):S2–S8.
87. Krolewski AS, Doria A, Magre J, et al: Molecular genetic approaches to the identification of genes involved in the development of nephropathy in insulin-dependent diabetes mellitus. *J Am Soc Nephrol,* 1992(suppl 4):S9–S17.
88. Bogardus C, Lillioja S, Nyomba BL, et al: Distribution of in vivo insulin action in Pima Indians as mixture of three normal distributions. *Diabetes* 1989;38:1423–1432.
89. Rich SS: Mapping genes in diabetes: Genetic epidemiological perspective. *Diabetes* 1990;39:1315–1319.
90. Martin BC, Warram JH, Rosner B, et al: Familial clustering of insulin sensitivity. *Diabetes,* to be published.
91. Stamler R, Stamler J, Gosch F, et al: Primary prevention of hypertension by nutritional-hygienic means. *JAMA* 1989;262:1801–1807.
92. Helmrich SP, Ragland DR, Leung RW, et al: Physical activity and reduced occurrence of non-insulin-dependent diabetes mellitus. *N Engl J Med* 1991;325:147–152.
93. Manson J, Nathan DM, Krolewski AS, et al: A prospective study of exercise and incidence of diabetes among U.S. male physicians. *JAMA* 1992;268:63–67.

Chapter 20

Clinical Picture and Therapy of Hypertension in Diabetes Mellitus

Susan Savage, MD, and Robert W. Schrier, MD

Epidemiology

Diabetes mellitus is an important cause of morbidity and mortality in the United States. The National Health Interview Survey reported that over 15 million Americans suffer from diabetes. Type I diabetic patients comprise 8.3% of the diabetic population, and type II patients comprise the remaining 91.7%.[1] The health care costs of treating this disease are estimated to be in excess of $14 billion annually. In a recent national health survey, it was estimated that 17% to 18% of the white population will develop diabetes between the ages of 65 and 74 years, with an even greater incidence in the black and Hispanic populations.[2] With the elderly population expected to increase from 11% to 20% in this country by the year 2020, the human and economic costs of the morbidity and mortality of type II diabetes mellitus are expected to increase drastically.[3]

Hypertension is known to substantially aggravate and contribute to diabetic vascular complications. The prevalence of hypertension associated with type I diabetic patients without microalbuminuria is comparable to that of the general population.[4] Once microalbuminuria and the progression to frank diabetic nephropathy with proteinuria occurs, subsequent increases in both diastolic and systolic blood pressure occur.[5] Among the long-term survivors of type I diabetes (duration over 30 years) who are without diabetic nephropathy, nearly all are found to be normotensive.[6] Conversely, type II diabetic patients are frequently hypertensive at the time of diagnosis. It has been estimated from several sources that the prevalence of hypertension among type II diabetic patients is in the range of 50% to 60%.[7-9] This association between diabetes and hypertension extends to patients with impaired glucose tolerance, as the Whitehall study demonstrated significant elevations of mean blood pressure in this population of patients.[10] Furthermore, essential hypertension has been shown to be an insulin-resistant state, suggesting that common pathophysiologic factors may be involved in both diabetes and essential hypertension.[11]

With regard to the overall morbidity and mortality in diabetes mellitus, several studies have shown that increases in blood pressure significantly enhance the risks for the development of diabetic vascular complications, particularly cardiovascular disease. Dupree and Meyer reported that mortality rates were four times greater among diabetics with systolic blood pressures (SBPs) greater than 160 mm Hg than among those subjects with SBPs less than 160 mm Hg.[12] The Whitehall study also demonstrated an increased relative risk of death if systolic hypertension (SBP greater than 160 mm Hg) occurred in the presence of diabetes mellitus. Conversely, patients with the longest survival almost universally demonstrate low diastolic blood pressures.

Irrespective of the type of diabetes, or the etiology of the hypertension that frequently accompanies diabetes, the presence of hypertension confers significant risks for the development and progression of many of the micro- and macrovascular complications associated with diabetes. In one study using multivariate analyses to determine the most powerful risk predictor for cardiovascular mortality among diabetics from a series of population-based studies, the presence of hypertension was the single most prominent factor, independent of the duration or the severity of the diabetic state.[13]

The impact of treatment of hypertension on cardiovascular mortality and morbidity in diabetes remains to be determined. Long-term, prospective clinical trials evaluating the impact of antihypertensive therapy on the outcome of diabetic vascular complications are necessary to address this issue.

Diabetes, Hypertension, and Diabetic Vascular Complications

Cardiovascular Disease

Cardiovascular disease is the number one cause of mortality among type II diabetic patients, and it is preceded only by death from renal failure among type I diabetic patients. Hypertension significantly contributes to the development of cardiovascular disease among both type I and type II diabetic patients. A cohort study from the Joslin Diabetes Center in Boston demonstrated that, among type I patients, the risk for coronary heart disease was increased sixfold among those patients with hypertension.[14] The risk of coronary artery disease was increased 15-fold in the presence of diabetic nephropathy, a condition that is almost invariably accompanied by hypertension. Similar results have been reported for patients with type II diabetes mellitus. Age-adjusted death rates among diabetic Pima Indians were nearly tripled when hypertension was present, and were increased nearly fivefold if hypertension and proteinuria were present.[15] The presence of microalbuminuria in type II diabetes may signify a marked risk for the development of future cardiovascular disease and death among type II diabetic patients. In one study, only 4.7% of type II diabetic patients with microalbuminuria were alive after a 10-year follow-up period, whereas 54% of age- and sex-matched type II patients without microalbuminuria were alive after 10 years.[16]

With regard to the prevalence of cardiovascular disease among diabetic subjects, data from the Framingham study offer some of the most conclusive evidence that cardiovascular disease is significantly more prevalent among diabetics. For females, cardiovascular disease was 2.7 time more prevalent among diabetics than nondiabetics, and for diabetic men, cardiovascular disease was

2.1 times more prevalent than for nondiabetic men.[17] The World Health Organization Multinational Study of Vascular Disease in Diabetes demonstrated an even greater risk for the development of cardiovascular disease among diabetic women, with a relative risk of 3.7 versus 2.2 for diabetic men.[18] A Finnish study examining middle-aged type II diabetics demonstrated even higher age-adjusted relative risks of coronary heart disease death in diabetic patients as compared to nondiabetics: among newly diagnosed diabetics, the risk was 2.0 for men and 4.1 for women; among previously known diabetics, it was 2.6 for men and 3.6 for women.[19] These three studies suggest that the relative risk for cardiovascular disease type II diabetics is greater for women than for men.

Congestive heart failure also has a higher incidence in the diabetic population according to the Framingham study, and both cardiomyopathy with left ventricular systolic[20] and diastolic[21] dysfunction have been reported as frequent complications of diabetes. Cardiomyopathy, a frequent complication of diabetes, carries a relative risk that is greater for diabetic women than diabetic men.[22] The role of high blood pressure in the pathogenesis of diabetic cardiomyopathy is unclear. Most studies of cardiomyopathy have specifically excluded hypertensive diabetics; however, there is autopsy evidence to suggest that hypertensive diabetics may have a substantially increased risk for the development of this disorder.[23]

With regard to the impact of hypertension on specific cardiovascular complications in the presence of diabetes, there is a close association between systolic hypertension and below-the-knee peripheral vascular disease.[24] Diabetic patients with hypertension also have a two- to six-fold increased frequency of transient ischemic attacks and cerebrovascular accidents compared with nondiabetic subjects. Hypertension may be the most potent risk factor for the development of cerebrovascular disease in diabetic patients, as its incidence is doubled in hypertensive as compared to normotensive diabetics.[25]

In diabetic patients with coronary artery disease, hypertension can increase the frequency and severity of either symptomatic or silent myocardial ischemia by increasing left ventricular wall stress. In diabetic patients with left ventricular systolic dysfunction, hypertension increases left ventricular afterload and exacerbates congestive heart failure symptoms. Hypertension is also frequently the cause of left ventricular diastolic abnormalities in diabetics.

The role of antihypertensive therapy in modifying these adverse effects of hypertension in the diabetic patient is unknown but, potentially, antihypertensive treatment could have significant positive influences on cardiovascular morbidity and mortality. Although the treatment of hypertension has not been shown to significantly reduce the incidence of coronary artery disease in nondiabetic populations, it may be that the choice of antihypertensive agents used in these studies was at fault.[26–29] Specifically, the β-blockers and diuretic agents that were used in these studies are known to adversely affect lipid profiles and glucose tolerance. Thus, the type of antihypertensive agent used in the treatment of hypertension associated with diabetes mellitus may be very important.

Diabetic Renal Disease

Diabetes mellitus is an important cause of end-stage renal disease (ESRD), presently contributing to 33% of ESRD cases. Moreover, because the proportion of ESRD secondary to diabetic nephropathy is increasing at 2% per year, 50% of the ESRD population will be composed of diabetic patients by the year 2000.[30] Because type II diabetes is more common than type I, approximately 65% of all maintenance dialysis diabetic patients are type II patients. The cost for treatment of diabetic patients with ESRD is estimated to be $2 billion per year, or one third of the $6 billion total cost of the ESRD program.[31]

The presence of microalbuminuria in type I patients is associated with a 15- to 20-fold increase in the incidence of ESRD.[32,33] Although tight glucose control has been suggested to decrease microalbuminuria, it does not alter the course of diabetic nephropathy once proteinuria intervenes.[34-38] However, the control of hypertension has been a major factor in slowing the progression of diabetic nephropathy once proteinuria occurs.[39-42] Diabetic patients with microalbuminuria are at risk for developing ESRD, cardiovascular disease, and retinopathy, but frequently have blood pressures that may be within normal range (less than 140/90 mm Hg). Their blood pressures, however, may be higher than those blood pressures among diabetic patients without microalbuminuria.[43] In addition, blood pressures of patients with microalbuminuria are frequently higher than their baseline blood pressures prior to the development of microalbuminuria.[5] Thus, hypertension, defined as that blood pressure at which end-organ damage occurs, may be lower in the diabetic than in the nondiabetic population.

The natural history of type II diabetic nephropathy is less well understood and less well studied than that of type I diabetic nephropathy. However, it appears that type II diabetics may develop ESRD at a rate comparable to type I diabetics. Walker et al.[44] focused on the degree of blood pressure control related to the appearance and progression of diabetic renal disease among both type I and type II diabetic patients. The primary outcome variable that was used to characterize the rate of change of renal function was derived from a plot of the reciprocal of the serum creatinine value versus time. Among type I patients, the rate of fall in renal function was 6% per year for those patients with SBPs greater than 140 mm Hg, and less than 1% per year for those patients with SBPs of 140 mm Hg or less. Among type II patients, the rate of loss of renal function was 13.5% per year for those patients with SBPs greater than 140 mm Hg and less than 1% per year for those patients with SBPs of 140 mm Hg or less.

Moreover, data derived from studies of the Pima Indian population demonstrated that the incidence of ESRD was similar in this population of type II diabetic patients to that in subjects with type I diabetes followed at the Joslin's Clinic in Boston.[15] In the Pima Indian diabetic population, the progression to ESRD was significantly accentuated by the presence of hypertension. Previous studies that have indicated a lower incidence of ESRD among type II patients versus type I patients have not accounted for the duration of diabetes mellitus. Since the Pima Indians with type II diabetes tend to develop diabetes at an earlier age, they are more likely to develop ESRD earlier in life. This earlier occurrence of ESRD with type II diabetes mellitus may also be true for the black and Hispanic populations in this country. Conversely, other populations (ie, caucasians) with type II diabetes tend to develop diabetes later and die from other causes (primarily cardiovascular disease) before developing ESRD. The incidence of type II diabetes will increase in the United States as the elderly population grows, and as improved survival occurs in the population, this will lead to an increased incidence of ESRD secondary to type II diabetes mellitus.

Diabetic Retinopathy

Retinopathy is a significant source of morbidity in the diabetic patient. Diabetic retinopathy is the leading cause of blindness in the United States in patients less than 65 years of age. The results of studies designed to demonstrate that tight glucose control prevents or diminishes the progression of diabetic retinopathy have been inconclusive.[45-48] Investigators therefore have begun to investigate other potential contributing factors for the development of diabetic retinopathy. Results of three independent studies have suggested that the incidence of diabetic retinopathy is greater in both type I and type II diabetic patients with hypertension than in the normotensive diabetic patient. Knowler et al demonstrated that the incidence of retinopathy among diabetic Pima Indians is increased in diabetic patients with systolic pressures greater than 145 mm Hg over those with systolic pressures less than 125 mm Hg.[49] Ishihara et al later demonstrated among 742 type II diabetic patients that SBP greater than 142 mm Hg was significant risk factor for the development of retinopathy.[50] Recently, Klein et al noted that SBP remained a significant predictor of the incidence of diabetic retinopathy.[51]

In spite of the accumulating evidence demonstrating that hypertension is a significant risk factor for the development and progression of diabetic retinopathy, very few studies have been conducted to assess the impact of antihypertensive therapy on diabetic retinopathy. In this regard, Parving et al[52] demonstrated that systemic blood pressure elevation contributed to the abnormal blood–retina barrier permeability to fluorescein characteristically found in diabetic background retinopathy. This abnormality was reversed during antihypertensive treatment, suggesting that antihypertensive therapy may be beneficial in diabetic retinopathy. However, before wide-reaching conclusions can be made regarding the benefit of antihypertensive therapy in the treatment of diabetic retinopathy, prospective clinical trials with adequate sample sizes will need to be conducted.

Diabetic Neuropathy

Morphologic examination of diabetic nerve biopsies and postmortem specimens suggests that an ischemic etiology is involved in the pathogenesis of diabetic polyneuropathy.[53] Proximal focal fascicular lesions characterized by a reduced density of myelinated axons with surrounding perineurial and epineural damage are virtually pathognomic of ischemia, and have been found in lumbosacral and tibial nerve postmortem specimens in diabetic patients.[54] This pattern of nerve damage is similar to that seen with vasculitides. Neuropathies with a known vascular basis, such as those related to vasculitis or small vessel occlusion, are characteristically multifocal, but they summate to produce symmetric distal distribution.[55]

To further support the role of hypoxia in the pathogenesis of diabetic peripheral neuropathy, oxygen tension in the sural nerve of diabetic subjects has been measured and observed to be lower than that found in the dorsal vein of the same subjects.[56] This finding suggests that peripheral nerves in diabetic patients with neuropathy are hypoxic.

Hypertension contributes to the development and the propagation of atherosclerosis in large vessels, and it also causes endothelial hyperplasia with small vessel occlusion in microvascular structures. In this regard, evidence for small vessel disease has been demonstrated in progressive diabetic neuropathy in both type I and type II diabetics with good metabolic control.[57] Sural nerve biopsies in these patients showed endothelial cell hyperplasia sufficient to occlude vessel lumina by degenerated cellular material and fibrin. This pattern of hyperplasia of endothelial cells is seen in hypertensive diabetic patients. With regard to epidemiologic evidence to support the role of hypertension in the development of diabetic neuropathy, in a recently published cross-sectional analysis from the Pittsburgh Epidemiology of Diabetes Complications Study, neuropathy was found to be significantly associated with hypertension.[58]

Taken together, all of the aforementioned findings suggest that ischemia is involved in the pathogenesis of diabetic neuropathy, and that hypertension contributes to the ischemic lesion. Since the pathologic lesion of diabetic neuropathy appears to be ischemic, and hypertension is known to contribute to the development of ischemia, an intervention study is necessary to evaluate the impact of antihypertensive therapy on this diabetic complication.

Therapy of Hypertension in Diabetes Mellitus

The choice of antihypertensive therapy in the diabetic patient should be based on a rational approach that takes into account the pathogenesis and characteristics of the disorder, in addition to efforts to minimize the adverse side effects of therapy. In this regard, a brief description of the characteristics of hypertension associated with both type I and type II diabetes mellitus is warranted. Although the etiology of hypertension in diabetes is in part speculative, some of the potential hypotheses are discussed.

Theories of Etiology

Renin-Angiotensin System

The renin-angiotensin system has been extensively studied in diabetes with variable results and conclusions. In general, most investigators have reported low to normal levels of plasma renin activity (PRA) in diabetic subjects without vascular complications.[59–62] Decreases in plasma concentrations of angiotensin II and PRA have been noted in patients with diabetic neuropathy and nephropathy.[63–65] A few reports have noted increases in plasma angiotensin II concentrations in patients with microvascular disease.[66,67] Many of these studies investigating the plasma renin and angiotensin concentrations are flawed by the failure to report or account for glucose control (which is an important variable in volume regulation) or sodium intake, and frequently no distinction has been made between type I and type II diabetes. From the results of these studies, however, it appears that the activity of the renin-angiotensin system may be affected by the stage of diabetes and the progression of vascular complications.

Perhaps more important than plasma angiotensin II levels in the pathogenesis of hypertension associated with diabetes are the actual tissue concentrations of angiotensin II distributed throughout the body. In this regard, increased angiotensin-converting enzyme distribution has been demonstrated in the proximal tubule and glomerular vessels of streptozotocin-induced diabetic rats.[68]

These findings suggest that increased intrarenal angiotensin II levels may contribute to the pathogenesis of diabetic nephropathy. Furthermore, preliminary evidence using mRNA polymerase chain reaction techniques have demonstrated that the renin-angiotensin system may be involved in the pathogenesis of diabetic proliferative microangiopathy by the known effects of angiotensin II on angiogenesis. In this study, intraocular production of renin was demonstrated using RNA polymerase chain reaction assays to detect renin mRNA expression in human ocular tissue.[69] Gene expression was highest in the regions of the pigment epithelium–choroid and retina, which are the most highly vascularized regions of the eye.

Total Body Sodium

In addition to investigating the renin-angiotensin system as a possible contributor to hypertension in diabetes mellitus, total body sodium homeostasis has been extensively studied. Numerous investigators have noted that total exchangeable body sodium is increased approximately 10% in diabetic patients.[70–75] The increase in total body sodium may be secondary to hyperinsulinemia, because insulin is known to cause enhanced resorption of sodium in the distal nephron. In spite of increases in exchangeable body sodium, it appears that, in the steady state, plasma volume is normal or decreased in diabetic patients.[70–75] Increases in total exchangeable body sodium may be associated with increases in intracellular sodium, which in turn may result in increases in intracellular calcium levels secondary to an effect on Na^+-Ca^{2+} exchange. Such an increase in intracellular calcium levels in vascular smooth muscle may enhance contractility, thereby increasing peripheral vascular resistance.[76]

Hyperinsulinemia has also been proposed to contribute to the hypertension associated with diabetes mellitus by mechanisms other than its effect to enhance tubular sodium resorption. Insulin is known to stimulate sympathetic nervous system activity.[77] In addition to the absolute increase in plasma catecholamine levels, patients with diabetes may exhibit enhanced pressor responses to adrenergic stimulation.[78]

Insulin is also known to stimulate the Na^+-H^+ exchanger in the cell membrane.[79] Na^+-H^+ exchange maintains intracellular pH, and is linked with calcium exchange.[80] Thus, increases in the activity of the Na^+-H^+ pump could lead to increases in intracellular sodium, pH, and calcium. As noted earlier, an increase in intracellular calcium may enhance vascular tone and increase systemic blood pressure. In addition, an alkaline, intracellular pH may serve as a signal for the promotion of vascular smooth muscle cell growth and proliferation.[81] The resultant vascular smooth muscle cell proliferation could also increase vascular resistance and thus cause systemic hypertension.

Summary

Several theories for the pathogenesis of hypertension associated with diabetes have been discussed. The treatment of hypertension in the diabetic subject may therefore follow an approach based on several characteristics of this disorder.

General Measures

Obesity is a major contributor to the hypertension associated with type II diabetes mellitus. This may be related to the insulin resistance and consequent hyperinsulinemia that occurs in obesity. Nevertheless, weight loss is associated with reductions in blood pressure,[82] and it has been suggested that the hypertension associated with obesity is one form of salt-sensitive blood hypertension.[83] In this regard, of the nonpharmacologic measures that should be instituted in the treatment of hypertension associated with diabetes, weight loss and reduction of sodium intake (80 mmol/d) should be emphasized. Frequently, however, long-term compliance with either dietary recommendation is poor, and pharmacologic therapy is necessary.

Pharmacologic Therapy

Hypertension is a significant risk factor for the development of diabetic vascular complications, including nephropathy, cardiovascular disease, retinopathy, and possibly neuropathy. Thus, the treatment of hypertension associated with diabetes should be instituted early and vigorously. Of the many antihypertensive agents that are available on the market, the choice of therapy has been proposed to be based on the pathophysiology of the hypertension and the potential side effects of the drug concerned.

Angiotensin-Converting Enzyme Inhibitors

For several reasons, the angiotensin-converting enzyme (ACE) inhibitors are becoming one of the primary agents of choice for the treatment of hypertension associated with diabetes mellitus. Unlike the β-blockers and thiazide diuretics, which adversely affect lipid profiles and aggravate glucose intolerance, the ACE inhibitors are metabolically neutral, and they may actually enhance insulin sensitivity. Using the glucose clamp technique, the ACE inhibitor captopril has been shown to enhance insulin sensitivity of skeletal muscle glucose uptake with improvement in glycemic control.[84]

In diabetic patients with renal disease, ACE inhibitors have been shown to decrease the excretion of microalbumin in several independent studies.[40,41,85-87] This may be a consequence of the unique renal protective effects afforded by ACE inhibitors, which decrease intraglomerular hypertension in animal models by preferentially dilating the efferent arteriole of the glomerulus.[88] However, because it is impossible to perform micropuncture studies in humans, it is difficult to differentiate the effects of ACE inhibition in lowering systemic blood pressure from its unique effects of glomerular hemodynamics observed in experimental animal models.[89] The possibility also exists that diabetic complications can benefit from lowering blood pressure regardless of the specific antihypertensive agent that is used.[90] Long-term prospective clinical trials comparing the effects of ACE inhibition to those of other antihypertensive agents that do not have adverse metabolic effects are therefore necessary before conclusions can be reached regarding the renal protective effects of ACE inhibition therapy in the hypertension associated with diabetes.

As aforementioned, the PRA and serum angiotensin concentrations tend to be low in the diabetes associated with hypertension. In spite of this finding, ACE inhibition therapy is clearly efficacious in the treatment of hypertension associated with diabetes. This is most likely due to the effects of ACE inhibitors on the intravascular renin-angiotensin system at the tissue level. In this regard, all ACE inhibitor agents decrease total peripheral vascular resistance by blocking the conversion of angiotensin I to angiotensin II and perhaps by potentiating the effects of bradykinin. In addition to the above reasons for choosing ACE inhibitors as the first-line therapy for the treatment of hypertension associated with diabetes, ACE inhibitors also have a relatively low side effect profile when compared with other classes of antihypertensive agents. However, there are circumstances in which ACE inhibitors should be used with caution. These situations include bilateral renal artery stenosis or stenosis in a solitary functioning kidney, as well as situations in which hyperkalemia is likely to occur, including severe sodium restriction, advanced renal failure, severe congestive heart failure, type IV renal tubular acidosis associated with diabetes mellitus, and the concomitant administration of potassium-sparing diuretics, potassium supplements, or nonsteroidal anti-inflammatory agents.

Calcium Channel Blockers

Similar to the ACE inhibitors, calcium channel blockers are becoming popular in the treatment of hypertension associated with diabetes because they do not adversely affect lipid or glucose profiles. A recent review of 35 published reports concluded that calcium channel blockers had no untoward effects on blood glucose concentrations, insulin response, hemoglobin A_{1c} levels, or lipid profiles.[91] Common side effects of the dihydropyridine family of calcium channel blockers are peripheral edema, headaches, and constipation.

With regard to the treatment of hypertension associated with diabetic renal disease, the effects of calcium channel blockers on microalbuminuria and renal function are conflicting. Numerous short-term studies have been conducted to assess the effects of different classes of calcium channel blockers on microalbumin excretion and glomerular filtration rate. In general, the majority of these studies demonstrated that the dihydropyridine compound nifedipine frequently worsened microalbuminuria and, in some circumstances, decreased creatinine clearance.[87,92–94] Conversely, studies designed to assess the effects of other classes of calcium channel blockers, such as verapamil and diltiazem, have demonstrated decreases in microalbumin excretion and preservation of renal function.[92,95] In this regard, Baba et al demonstrated that both enalapril and nicardipine significantly reduced microalbumin excretion in a group of eight hypertensive type II diabetic individuals.[94] Recent studies by DeMarie and Bakris in diabetic patients who were treated with both diltiazem and verapamil demonstrated a reduction in urinary albumin excretion and preservation of renal function.[92] Finally, recent clinical evidence suggests that the concomitant use of calcium channel blockers and ACE inhibitors may potentiate the antiproteinuric effects of either agent used independently. In a small short-term study, Valentino et al demonstrated that the addition of verapamil to lisinopril in a group of type II diabetic patients diminished microalbuminuria without additional decreases in arterial blood pressure.[96]

To date, it is difficult to assess fully the effects of calcium channel blockers on microalbuminuria and renal function, because most of the studies designed to analyze the effects of these agents in the hypertensive diabetic population have involved small numbers of patients, and follow-up has been for short durations of time. Large-scale, prospective, randomized, double-blinded clinical trials are necessary before these issues can be definitively answered.

For several theoretical reasons, the calcium channel blockers are reasonable agents for the treatment of hypertension associated with diabetes mellitus.[97] Type II diabetic patients have an increase in total exchangeable body sodium content, and calcium channel blockers are known to have natriuretic effects. In addition, the major effect of these agents is to prevent the accumulation of intracellular calcium by blocking the potential-activated calcium channels in vascular smooth muscle. Thus, calcium channel blockers may act by decreasing intracellular calcium, thereby decreasing peripheral vascular resistance, and by decreasing total body sodium by acting as a natriuretic agent.

Diuretics

Diuretics have been shown to adversely affect cardiovascular risk factors, including cholesterol and glucose levels. In type II diabetic patients, diuretic-induced hypokalemia can impair insulin release and worsen glucose tolerance.[98] In addition, hypokalemia may predispose the diabetic patient to the development of ventricular ectopy. However, when diuretics are used in conjunction with ACE inhibitors, which are potassium sparing, diuretic-induced hypokalemia is unusual.

In a recently published retrospective analysis from the Joslin Clinic, an excess cardiovascular mortality was demonstrated for hypertensive diabetic patients treated with diuretics alone.[99] After adjusting for differences in risk factors, cardiovascular mortality was 3.8 times higher in patients treated with diuretics alone than in patients with untreated hypertension. Because the study is retrospective, it is difficult to derive definitive conclusions regarding the further use of diuretics alone in the treatment of hypertension associated with diabetes mellitus. However, diuretics can also produce elevation of low-density lipoprotein cholesterol and reductions in high-density lipoprotein cholesterol, which are disadvantageous in the diabetic patient, who already has baseline lipid abnormalities.

β-Adrenergic Blocking Agents

As a class of antihypertensive agents, the β-blockers may adversely affect lipid profiles. Both cardioselective and nonselective β-blockers have been shown to elevate plasma very-low-density lipoprotein triglycerides and reduce high-density lipoprotein concentrations. The β-adrenergic–mediated responses to hypoglycemia may be inhibited by β-blockers. Moreover, β-blockers also prolong the time necessary to restore euglycemia after an episode of hypoglycemia. For these reasons, β-blockers should be used very carefully in the diabetic population. Furthermore, because β-blockers lower blood pressure by decreasing cardiac output and the activity of the renin-angiotensin system, they may be less effective than other agents in the diabetic population.[100]

Central-Acting Agents

The central-acting agents have the primary side effects of dry mouth, a high incidence of orthostatic hypotension, sedation, and frequent impotence in men. These effects may be accentuated in diabetic patients who have clinical or subclinical autonomic insufficiency. These side effects commonly place the central-acting agents as second- or third-line therapy in the diabetic population.

α-Adrenergic Blocking Agents

The most frequently prescribed α-adrenergic blocking agent, prazosin, commonly results in first-dose orthostatic hypotension, sodium retention, and tachyphylaxis. However, these agents do not result in altered metabolic disturbances, and therefore they are commonly prescribed in the diabetic population when there is evidence of autonomic insufficiency.

Direct Vasodilators

Minoxidil and hydralazine are potent direct vasodilators that are usually reserved for severe, refractory hypertension. Because these agents cause reflex tachycardia and sodium retention, they should be prescribed in conjunction with a diuretic and a β-blocker. In females, minoxidil has the disadvantage of causing hirsutism; however, in balding males this may be a benefit.

Conclusion

Hypertension is a frequent occurrence in the diabetic population and places the diabetic patient at risk for the development of cardiovascular disease, diabetic nephropathy, retinopathy, and possibly neuropathy. Long-term, prospective clinical trials are necessary before the effects of antihypertensive therapy on the various diabetic vascular complications can be fully determined. The ACE inhibitors and calcium channel blockers are emerging as the agents of choice, given their efficacy and low side effect profiles in the diabetic population.

References

1. National Diabetes Data Group: *Classification of Diabetes Mellitus and Other Categories of Glucose Intolerance*. Bethesda, MD, National Institutes of Health, 1978.
2. Harris MI, Hadden WC, Knowler WC, et al: Prevalence of diabetes and impaired glucose tolerance and plasma glucose levels in U.S. population aged 20–74 years. *Diabetes* 1987;36:523–534.
3. Jahningen DW, Schrier RW: The doctor-patient relationship in geriatric care, in Jahnigen DW, Schrier RW (eds): *Geriatric Clinics; Ethical Issues in the Care of the Elderly*. Philadelphia, WB Saunders, 1986, pp 457–464.
4. Modan M, Halkin H, Almog S, et al: Hyperinsulinemia: A link between hypertension, obesity and glucose intolerance. *J Clin Invest* 1985;75:809–817.
5. Mathiesen ER, Ronn B, Deckert T, et al: Relationship between blood pressure and urinary albumin excretion in development of microalbuminuria. *Diabetes* 1990;39:245–249.
6. Borch-Johnson K, Nissen H, Nerup J: Blood pressure after forty years of insulin dependent diabetes. *Diabetic Nephrop* 1985;4:5–11.
7. Pell S, Donzo CA: Some aspects of hypertension in diabetes mellitus. *JAMA* 1967;202:104–110.
8. Fuller JH: Epidemiology of hypertension associated with diabetes mellitus. *Hypertension* 1985;7(suppl 2):113–117.

9. Panzram G: Mortality and survival in type II diabetes mellitus. *Diabetologia* 1987; 30:123–131.
10. Fuller JH, Shipley MJ, Rose G, et al: Mortality from coronary heart disease and stroke in relation to degree of glycemia: The Whitehall Study. *BMJ* 1983;287:867–870.
11. Ferrannini E, Buzzigoli G, Bonadonna R, et al: Insulin resistance in essential hypertension. *N Engl J Med* 1987;317:350–357.
12. Dupree EA, Meyer MB: Role of risk factors in the complications of diabetes mellitus. *Am J Epidemiol* 1980;112:100–112.
13. Janka HU, Dirschedl P: Systolic blood pressure as a predictor for cardiovascular disease in diabetes: A five year longitudinal study. *Hypertension* 1985;7(suppl II):II-90–II-94.
14. Krolewski AS, Kosinski DJ, Warram JH, et al: Magnitude and determinants of coronary artery disease in juvenile-onset, insulin-dependent diabetes mellitus. *Am J Cardiol* 1987;59:750–755.
15. Nelson RG, Newman JM, Knowler WC, et al: Incidence of end-stage renal disease in type II diabetes mellitus in Pima Indians. *Diabetologia* 1988;31:730–746.
16. Mogensen CE: Microalbuminuria predicts clinical proteinuria and early mortality in maturity-onset diabetes. *N Engl J Med* 1984;310:356–360.
17. Kannel WB, McGee DL: Diabetes and glucose tolerance as risk factors for cardiovascular disease, The Framingham Study. *Diabetes Care* 1979;2:120–126.
18. Fuller JH, Stevens LK: Epidemiology of hypertension in diabetic patients and implications for treatment. *Diabetes Care* 1991;14(suppl 4):8–12.
19. Pyorala K: Diabetes and heart disease, in Mogensen CE (ed): *Prevention and Treatment of Diabetic Late Complications*. Berlin: New York, DeGruyter Publishing, 1989.
20. Fein FS, Sonnenblick DH: Diabetic cardiomyopathy. *Prog Cardiovasc Dis* 1985;27:255–270.
21. Takenaka K, Sakamoto T, Amano K, et al: Left ventricular filling determined by Doppler echocardiography in diabetes mellitus. *Am J Cardiol* 1988;61:1140–1143.
22. Kannel WB, McGee DL: Diabetes and cardiovascular disease. *JAMA* 1979;241:2035–2038.
23. Factor SM, Minase T, Sonnenblick EH: Clinical and morphological features of human hypertensive-diabetic cardiomyopathy. *Am Heart J* 1980;99:446–458.
24. Tuck ML: Diabetes and hypertension. *Postgrad Med J* 1988;64(suppl 3):76–83.
25. Kuller LH, Dorman JS, Wolf PA: Cerebrovascular disease and diabetes, in *Diabetes in America*, publication no. 85-1468. Washington, DC, US Department of Health and Human Services, 1985, pp 1–18.
26. Veterans Administration Cooperative Study Group on Antihypertensive Agents: Effects of treatment on morbidity in hypertension. *JAMA* 1970;213:1143–1152.
27. Medical Research Council Working Party: MRC trial of treatment of mild hypertension: Principal results. *BMJ* 1985;291:97–104.
28. Wikstrand J, Warnold I, Olsson G: Primary prevention with metoprolol in patients with hypertension: Mortality results from the MAPHY study. *JAMA* 1988;259:1976–1982.
29. MacMahon S, Cutler JA, Stamler J: Antihypertensive drug treatment: Potential, expected, and observed effects on stroke and on coronary heart disease. *Hypertension* 1989;13(suppl I):I-45–I-50.
30. NIH Task Force on Kidney Disease of Diabetes: Kidney Disease of Diabetes. Bethesda, MD, National Institutes of Health, 1986.
31. United States Renal Data System: Annual Data Report. Bethesda, MD, National Institutes of Health, 1991.
32. Mogensen CE, Christensen CK: Predicting diabetic nephropathy in insulin-dependent patients. *N Engl J Med* 1984;311:89–93.
33. Viberti GC, Garrett RJ, Mahmud U, et al: Microalbuminuria as a predictor of clinical nephropathy in insulin-dependent diabetes mellitus. *Lancet* 1982;1:1430–1432.

34. Viberti GC, Mackintosh D, Bilous RW, et al: Proteinuria in diabetes mellitus: Role of spontaneous and experimental variation of glycemia. *Kidney Int* 1982;21:714–720.

35. Viberti GC, Bilous RW, Mackintosh D, et al: Long-term correction of hyperglycemia and progression of renal failure in insulin dependent diabetes. *BMJ* 1983;286:598–602.

36. Bending JJ, Viberti GC, Watkins PJ, et al: Intermittent clinical proteinuria and renal function in diabetes evolution and the effect of glycemic control. *BMJ* 1986;292:83–86.

37. Bending JJ, Viberti GC, Bilous RW, et al: Eight-month correction of hyperglycemia in insulin-dependent diabetes mellitus is associated with a significant and sustained reduction of urinary albumin excretion rates in patients with microalbuminuria. *Diabetes* 1985;34(suppl 3):69–73.

38. Dahl-Jorgensen K, Brinchmann-Hansen O, Hanssen K, et al: Effect of near normal glycemia for two years on progression of early diabetic retinopathy, nephropathy and neuropathy: The Oslo Study. *BMJ* 1986;293:1195–1199.

39. Mogensen CE: Progression of nephropathy in long-term diabetics with proteinuria and effect of initial antihypertensive treatment. *Scand J Clin Lab Invest* 1976;36:384–388.

40. Parving HH: Early aggressive antihypertensive treatment reduces rate of decline in kidney function in diabetic nephropathy. *Lancet* 1983;1:1175–1177.

41. Parving HH: Effects of long-term antihypertensive treatment on kidney function in diabetic nephropathy. *Hypertension* 1985;7:114–117.

42. Parving HH, Andersen AR, Smidt UM, et al: Effect of antihypertensive treatment on kidney function in diabetic nephropathy. *BMJ* 1987;294:1443–1447.

43. Parving HH, Viberti GC, Keen H, et al: Hemodynamic factors in the genesis of diabetic microangiopathy. *Metabolism* 1983;32:943–949.

44. Walker WG, Hermann J, Murphy R, et al: Elevated blood pressure and angiotensin II are associated with accelerated loss of renal function in diabetic nephropathy. *Trans Am Clin Climatol Assoc* 1985;97:94–104.

45. Lauritzen T, Larsen HW, Frost-Larsen K, et al: The Steno Study Group: Effect of one year of near-normal blood glucose levels on retinopathy in insulin dependent diabetics. *Lancet* 1983;1:200–204.

46. Dahl-Jorgensen K, Brinchmann-Hanssen O, Hanssen KF, et al: Aker Diabetes Group: Rapid tightening of blood glucose control leads to transient deterioration of retinopathy in insulin dependent diabetes mellitus. *BMJ* 1985;290:811–815.

47. Kroc Collaborative Study Group: Blood glucose control and the evolution of diabetic retinopathy and albuminuria. *N Engl J Med* 1984;311:365–372.

48. Ramsay RC, Goetz FC, Sutherland DE, et al: Progression of diabetic retinopathy after pancreas transplantation for insuln dependent diabetes mellitus. *N Engl J Med* 1988;318:208–214.

49. Knowler WC, Bennett PH, Ballintine EJ: Increased incidence of retinopathy in diabetics with elevated blood pressure. *N Engl J Med* 1980;302:645–650.

50. Ishihara M, Yukimura Y, Aizawa T, et al: High blood pressure as risk factor in diabetic retinopathy development in NIDDM patients. *Diabetes Care* 1987;10:20–25.

51. Klein R, Klein BE, Moss SE, et al: Is blood pressure a predictor of the incidence or progression of diabetic retinopathy? *Arch Intern Med* 1989;149:2427–2432.

52. Parving H, Larsen M, Hommel E: Effect of antihypertensive treatment on blood-retinal barrier permeability of fluorescein in hypertensive type I diabetic patients. *Diabetologia* 1989;32:440–444.

53. Dyck P, Karnes J, O'Brien P: The spacial distribution of fiber loss in diabetic polyneuropathy suggests ischemia. *Ann Neurol* 1986;19:440–449.

54. Johnson PC, Doll SC, Cromey DW: Pathogenesis of diabetic neuropathy. *Ann Neurol* 1986;19:450–457.

55. Thomas PK: Vascular factors in the causation of diabetic neuropathy. *TINS* 1987;10:6–8.

56. Dyck PJ: Hypoxic neuropathy: Does hypoxia play a role in diabetic neuropathy? *Neurology* 1989;39:111–118.

57. Timperley WR, Bouton A, Davies-Jones CT, et al: Small vessel disease in progressive diabetic neuropathy associated with good metabolic control. *J Clin Pathol* 1985;38: 1030–1038.

58. Maser R, Steenkisste A, Dorman J, et al: Epidemiological correlates of diabetic neuropathy. *Diabetes* 1989;38:1456–1461.

59. Christleib AR: Renin-angiotensin-aldosterone system in diabetes mellitus. *Diabetes* 1976;25(suppl 2):820–825.

60. De Chatel R, Weidmann P, Flammer J, et al: Sodium, renin, aldosterone, catecholamines, and blood pressure in diabetes mellitus. *Kidney Int* 1977;12:412–421.

61. Christlieb AR, Kaldany A, D'Elia JA: Plasma renin activity and hypertension in diabetes mellitus. *Diabetes* 1976;25:969–974.

62. Sundkvist G, Bergstrom B, Bramnert M: The activity of the renin-angiotensin-aldosterone system before and during submaximal bicycle exercise in relation to circulatory catecholamines in patients with type I diabetes mellitus. *Diabetologia* 1990;33:148–151.

63. Ferriss JB, Sullivan PA, Gonggrijp H, et al: Plasma angiotensin II and aldosterone in unselected diabetic patients. *Clin Endocrinol* 1982;17:261–269.

64. Fernandez-Cruz A, Noth RH, Lassman MN: Low plasma renin activity in normotensive patients with diabetes mellitus: Relationship to neuropathy. *Hypertension* 1981;3: 87–92.

65. Tomita K, Matsuda O, Ideura T, et al: Renin-angiotensin-aldosterone system in mild diabetic nephropathy. *Nephron* 1982;31:361–367.

66. Drury PL, Bodansky HJ, Oddie CJ, et al: Increased plasma renin activity in type I diabetes with microvascular disease. *Clin Endocrinol* 1982;16:453–461.

67. Burden AC, Thurston H: Plasma renin activity in diabetes mellitus. *Clin Sci* 1979;56: 255–259.

68. Jung F, Anderson S, Ingelfinger J: Increased intrarenal antiotension converting enzyme distribution in streptozotocin diabetes prevented by interruption of renin angiotensin system. Abstract, Third International Symposium Hypertension Associated with Diabetes, 1991, Boston, MA.

69. Wagner J, Danser AJ, Paul M: Demonstration of renin-angiotensin and converting enzyme-mRNA expression in human eyes by the polymerase chain reaction. Abstract, Third International Symposium Hypertension Associated with Diabetes Mellitus, 1991, Boston, MA.

70. Weidmann P, Beretta-Piccoli C, Keusch G, et al: Sodium-volume factor, cardiovascular reactivity and hypotensive mechanism of diuretic therapy in mild hypertension associated with diabetes mellitus. *Am J Med* 1979;67:779–784.

71. O'Hare JP, Anderson JV, Millar ND: The relationship of the renin-angiotensin-aldosterone system to atrial natriuretic peptide and the natriuresis of volume expansion in diabetics with and without proteinuria. *Postgrad Med J* 1988;64:35–38.

72. Wiseman MJ: Plasma renin activity in insulin dependent diabetics with raised glomerular filtration rate. *Clin Endocrinol* 1984;21:409–414.

73. Feldt-Rasmussen B, Mathiesen ER, Deckert T: Central role for sodium in the pathogenesis of blood pressure changes independent of angiotensin, aldosterone and catecholamines in type I diabetes mellitus. *Diabetologia* 1987;30:610–617.

74. O'Hare JP: Exchangeable sodium and renin in hypertensive diabetic patients with and without nephropathy. *Hypertension* 1985;7(suppl II):II-43–II-48.

75. Beretta-Piccoli C: Body sodium and renin activity in diabetes mellitus. *Diabete Metab* 1989;15:296–299.

76. Blaustein M: Sodium transport inhibition, cell calcium and hypertension: The natriuretic hormone/Na^+-Ca^{++} exchange/hypertension hypothesis. Am J Med 1984; 77(4A):45–48.

77. Rowe JW, Young JB, Minaker DL, et al: Effect of insulin and glucose infusions on sympathetic nervous system activity in normal man. *Diabetes* 1981;30:219–225.
78. Weidmann P, Beretta-Piccoli C, Trost BN: Pressor factors and responsiveness in hypertension accompanying diabetes mellitus. *Hypertension* 1985;5(suppl II):II-33–II-42.
79. Mahnensmith RL, Aronson PS: The plasma membrane sodium-hydrogen exchanger and its role in physiological and pathophysiological processes. *Circ Res* 1985;56:773–778.
80. Blaustein MP: Sodium ions, calcium ions, blood pressure regulation, and hypertension: A reassessment and hypothesis. *Am J Physiol* 1977;232:C165–C173.
81. Moolenaar WH: Effects of growth factors on intracellular pH regulation. *Annu Rev Physiol* 1986;48:363–376.
82. Tuck MC, Sowers J, Dornfidd L: The effect of weight reduction on blood pressure, plasma renin activity and plasma aldosterone levels in obese patients. *N Engl J Med* 1981;304:930–933.
83. Rocchini A, Katch V, Kelch R, et al: Insulin and blood pressure during weight loss in obese adolescents. *Hypertension* 1989;10:267–273.
84. Martz K, Jauch KW, Wicklmayr M, et al: Angiotensin converting enzyme inhibitors in diabetes: Experimental and human experience. *Postgrad Med J* 1986;62(suppl 1):59–64.
85. Taguma Y, Kitamoto Y, Futaki G, et al: Effect of captopril on heavy proteinuria in azotemic diabetes. *N Engl J Med* 1985;313:1617–1620.
86. Marre M, Leblanc H, Suareq L, et al: Converting enzyme inhibition and kidney functioning in normotensive diabetic patients with persistent proteinuria. *BMJ* 1987;294:1448–1452.
87. Mimran A, Insua A, Ribstein J, et al: Comparative effect of captopril and nifedipine in normotensive patients with incipient diabetic nephropathy. *Diabetes Care* 1988;11:850–853.
88. Zatz R, Dunn BR, Brenner B, et al: Prevention of diabetic glomerulopathy by pharmacological amelioration of glomerular capillary hypertension. *J Clin Invest* 1986;77:1925–1930.
89. Schrier RW, Holzgreve H: Hemodynamic factors in the pathogenesis of diabetic nephropathy. *Klin Wochenschr* 1988;66:325–331.
90. Savage S, Schrier RW: Progressive renal insufficiency: The role of angiotensin converting enzyme inhibitors. *Adv Intern Med* 1992;37:85–101.
91. Trost BN, Weidman P: Effects of calcium antagonists on glucose homeostasis and serum lipids in non-diabetic and diabetic subjects—a review. *J Hypertens* 1987;5(suppl 4):S81–S104.
92. DeMarie BK, Bakris GL: Different effects of calcium antagonists on proteinuria in diabetic man. *Ann Intern Med* 1990;113:987–988.
93. Fuder L, Daccorditt G, Mentello M, et al: ACE inhibitors versus calcium antagonists in the treatment of diabetic hypertensive patients. *Hypertens Abstr* 1991;45:17.
94. Baba T, Murabayashi Y, Takebe K: Comparison of the renal effects of angiotensin converting enzyme inhibitor and calcium antagonist in hypertensive type II diabetic patents with microalbuminuria: A randomized controlled trial. *Diabetologia* 1989;32:40–44.
95. Bakris GL: Effects of diltiazem or lisinopril on massive proteinuria associated with diabetes mellitus. *Ann Intern Med* 1990;112:707–708.
96. Valentino V, Wilson M, Bakris GL, et al: A perspective on converting enzyme inhibitors and calcium channel antagonists in diabetic renal disease. *Arch Intern Med* 1991;151:2367–2372.
97. Savage S, Miller L, Schrier RW: The future of calcium channel blockers in diabetes mellitus. *J Cardiovasc Pharmacol* 1991;18:519–524.
98. Conn JW: Hypertension, the potassium ion and impaired carbohydrate tolerance. *N Engl J Med* 1983;21:1135–1143.

99. Warram J, Laffel L, Krolewski A, et al: Excess mortality associated with diuretic therapy in diabetes mellitus. *Arch Intern Med* 1991;151:1350–1356.
100. Elving LD, de Nobel E, Thein TH: Comparison of captopril and atenolol in the treatment of hypertension in patients with diabetes mellitus. *Postgrad Med J* 1988; 64(suppl 3):75.

Index